PREPARE FOR THE UNEXPECTED

Prostate biopsy . . . breast biopsy . . . stress test . . . amniocentesis . . . drug testing . . . lipid profile . . . Lyme disease antibody . . . MRI . . .

Every day physicians prescribe diagnostic tests, often inadequately preparing their patients for what is to come. Here, at last, is an award-winning doctor's prescription: **knowledge,** to ease your anxiety and keep you fully informed. In these pages you will learn everything you need to know about any test you're ever likely to need, including:

- Alternate names of tests
- A definition of the test and the indications for its use
- How the test works, in layman's language, including what it feels like (in other words, does it hurt?)
- How to prepare in order to get accurate results
- What to expect following the test, including complications and risks
- The meaning of negative and positive test results, and other tests that may be helpful

How accurate are the tests? How invasive? What are your options? What constitutes a good workup? The answers are here, and more in

The Encyclopedia of
Medical Tests

The ENCYCLOPEDIA of MEDICAL TESTS

MICHAEL B. BRODIN, M.D.

POCKET BOOKS

New York   London   Toronto   Sydney   Tokyo   Singapore

The ideas, procedures, and suggestions in this book are not intended as a substitute for the medical advice of a trained health professional. All matters regarding your health require medical supervision. Consult your physician before adopting the suggestions in this book, as well as about any condition that may require diagnosis or medical attention. In addition, the statements made by the author regarding certain products and services represent the views of the author alone, and do not constitute a recommendation or endorsement of any product or service by the publisher. The author and publisher disclaim any liability arising directly or indirectly from the use of the book, or of any products mentioned herein.

An *Original* Publication of POCKET BOOKS

POCKET BOOKS, a division of Simon & Schuster Inc.
1230 Avenue of the Americas, New York, NY 10020

ISBN: 0-671-53537-4

First Pocket Books printing September 1997

10 9 8 7 6 5 4

POCKET and colophon are registered trademarks of Simon & Schuster Inc.

This book is a creation of Siegel & Siegel Ltd.

Front cover photo ©1992 Michael W. Thomas/PNI

Printed in the U.S.A.

Notice

The purpose of this book is education. It is not intended as a substitute for the advice of a physician or as a handbook for self-diagnosis.

For Laura, Heather, and Ashley
With immeasurable love

Acknowledgments

I would like to express my deep gratitude to the physicians who served on the advisory board for taking time from their busy lives to provide me with their expertise. Thanks also to Carole and Pam for their helpful suggestions.

Very special thanks go to Scott and Barbara Siegel, who, besides being my terrific agents and good friends, have given me much support, encouragement, and advice. Without them this book would not have come into being.

Contents

□ □ □

How to Use This Book
xiii

Advisory Board
xv

Introduction
xvii

Test Listings
1

Cross-reference Tables
481

Glossary
493

Synonyms and Included Tests Index
505

xi

How to Use This Book

Although browsers are welcome, this book is of greatest value when your doctor has told you that you need "some tests." Here, humanity diverges into two broad camps: those who want to be put to sleep at once, only to be revived when the process has been completed, and those who want to know more. The difficulty for the latter group is that because of automated technology and the wide variety of available diagnostic procedures—over 435 are described in this volume—there will more than likely be a battery of tests, and it is quite impossible for medical personnel to give you a complete rundown on each one. It is at this point that this book can be of most value: All you need is the name of the test, and you can look up the details. You can use the information in talking to your doctor before deciding to have it, to help prepare for it, and in monitoring possible complications after it. You can also learn about complementary tests.

The format for each test entry is:

WHAT IT IS AND WHY IT'S OBTAINED
A definition of the test and the indications for its use.
HOW IT WORKS
The technical details, including what it feels like.
BEFORE THE TEST
Preparation which is desirable or crucial for accurate results.
AFTER THE TEST
What to expect following the test, including complications and risks.

SIGNIFICANCE OF RESULTS

What a negative test means and what a positive test means. Other tests which may be helpful are included here.

SYNONYMS AND INCLUDED TESTS

Alternate names and variants.

If you can't find the test in question in the alphabetical listing, look in the index, since many are known by more than one name. If you still can't find it, try the cross-reference tables under the heading most closely related to your problem. Tests are grouped in several ways: by general subject, by organ system, and by disease.

An asterisk (*) means that a word or term is defined in the glossary.

Bold print means that there is a test entry of that name.

Although this book has been designed to provide comprehensive information for each test in order to make you a more informed partner in the healing process, it is no substitute for obtaining medical care under a good diagnostician.

Advisory Board

Melvin H. Becker, M.D. (Radiology), Gouverneur Hospital and New York University Medical Center.

Kenneth Brookler, M.D. (Otolaryngology), Lenox Hill Hospital and the Manhattan Eye and Ear Infirmary.

Valentine Burroughs, M.D. (Endocrinology), St. Lukes-Roosevelt Hospital Center.

Joseph Cleary, M.D. (Surgery), Beth Israel Medical Center and Westchester County Medical Center.

Susan Frye, M.D.. (Urology), Beth Israel Medical Center.

Jonas Goldstone, M.D. (Hematology and Oncology), The Presbyterian Hospital in the City of New York and St. Lukes-Roosevelt Hospital Center.

Elliott Howard, M.D. (Cardiology), Lenox Hill Hospital.

Donald Morris, M.D. (Ophthalmology), The New York Eye and Ear Infirmary.

Richard Pierson, M.D. (Nuclear Medicine), The Presbyterian Hospital in the City of New York and St. Lukes-Roosevelt Hospital Center.

Michael Rehmar, M.D. (Internal Medicine)

Michael Ruoff, M.D. (Gastroenterology), New York University Medical Center.

Jay Alan Rosenblum, M.D. (Neurology), New York University Medical Center and Beth Israel Medical Center.

Michael Strongin, M.D. (Obstetrics and Gynecology), Lenox Hill Hospital and Beth Israel Hospital Center.

Introduction

> *"I ordered every test I could think of*
> *on every patient I had . . ."*
> SAMUEL SHEM, The House of God

Most doctors don't practice like the protagonist in *The House of God,* an intern who is trying to please a resident physician who is his superior. Yet there are doctors who routinely order many more tests than are needed. The habit most often stems from a desire to cover every possibility, to avoid missing something. But sometimes it comes from pressure to "do something." Sometimes it comes from fear of litigation, to produce documents which look good in court. Sometimes it comes from ignorance, and, rarely, sometimes from a desire to make money. Inconvenience and waste of money, however, are the least of one's problems with overtesting. Listen to what happens next in *The House of God* to one of the narrator's patients:

". . . every organ system crumpled: in a domino progression the injection of radioactive dye for her brain scan shut down her kidneys, and the dye study of her kidneys overloaded her heart, and the medication for her heart made her vomit, which altered her electrolyte balance in a life-threatening way, which increased her dementia and shut down her bowel, which made her eligible for the bowel run, the cleanout for which dehydrated her and really shut down her tormented kidneys, which lead to infection, the need for dialysis, and big-time complications of these big-time diseases.

She and I both became exhausted, and she became very sick."

The House of God is a novel of farce and exaggeration, but it rings true. It is an old medical maxim that nobody could survive a complete workup (diagnostic evaluation). As one might discover from browsing through the entries in this book, it would require much time, discomfort, and risk.

To many, one answer to the high price of overtesting is managed care. By putting businessmen, accountants, and entrepreneurs in charge of medical expenditures it is hoped that costs will come down. Will they? For a time they will. They will come down just the way they always do when anything is rationed and doled out piecemeal. It remains to be seen, however, whether this will translate into quality of care, that very difficult and elusive term which everyone is fond of throwing about. It should be remembered that the legal, ethical, and moral obligation of the managed care insurance company is to do the best it can for its shareholders. The legal, ethical, and moral obligation of your doctor is to do the best he or she can for you.

I don't know how best to deliver medical care, whether it's fee for service, managed care, or government-run single-payer. I suspect that no society will ever achieve the perfect system, and in the end we may very well find that a hybrid, or a mixture of systems, satisfies most people. And although we are bombarded with advertising propaganda extolling the virtues of U.S. Healthcare versus Kaiser Foundation versus the Harvard Community Health Plan, I do know that nothing beats a good doctor, no matter what your health plan says. And the "good doctor" knows that the first step toward getting you better is to make the right diagnosis, to find out what's wrong in the quickest, safest, and most comfortable way possible.

The workup

The good doctor does not leap from complaint to treatment. People sometimes pose questions like, "What's good for the skin?" or, "What's good for arthritis?" One might even say, "What's good for a stomachache?" without first giving thought as to the cause of that stomachache. Was it something you ate? Appendicitis? Gallstones? Ulcers? Cancer?

To this end the good doctor can only go so far by listening to your symptoms. More often than not one or more tests is called for. It is at this point that this book can be of value by helping you to become a partner in the process. If it is simply a matter of providing a sample for a routine **urinalysis** or drawing some blood for a **sequential multiple analyzer** battery you needn't worry. The risks of not having these screening tests are worse than the remote possibility of a complication. But what if the tests are abnormal, or questionable, or if others are called for? You'll fare better if you understand fully what's going on.

The way the good doctor goes about trying to find out what ails you is called the diagnostic workup, or, simply, the workup. One can "work up" high blood pressure, constipation, hair loss, or any of the scores of problems that might lead you to seek medical care. The first part of the workup is the history and physical examination.

This phase of the process must never be neglected. The history has to include the nature, duration, location, and characteristics of your symptoms. It has to include any medications you are taking. It has to include your past history, family history, social history, and occupation. It also has to include features in your personal life, such as major life changes or stressful situations, which might be significant. The physical examination may be complete or focused, depending upon circumstances.

After a list of possible conditions—the "differential diagnosis"—has been drawn up, a logical plan of investigation should be launched. Although the tests in this book are arranged alphabetically, the procedure in the mind of the diagnostician is much different. The tests and the order in which the good doctor orders them has to take into account factors such as the probability of yielding useful information, safety, cost, and certain technical matters, such as making certain that one test does not interfere with a subsequent one. One hypothetical example is what might happen if you come to the doctor with the very common complaint of fatigue.

After a thorough history and physical examination, the

doctor may conclude that one possibility is anemia, owing to, say, iron deficiency from a heavy menstrual flow and a poor diet. The first test would typically be a **complete blood count,** which includes a **hemoglobin.** If the hemoglobin is within normal limits, anemia is not the cause of the fatigue, and some other reason must be found. If hemoglobin is low, however, one would next look to the **red blood cell indices,** which can reveal several patterns of abnormality. Depending upon the characteristics of the red blood cells one might next look at the **red blood cell count, reticulocyte count, Coombs' test, ferritin,** or **folate.** The results of these will lead to other investigations, possibly an **iron and iron binding capacity,** or a **bone marrow.** One may indeed end up with a diagnosis of iron deficiency anemia, but sickle cell anemia, pernicious anemia, or an underlying chronic disease may be the culprit. The manner of progessing through this series of tests is often represented by a flowchart which includes decision trees. These usually work well, but the human machine, particularly when malfunctioning, is sufficiently complex so that it does not always follow the rules we lay down for it. Futhermore, the situation may be complicated by more than one cause of anemia being present, such as iron deficiency anemia and sickle cell anemia. There are similar flowcharts for other complaints, whether they be sore throat, headache, shortness of breath, or decreased sexual drive.

I haven't included any flowcharts in this book because that is your doctor's job, and you should not try to be your own doctor. When you're in trouble you need the objective and seasoned eye of a professional. You can use this book to make an informed decision as whether to consent to the **barium enema** or **prostate biopsy** or **stress test,** but you need someone to give you professional guidance along the way. It's not smart trying to be your own doctor, *even if you are a doctor,* but I am convinced that the more you know that is accurate and the more objective you can be, the better off you are. One part of that knowledge is understanding something about the limitations of medical diagnostic testing, specifically what is meant by the terms "false negative" and "false positive."

The results of medical tests come in various forms. In some, such as the **pregnancy test,** the answer is "positive" or "negative"; either you are, or you're not. In others, such as a **hearing test** or **visual acuity test,** there are gradations. And in others, such as **cholesterol** or blood **glucose,** there are both gradations and levels which are considered "high" or "low." In most cases, however, it is the simple positive or negative result which is most desirable. Unfortunately, nothing is perfect, and an important part in interpreting any test is knowing how accurate it is.

Medical science recognizes the inherent imperfections in testing by devising statistics to quantify the problem. There are generally two types of inaccuracies, false negatives and false positives.

A false negative means that you have a certain disease, but the test says you don't.

A false positive means that you don't have a certain disease, but the test says you do.

Most tests suffer a little bit from both. This is why confirmatory tests or repeat tests are advisable in cases of doubt.

Additional terms derived from the above are "sensitivity" and "specificity."

Sensitivity means how well a test is able to detect a disease; a test is sensitive if the false negative rate is low.

Specificity means how well a test is able to rule out a disease; a test is specific if the false positive rate is low.

Another term is called "predictive value." This takes into consideration both the sensitivity and specificity, and the prevalence of the disease (how many cases exist in a given area at any one time). Ideally, tests should be sensitive, specific, and predictive.

But even if you know the figures you can be misled. A certain test may be touted as 99 percent predictive. This is very high indeed, but if many tests are done, that one error in a hundred can add up. If the airline industry, for instance, operated at 99 percent efficiency there would be two crashes a day at Chicago's O'Hare airport alone.

Being able to have an intelligent discussion about statistics with your doctor, however, is only part of the battle: you still want to get over your illness as quickly as you can. To this end I offer the following advice:

• If you adhere to the principle of using a "good doctor," you are not likely to go wrong.

- The doctor should treat you, not the laboratory. There are many cases where people live long, healthy lives with one or more "abnormal" test results which are never adequately explained. Few tests, taken by themselves, are so predictive that they signify without doubt the presence of disease.

- When in doubt as to the significance of a test result, repeat the test. Unless it's a brain or heart biopsy, nothing much is lost.

- If there is a question as to whether or not to have a certain test because of possible *risk,* your doctor and you should ask yourselves this question: Will the result, positive or negative, change any decision I have to make? If it won't, then the test doesn't matter, no matter what it shows.

- Always bring your own reading material to the doctor's office or to the testing facility. It is in the nature of medicine for complications to develop and for emergencies to pop up.

- Dealing with pain is easier for some people than for others. Some tests are uncomfortable, embarrassing, or both. Always remember that the pain is *temporary* and will not represent a constant feature in your life. It is good to come right out with your fears and apprehensions. Many patients tell me that they are "no good with needles," and this helps both of us, because it's perfectly normal.

- Many tests are available for use at home. There is nothing wrong with this, and some are particularly valuable, such as blood or urine **glucose** tests for those with diabetes, and **pregnancy tests.** In most other cases, however, it is best to rely upon a doctor's guidance.

- Remember, if you need a test, you need it. If you're worried about finances and don't have insurance, ask the doctor or call the lab or X-ray facility directly to see how much it will cost.

- As far as diagnosis is concerned, it is better to overtest rather than undertest, because most errors are those of omission. The fact remains that most tests turn up negative, not positive.

- There are some screening tests which should be performed at intervals even if you are feeling perfectly well. These include **cholesterol, glucose, stool for occult blood,** and **colonoscopy.** In addition men should have a **prostate specific antigen** and women should have a **mammogram** and **Pap smear.**

- The wide variety of tests described here cover every organ system and range from those over a hundred years old to those which have been described only in the past few years. Each has been reviewed for accuracy and suitability for inclusion by at least one physician member of the board of advisors, and the material should cover well over 99 percent of the diagnostic procedures you are likely to encounter. Still, highly trained specialists in any field have cutting-edge techniques and tools at their disposal which may not be mentioned because they are performed so rarely or are so esoteric. Futhermore, things change rapidly. At any one time we are in a "state of the art," and what is adequate today might be completely outmoded tomorrow. In a few years the human genome will be completely mapped and a whole new series of tests will be available.

Test Listings

☐ Acetylcholine receptor antibody

WHAT IT IS AND WHY IT'S OBTAINED

Acetylcholine is a substance which helps transmit impulses across nerve junctions by attaching itself to a "receptor" on nerve cells. Blood levels of antibodies (blood proteins which are an important part of the immune system) to this receptor are used to diagnose myasthenia gravis, a disease which causes weakness and fatigue.

HOW IT WORKS

You will be asked to provide a **venous blood sample** from which serum* will be separated. Immunoassay* is used for the laboratory analysis.

BEFORE THE TEST

No special preparation is required.

AFTER THE TEST

Follow **venous blood sample** aftercare.

SIGNIFICANCE OF RESULTS

High levels of acetylcholine receptor antibody are found in most people with myasthenia gravis, but not all. This test must be interpreted along with your symptoms and signs.

☐ ☐ ☐

☐ Acid fast smear

WHAT IT IS AND WHY IT'S OBTAINED

"Acid fast" bacteria are usually those which cause tuberculosis. Thus, any body sample which contains them is taken to mean that there is active tuberculous infection.

HOW IT WORKS

Specimens may be taken from anywhere, but most commonly the sputum. You will be given a plastic container in which to place sputum that you cough up over a period of time. Sputum should be from a deep cough. The material will be spread on a glass slide, stained, and examined under a microscope.

BEFORE THE TEST

No special preparation is required.

AFTER THE TEST

No special aftercare is needed.

SIGNIFICANCE OF RESULTS

A positive result means active tuberculosis. Further testing, such as **bacterial culture,** will be necessary to confirm the diagnosis and determine the best treatment. A negative result means that no organisms were found but repeat examinations are advisable if your symptoms strongly suggest tuberculosis. **Sputum induction** may be helpful if you have trouble providing a suitable specimen.

□ □ □

□ Acid phosphatase

WHAT IT IS AND WHY IT'S OBTAINED

Acid phosphatase (AP) is an enzyme found mostly in the prostate gland of men. Blood levels are used mainly to evaluate and monitor prostate carcinoma. It is sometimes measured in vaginal specimens in cases of suspected rape.

HOW IT WORKS

You will be asked to provide a **venous blood sample** from which serum* will be separated. There are many laboratory methods for measuring this enzyme.

BEFORE THE TEST

AP levels should not be obtained immediately after a rectal examination or prostatic massage since both of these procedures may falsely increase levels.

AFTER THE TEST

Follow **venous blood sample** aftercare.

SIGNIFICANCE OF RESULTS

A negative test means that AP levels were within normal limits or decreased. Elevated levels of AP are found in prostate carcinoma, prostate infarction (local tissue death caused by an interruption of the blood supply), prostate injury, certain diseases of the bones, and certain diseases of the liver. When used to monitor therapy for prostate cancer it should decrease to normal levels shortly after treatment. Failure to become normal may indicate spread of the cancer. Unlike **prostate specific antigen,** AP is *not* useful to screen for prostate cancer.

SYNONYMS AND INCLUDED TESTS

Prostatic acid phosphatase, PAP.

□ □ □

□ Acid reflux test

WHAT IT IS AND WHY IT'S OBTAINED

The acid reflux test is used to evaluate heartburn or "reflux esophagitis," caused by upward leakage of stomach acid.

HOW IT WORKS

The procedure is usually performed in a special procedure room or laboratory. Your pulse and blood pressure will be taken and the blood pressure cuff kept in place on your arm. A flexible lubricated tube will be inserted into one of your nostrils and guided to the back of your throat. Follow instructions regarding swallowing and do not fight the tube. You may feel the urge to gag but this will pass. The tube will be advanced into your stomach and an electrode designed to detect acidity will be threaded down through it. Acidity will be tested in your stomach and lower esophagus and the two readings compared, the stomach normally being much more acid. Depending upon the initial findings you may be asked to swallow repeatedly and to perform several straining maneuvers, such as trying to exhale with your mouth closed, trying to inhale with your mouth closed, and raising your legs. During this time the acidity of the esophagus will continue to be monitored. If no abnormalities are detected, a dilute solution of hydrochloric acid will be dripped into your stomach and the previous maneuvers repeated.

BEFORE THE TEST

You should fast overnight and follow specific instructions carefully regarding medications, particularly antacids and drugs affecting acidity in the stomach, such as omeprazole, lansoprazole, famotidine, cimetidine, and ranitidine.

AFTER THE TEST

You may have a sore throat for a day or two. Serious complications are rare.

SIGNIFICANCE OF RESULTS

A negative test means that your lower esophagus remained less acid than your stomach. A positive test is good evidence for the presence of esophageal reflux. Other tests for esophageal reflux are the **Bernstein test, esophageal motility,** and the **esophageal pH study.**

SYNONYMS AND INCLUDED TESTS

Standard acid reflux test, Tuttle test.

□ □ □

☐ Acoustic admittance test

WHAT IT IS AND WHY IT'S OBTAINED

The acoustic admittance test is used to evaluate hearing. Unlike a **hearing test,** the acoustic admittance test provides more scientific and objective information. "Admittance" refers to the ability of the eardrum to respond to sound.

HOW IT WORKS

There are two parts to the test, *tympanometry,* which measures the response of the eardrum to air pressure changes, and *acoustic reflexes,* which measures the response of the eardrum to sound. You will be seated in a chair in a special room. **Otoscopy** will first be performed to check for the presence of excessive ear wax or other problems in your ear canal. Your ear will then be pulled upward and backward and a tube of the proper size, called a probe, will be inserted and wedged into your ear canal to form an airtight seal. The probe contains a tiny sound generator, a pressure sensor, channels to change air pressure, and a microphone to record sound. For tympanometry you will be told when the test is to begin and will experience a change in the pressure in your ear. Your eardrum may "pop," but there is no real pain. A series of pressure changes and measurements will be conducted. Follow instructions carefully and do not swallow or move as the test proceeds. For acoustic reflexes, a loud sound will be generated within your ear. You will be told when this is about to occur so as not to be startled. Again the sound will be repeated at different levels as measurements are made. In all cases tracings are produced which are analyzed.

BEFORE THE TEST

No special preparation is required.

AFTER THE TEST

No special aftercare is needed.

SIGNIFICANCE OF RESULTS

The interpretation of the acoustic admittance test will be performed by your doctor. Abnormal tracings may be found with a perforated or scarred eardrum, fluid in the middle ear, wax buildup, disease of the bones in the middle ear, tumors, or nerve damage.

SYNONYMS AND INCLUDED TESTS

Acoustic immitance, impedance audiometry, tympanometry, acoustic reflexes.

□ □ □

□ Activated clotting time

WHAT IT IS AND WHY IT'S OBTAINED

The activated clotting time (ACT) is used to evaluate bleeding disorders and to monitor treatment with the anticoagulant called heparin, which is usually given intravenously in a hospital.

HOW IT WORKS

You will be asked to provide a **venous blood sample,** which will be drawn into or added to a tube containing an activator which enhances clotting, such as powdered glass. The tube is kept at body temperature and tilted every thirty seconds until a clot forms, at which point the time is noted. The tilting and observation may be done by hand or machine.

BEFORE THE TEST

No special preparation is required.

AFTER THE TEST

Follow **venous blood sample** aftercare.

SIGNIFICANCE OF RESULTS

A prolonged ACT is found in any case where there is some interference with blood clotting. Although this is most commonly found when heparin is being given, it should be noted that this test evaluates overall clotting ability.

SYNONYMS AND INCLUDED TESTS

Activated coagulation time, ground glass clotting time.

□ □ □

□ Adrenal antibody

WHAT IT IS AND WHY IT'S OBTAINED

Blood levels of adrenal antibody (a blood protein which is an important part of the immune system) are used to evaluate insufficiency of the adrenal gland (Addison's disease), which causes weakness and low blood pressure.

HOW IT WORKS

You will be asked to provide a **venous blood sample** from which serum* will be separated. Immunoassay* is used for the laboratory analysis.

BEFORE THE TEST

No special preparation is required.

AFTER THE TEST

Follow **venous blood sample** aftercare.

SIGNIFICANCE OF RESULTS

Adrenal antibodies in the blood are found in most cases of Addison's disease but may also be present in adrenal gland infections, in hypoparathyroidism*, and in Hashimoto's thyroiditis*. Urine **cortisol** is a good indicator of adrenal gland function.

□ □ □

□ Adrenocorticotropic hormone

WHAT IT IS AND WHY IT'S OBTAINED

Adrenocorticotropic hormone (ACTH) is a hormone produced by the pituitary gland which stimulates the adrenal gland to produce **cortisol.** Blood levels of ACTH are mainly used to diagnose Cushing's syndrome*, a disease which causes acne, fat accumulations of the face ("moon face") and upper back ("buffalo hump"), high blood pressure, and diabetes.

HOW IT WORKS

You will be asked to provide a **venous blood sample,** with care being taken to use a chilled syringe. The serum* will be separated and frozen immediately. Immunoassay* is used for the laboratory analysis. Because ACTH levels normally vary during the day, at least two samples are obtained, one in the morning and one in the evening. Cortisol levels are usually obtained simultaneously for comparison.

BEFORE THE TEST

You should fast overnight.

AFTER THE TEST

Follow **venous blood sample** aftercare.

SIGNIFICANCE OF RESULTS

ACTH levels are usually obtained as part of a battery of endocrine tests and must be interpreted along with them. Decreased levels of ACTH are found in pituitary insufficiency, Cushing's syndrome from an adrenal tumor, and steroid intake. Increased levels are found in adrenal insufficiency (Addison's disease), congenital adrenal hyperplasia*, Cushing's syndrome from pituitary gland tumors, and some nonpituitary cancers, such as lung cancer. In the last named case the level of ACTH is often markedly elevated. ACTH production may be measured in the **dexamethasone suppression test.**

SYNONYMS AND INCLUDED TESTS

Corticotropin.

□ □ □

□ Alanine aminotransferase

WHAT IT IS AND WHY IT'S OBTAINED

Alanine aminotransferase (ALT) is an enzyme prevalent in the liver. Blood levels are used to detect liver disease.

HOW IT WORKS

You will be asked to provide a **venous blood sample** from which serum* will be separated. Spectrophotometry* is used for the analysis.

BEFORE THE TEST

No special preparation is required.

AFTER THE TEST

Follow **venous blood sample** aftercare.

SIGNIFICANCE OF RESULTS

A very high ALT suggests severe viral or drug-induced hepatitis and is interpreted in conjunction with other **liver function tests** and **hepatitis screening tests.** A negative result is evidence against viral hepatitis. Smaller elevations may be seen in other types of liver disease, heart failure, heart attacks, and infectious mononucleosis.

SYNONYMS AND INCLUDED TESTS

Serum glutamic pyruvate transaminase, SGPT.

❑ ❑ ❑

❑ Albumin

WHAT IT IS AND WHY IT'S OBTAINED

Albumin is a **protein** found in most plants and animals. Blood levels are used to evaluate nutritional status, particularly in kidney diseases and other chronic diseases.

HOW IT WORKS

You will be asked to provide a **venous blood sample** from which serum* will be separated. Of the several methods of laboratory evaluation, bromcresol green is most commonly used.

BEFORE THE TEST

No special preparation is required.

AFTER THE TEST

Follow **venous blood sample** aftercare.

SIGNIFICANCE OF RESULTS

Low albumin levels are found in a wide variety of circumstances, including malnutrition, burns, infections, cancer, pregnancy, and in those taking birth control pills. Chronic diseases of the liver, kidney, and heart also depress albumin levels. Other tests of nutritional status which may prove useful are **iron and iron binding capacity, transferrin, vitamin B$_{12}$** and **folic acid.** High albumin is seen in dehydration.

❑ ❑ ❑

❑ Albumin/globulin ratio

WHAT IT IS AND WHY IT'S OBTAINED

The albumin/globulin (A/G) ratio is a number derived from the blood levels of two components of **protein, albumin** and globulin. It is used to evaluate a variety of diseases.

HOW IT WORKS

The A/G ratio is calculated by subtracting the serum* albumin from the total protein to obtain the globulin level, then dividing the albumin by the globulin.

BEFORE THE TEST

No special preparation is required.

AFTER THE TEST

No special aftercare is needed.

SIGNIFICANCE OF RESULTS

A high A/G ratio is not significant. Low A/G ratios are found in liver disease, kidney disease, sarcoidosis*, autoimmune diseases, severe infections, burns, and ulcerative colitis. More accurate information about the state of the blood proteins can be obtained by a **protein electrophoresis.**

❑ ❑ ❑

❑ Aldolase

WHAT IT IS AND WHY IT'S OBTAINED

Aldolase is an enzyme which is widely distributed in the body. Blood levels are used to evaluate diseases of muscle degeneration.

13

HOW IT WORKS

You will be asked to provide a **venous blood sample** from which serum* will be separated. There are several laboratory methods for determining aldolase levels.

BEFORE THE TEST

You should fast overnight.

AFTER THE TEST

Follow **venous blood sample** aftercare.

SIGNIFICANCE OF RESULTS

Elevated aldolase levels are found in the early stages of some muscle diseases, such as muscular dystrophy. As the disease progresses, aldolase levels tend to decrease. Aldolase, however, may be high in liver disease, after heart attacks, and with certain types of cancer. **Creatine kinase** is a better test for muscle degeneration.

□ □ □

□ Aldosterone

WHAT IT IS AND WHY IT'S OBTAINED

Aldosterone is a hormone produced by the adrenal gland which affects excretion of **electrolytes** by the kidneys. Blood levels are obtained to evaluate high blood pressure.

HOW IT WORKS

You will be asked to provide a **venous blood sample** from which serum* will be separated. Immunoassay* is used for the laboratory analysis. The blood sample is best taken under controlled conditions, while you are lying on your back in the early morning before you rise.

14

BEFORE THE TEST

Blood pressure medications, diuretics, licorice, and hormones such as birth control pills or steroids should be discontinued at least two weeks prior to the test.

AFTER THE TEST

Resume medications as directed and follow **venous blood sample** aftercare.

SIGNIFICANCE OF RESULTS

High aldosterone may be seen in primary aldosteronism (Conn's syndrome) and in high blood pressure from other causes. Conn's syndrome also causes low **potassium**. Decreased levels of aldosterone may be seen in Cushing's syndrome*, licorice ingestion, with certain steroids, and in congenital adrenal hyperplasia*. The blood **renin** is usually taken simultaneously and its level should be taken into consideration.

□ □ □

□ Alkaline phosphatase

WHAT IT IS AND WHY IT'S OBTAINED

Alkaline phosphatase (ALP) is an enzyme which is widely distributed in the body. Blood levels are used to evaluate diseases of liver and bone.

HOW IT WORKS

You will be asked to provide a **venous blood sample** from which serum* will be separated. There are many assay methods available.

BEFORE THE TEST

You should fast overnight.

AFTER THE TEST

Follow **venous blood sample** aftercare.

SIGNIFICANCE OF RESULTS

High levels of ALP are found in liver disease, particularly in those which are characterized by an obstruction to the normal flow of bile*, such as occurs with gallstones or liver cancer. It is also increased in many bone diseases, especially Paget's disease of bone. High levels of ALP occur in the last trimester of pregnacy, and as a side effect of many drugs, including birth control pills. A certain number of people normally have high levels of ALP, which is inherited and does not signify disease. A **gamma glutamyl transferase** (GGT) may help distinguish between liver and bone disease if ALP is high: if the GGT is elevated, liver disease is indicated, whereas if it is normal, skeletal disease is more likely. If the cause of a high ALP still cannot be found ALP isoenzyme studies may help. Low levels of ALP are uncommon but may occur in excess vitamin D ingestion, the milk-alkali syndrome, hypophosphatasia, hypothyroidism*, pernicious anemia*, and malnutrition.

SYNONYMS AND INCLUDED TESTS

Alk phos.

□ □ □

□ Allergic lung antibodies

WHAT IT IS AND WHY IT'S OBTAINED

Allergic lung antibodies are blood proteins in the immune system which act against various molds. Blood levels of them are used to evaluate symptoms of asthma, which may include shortness of breath and wheezing.

HOW IT WORKS

You will be asked to provide a **venous blood sample** from which serum* will be separated. Immunoassay* is used for the laboratory analysis.

BEFORE THE TEST

No special preparation is required.

AFTER THE TEST

Follow **venous blood sample** aftercare.

SIGNIFICANCE OF RESULTS

A positive test suggests but does not prove that your breathing difficulties are due to an allergy to molds. A lung biopsy is sometimes performed to establish the diagnosis.

SYNONYMS AND INCLUDED TESTS

Hypersensitivity pneumonitis serology, farmer's lung disease, air conditioner lung test.

□ □ □

□ Allergy skin testing

WHAT IT IS AND WHY IT'S OBTAINED

Allergy skin testing is used to evaluate allergic symptoms such as hay fever, asthma, and hives. Skin testing may also be used to detect allergies to certain drugs, such as penicillin, prior to instituting treatment with them.

HOW IT WORKS

The substances used for skin testing are liquid extracts of trees, molds, grasses, dander, dust, mites, foods, and insect venoms. Hundreds of possibilities exist, depending upon your geographical location, occupation, or symptoms. There are three general methods of testing: prick tests, scratch tests, and intradermal tests. In the *prick* test a drop of the suspect substance (allergen) will be placed on your back or forearm and a sterile needle passed through the liquid and into your skin just beneath the epidermis, superficially enough not to cause bleeding. After a period of time ranging from one to twenty minutes (depending upon your doctor's preference), the liquid is wiped off. In fifteen or twenty minutes the test site is examined for a reaction and the intensity of the reaction (a wheal and redness) is noted. It is common to do multiple tests at the same time. The *scratch* test is similar except that instead of your skin's being pricked by the needle, it will be scratched. The prick test is generally considered superior because it is less traumatic. In the *intradermal* test the allergen will be injected into your skin through a needle. The choice of which test to use is arbitrary. Some allergists prefer to use the intradermal test to confirm equivocal prick or scratch tests; others use one method exclusively.

BEFORE THE TEST

Because there are so many substances available for testing, a thorough history of your problem should be taken and a physical examination should be performed prior to testing in order to narrow the possibilities. Antihistamines other than hydroxyzine should be discontinued for two days prior to testing. Because of its potency, hydroxyzine should be discontinued for one week prior to testing. Discontinue nonessential medications or others as directed by your doctor.

AFTER THE TEST

Keep the test sites clean by washing daily with soap and water. Report immediately shortness of breath, wheezing, itching, or dizziness which occur later in the day of testing. Late allergic reactions occur but are rare.

SIGNIFICANCE OF RESULTS

Interpreting skin test results, as is the case with all diagnosis in allergy, is very difficult and subject to much variation. Unfortunately, in the mind of the public, almost any symptom may be attributed to an allergy, and this has led to abuse of allergy testing. Many opportunities for false positives and false negatives exist. Studies have shown that individuals who have no symptoms whatsoever may have positive skin tests and vice versa. An individual positive test to pecan, for example, even if strongly positive, may be meaningless in your case, whereas a negative reaction to house dust may overlook a potential cause for your asthma. False negatives may be due to a poorly prepared test liquid, inadequate penetration of the needle, or misreading of a result. Some tranquilizers may also cause false negative testing. Intradermal skin testing is somewhat more specific than either the scratch or prick tests. The **radioallergosorbent test** may help clarify your problem.

□ □ □

□ Alpha fetoprotein

WHAT IT IS AND WHY IT'S OBTAINED

Alpha fetoprotein (AFP) is a **protein** found in fetuses and in certain tumors. Blood levels are used in men and nonpregnant women to screen for liver cancer in those at high risk, such as alcoholics and those with liver disease. It is also of value in monitoring the course and treatment of liver cancer.

HOW IT WORKS

You will be asked to provide a **venous blood sample** from which serum* will be separated. Immunoassay* is used for the laboratory analysis.

BEFORE THE TEST

No special preparation is required.

AFTER THE TEST

Follow **venous blood sample** aftercare.

SIGNIFICANCE OF RESULTS

High levels of AFP are found in those with liver or testicular cancer, although in the latter case the test is not so sensitive In general, the AFP level corresponds to how large the tumor is, so that AFP is useful in determining response to treatment. Liver **ultrasound** is often used along with AFP to screen for liver cancer.

SYNONYMS AND INCLUDED TESTS

Alpha fetoprotein tumor marker.

□ □ □

□ Alpha₁-antitrypsin

WHAT IT IS AND WHY IT'S OBTAINED

Alpha₁-antitrypsin is an enzyme which has several important body functions. Blood levels are used to diagnose alpha₁-antitrypsin deficiency, a hereditary disease, which produces emphysema and liver disease, and to detect hidden inflammation.

HOW IT WORKS

You will be asked to provide a **venous blood sample** from which serum* will be separated. Immunoassay* is used for the laboratory analysis.

BEFORE THE TEST

No special preparation is required.

AFTER THE TEST

Follow **venous blood sample** aftercare.

SIGNIFICANCE OF RESULTS

Low levels indicate alpha₁-antitrypsin deficiency. Detection is important, since the disease can be treated by replacing the enzyme. High levels are seen in chronic inflammation of various types such as cancer, autoimmune disease (where the immune system acts against the body's own tissues), and infections.

Acute phase proteins, A_1 AT.

◻ ◻ ◻

◻ Aluminum

WHAT IT IS AND WHY IT'S OBTAINED

Blood and bone levels of aluminum are obtained in situations in which aluminum toxicity tends to develop, such as kidney failure and industrial exposure.

HOW IT WORKS

You will be asked to provide a **venous blood sample** from which serum* will be separated. A special aluminum-free needle will be used. Atomic absorption is used for the assay. Bone levels of aluminum may be obtained by taking a **bone biopsy** after your have been given oral doses of tetracycline and demeclocycline.

BEFORE THE TEST

No special preparation is required.

AFTER THE TEST

Follow **venous blood sample** aftercare.

SIGNIFICANCE OF RESULTS

High levels of aluminum can cause disease of the bones (osteomalacia), nervous system, muscles, and blood. It also predisposes one to infection. The "desferrioxamine infusion test" for aluminum toxicity is controversial because of possible side effects.

◻ ◻ ◻

◻ Amino acid screening

WHAT IT IS AND WHY IT'S OBTAINED

Amino acids are the building blocks of **protein.** Of the approximately 300 of them which are known, twenty are found in humans. Of these twenty, ten are "essential" and must be ingested in food, since they cannot be manufactured by the body. The proper production of protein depends upon an intricate system of enzymes and problems can occur at any of a number of steps. Amino acid screening on blood or urine is used to detect diseases in which an enzyme deficiency or kidney disease produces abnormal amino acid metabolism and thus abnormal protein synthesis.

HOW IT WORKS

Either blood or urine can be tested. Most information is obtained with both, but of the two, blood levels are the more accurate. Most of the time testing is performed on infants using a **heelstick blood sample.** Alternatively, a random sample of urine may be used. If you are an adult you will be asked to provide a **venous blood sample** from which serum* will be separated. There are several methods used for the laboratory assay.

BEFORE THE TEST

Infants should be fasting for four hours before the test.

AFTER THE TEST

Follow **heelstick blood sample** or **venous blood sample** aftercare.

SIGNIFICANCE OF RESULTS

A negative test means that the amino acids were found in normal amounts. If one or more amino acids either in the blood or urine are found to be elevated, further testing is performed. For example, if the screen for cystine is positive, urine is analyzed in detail for cystine. The multiple diseases included in the general classification called "inborn errors of metabolism" are important since early detection can prevent serious problems, such as mental retardation. Some of the diseases which can be detected with this test are:

Arginosuccinicaciduria
Citrullinuria
Congenital lysine
   intolerance
Cysinuria
Cystathionuria
Cystinosis
Fanconi syndrome
Galactosemia
Hartnup disease
Histidinemia
Homocystinuria
Hyperammonemia
Hyperargininemia

Hyperglycinemia
Hypervalinemia
Hyroxyprolinemia
Lowe's disease
Maple syrup urine disease
Ornithine transcarbamylase
   deficiency
Phenylketonuria
Prolinemia
Sarcosinemia
Tyrosinemia
Tyrosinosis
Wilson's disease*

SYNONYMS AND INCLUDED TESTS

Inborn errors of metabolism screen.

□ □ □

□ Ammonia

WHAT IT IS AND WHY IT'S OBTAINED

Ammonia is a waste product of **protein** metabolism. It is produced in the intestines by the breakdown of protein by bacteria, then absorbed into the bloodstream, and metabolized by the liver. This process fails in liver disease, causing blood ammonia to increase. Thus, blood ammonia is used to diagnose liver disease, particularly hepatic (liver) coma and Reye's syndrome. It is also indicated in infants with unexplained lethargy, vomiting, or deterioration.

HOW IT WORKS

You will be asked to provide a **venous blood sample** from which serum* will be separated. Many laboratory methods of analysis are available. Much care must be taken to avoid contamination by ammonia containing compounds. A **heel-stick blood sample** is used in infants.

BEFORE THE TEST

An overnight fast is recommended. Smoking should be avoided.

AFTER THE TEST

Follow **venous blood sample** aftercare.

SIGNIFICANCE OF RESULTS

Increased blood ammonia generally signifies severe liver dysfunction. In Reye's syndrome, a serious disease of children, three tests are commonly elevated, the blood ammonia, **aspartate aminotransferase**, and **alanine aminotransferase**. Blood ammonia is often used to diagnose and predict hepatic coma, but it is not always reliable.

□ □ □

□ Amniocentesis

WHAT IT IS AND WHY IT'S OBTAINED

Amniocentesis is the removal of a small portion of amniotic fluid—the liquid which cushions and protects the fetus during pregancy—for analysis. It can be performed after about fifteen weeks of pregnancy, when there is enough fluid. Amniocentesis is used to detect a variety of potential problems, various genetic and metabolic diseases, lung immaturity, Down's syndrome, and spina bifida. Amniocentesis is indicated if you are over thirty-five years old, if you have had a child with a genetic or chromosomal abnormality, or if there are diseases which run in your family. It should not be considered as a routine screening test in all pregnancies.

HOW IT WORKS

Amniocentesis is usually performed in a room devoted to the purpose. You will be asked to lie on your back with your hands behind your head. The position of your baby and the placenta is first determined by **ultrasound** and palpation, after which your skin will be swabbed with an antiseptic. A small amount of local anesthetic will then sting or burn slightly as it is injected into your skin. A needle will then be introduced through your skin and uterus and some amniotic fluid will be removed. This is sent to the laboratory. Many tests can be performed on the fluid, including spectral analysis (for hemolytic disease of the newborn), **creatinine** (for kidney maturity), lecithin/sphingomyelin ratio, phosphatidylglycerol, and pulmonary surfactant (for lung maturity), and chromosome analysis (for genetic disorders such as Down's syndrome). **Uric acid, estriol, estradiol,** various enzymes, and **alpha fetoprotein** may also be measured. The sex of your baby is determined with **chromosome analysis.** Cystic fibrosis, hemophilia, polycystic kidney disease, and sickle cell anemia*, among many other diseases can be detected.

BEFORE THE TEST

You should empty your bladder just before the procedure.

AFTER THE TEST

Your vital signs (pulse, blood pressure, respiration, and temperature) will be monitored frequently in a recovery area. You should report any vaginal bleeding or discharge, abdominal pain, cramping, chills, fever, or change in your baby's activity, either increased or decreased. Complications are rare. A Band-Aid will be applied to the puncture site and may be removed in a few hours.

SIGNIFICANCE OF RESULTS

A negative test means that all tests performed on the fluid were within normal limits and that the odds of your having a healthy baby are good.

If the fluid is *bloody* (which occurs about 10 percent of the time) an **Apt test** will be performed to see if the blood is from you or your baby. It is usually from you and carries no special significance except that it may interfere with some of the other tests. If from your baby it may signify damage to the umbilical cord or placenta.

The tests for lung and kidney maturity usually run in parallel and are useful in estimating the age of your baby and the maturity of the organs.

An increase in alpha fetoprotein may indicate spina bifida, in which the spinal column does not close properly.

The significance of other tests which can be run on amniotic fluid depends in large part on the information being sought. In cases of potential Rh incompatibility, which causes hemolytic diseases of the newborn, for example, **bilirubin** becomes important. On the other hand, if you carry an X-linked genetic disease (carried by the you but passed only to a baby boy), the sex of your baby is important.

Over 1,000 diseases can now be diagnosed by amniocentesis using a variety of methods, including chromosome analysis, biochemistry, and DNA testing. Genetic counseling before amniocentesis helps to determine what special tests are indicated. The **polymerase chain reaction** will further revolutionize prenatal diagnosis.

❏ Amsler grid test

WHAT IT IS AND WHY IT'S OBTAINED

The Amsler grid test is a vision test which screens for defects in the central visual field (scotomas) and distortions of central vision.

HOW IT WORKS

Each eye is tested independently. You will be handed a black card containing a grid of fine white lines; in the center of the grid there is a white dot. You will then be asked to answer questions about the chart: Can you see the dot? Can you see the edges and corners of the grid? Can you see all the lines? Are they straight? Is there any blurring or distortion? If there is an abnormality you may be asked to draw what you see. Results depend entirely upon your cooperation.

BEFORE THE TEST

Bring corrective lenses for near vision, if you have them.

AFTER THE TEST

No special aftercare is needed.

SIGNIFICANCE OF RESULTS

There are many causes for the defects and distortions which may be detected by this test. Abnormal results may be further studied with **visual fields, ophthalmoscopy,** and **fluorescein angiography.**

❏ ❏ ❏

❏ Amylase

WHAT IT IS AND WHY IT'S OBTAINED

Amylase is a digestive enzyme secreted by the pancreas and salivary glands. Blood or urine levels of it are used to evaluate abdominal symptoms such as pain, nausea, and vomiting in order to diagnose pancreatitis (inflammation of the pancreas).

HOW IT WORKS

You will be asked to provide a **venous blood sample** from which serum* will be separated. To test urine you will be given a plastic container to collect a two-hour specimen. Many laboratory methods are available for the analysis.

BEFORE THE TEST

No special preparation is required.

AFTER THE TEST

Follow **venous blood sample** aftercare.

SIGNIFICANCE OF RESULTS

Increased amylase is found in pancreatitis and in other diseases of the pancreas, such as injuries or abscesses. It is also increased in stomach ulcers, intestinal obstruction, gall bladder disease, peritonitis, appendicitis, kidney disease, and salivary gland diseases such as mumps. An increased amylase, therefore, is not specific for pancreatitis, and diagnosis of this disease must be made in conjuction with your symptoms and with other laboratory tests, most notably **lipase.** Amylase may be increased by a number of substances which may cause inflammation of the pancreas, such as diuretics, birth control pills, and alcohol. Amylase is also increased in "macroamylasemia," a benign condition in which amylase combines with a blood **protein.**

□ □ □

□ Anal rectal motility

WHAT IT IS AND WHY IT'S OBTAINED

This test measures the ability of the anal sphincter—the muscle which surrounds the anus—to contract. It is used to evaluate incontinence and Hirschsprung's disease, in which the colon is enlarged. It is also used in biofeedback treatments for incontinence.

HOW IT WORKS

There are several devices which may be used, all of which involve the insertion of a tube into the rectum, the inflation of a balloon or balloons, and the measurement of pressures. You will be asked to undress from the waist down, to put on a hospital gown, and to lie on a table, either on your back or left side. You will feel some pressure as the tube is inserted into your anus and rectum but there is no real pain. At times you will be asked to report when you feel the urge to defecate and to squeeze your anal sphincter as hard as you can. This may be repeated as the balloon is inflated and moved and as pressures are recorded.

BEFORE THE TEST

Preparation varies according to the doctor who performs the test. Some gastroenterologists prefer preparation with laxatives and enemas whereas others do not. Follow instructions carefully.

AFTER THE TEST

No special aftercare is needed.

SIGNIFICANCE OF RESULTS

The results of this test will be used in conjunction with your symptoms and history to pinpoint the cause of your fecal incontinence or large colon. Possibilities for incontinence include injury, nerve disease, muscle disease, anal sphincter dysfunction, hyperthyroidism*, and diabetes mellitus*. An enlarged colon may be congenital or acquired, sometimes as the result of chronic constipation.

SYNONYMS AND INCLUDED TESTS

Anorectal manometry, ARM, balloon manometry.

□ □ □

☐ Androstenedione

WHAT IT IS AND WHY IT'S OBTAINED

Androstenedione is a hormone which is produced by the adrenal glands in men, and in both the adrenal glands and ovaries in women. Although it is a male hormone, its effects in men are overshadowed by **testosterone.** In women, however, androstenedione, and the testosterone and **dehydroepiandosterone** which are formed from it can cause male characteristics to appear. Thus, blood levels are used in women to evaluate virilization or masculinization.

HOW IT WORKS

You will be asked to provide a **venous blood sample** from which serum* will be separated. Immunoassay* is used for the laboratory analysis.

BEFORE THE TEST

The test should be taken one week before or after your menstrual period, early in the morning and after an overnight fast.

AFTER THE TEST

Follow **venous blood sample** aftercare.

SIGNIFICANCE OF RESULTS

Elevated levels are found in idiopathic* hirsutism, polycystic ovary syndrome (Stein-Leventhal syndrome), Cushing's syndrome*, **adrenocorticotropic hormone**–producing tumors, adrenal tumors, ovarian tumors, and congenital adrenal hyperplasia*. Other tests which may be helpful are **testosterone, dehydroepiandosterone,** and **17-hydroxyprogesterone.**

☐ ☐ ☐

❑ Anergy skin testing

WHAT IT IS AND WHY IT'S OBTAINED

Anergy refers to failure of the immune system, either total or partial. Anergy skin testing is performed to evaluate the immune system.

HOW IT WORKS

This test is not standardized, and individual doctors have different preferences. The general procedure is to inject substances into the skin of your forearm and note any reaction one, two, and three days afterward. The substances selected are those to which most people have had exposure, and so would be expected to react to. These include antigens* from *Streptococcus, Candida, Trichophyton, Histoplasma,* tetanus, diphtheria, and mumps, among others. The technique is identical to that used for the **tuberculin skin test,** except that multiple injections are made. Commercial kits are available, such as Multitest CMI, in which all the injections are made at the same time by means of a plastic strip.

BEFORE THE TEST

No special preparation is required.

AFTER THE TEST

Keep the site open; do not cover with a Band-Aid. Wash normally and pat dry. Don't scratch or manipulate the test site. If it itches put a plain tap water compress on it.

SIGNIFICANCE OF RESULTS

Normally you should have a positive reaction to one or more of the antigens. A completely negative test implies a problem with your immune system, specifically with your T cell lymphocytes. Further testing is then indicated and will usually include **lymphocyte typing.** There are numerous causes for defective immunity besides AIDS. These include infections, hereditary dysfunction, cancer, autoimmune disease (where the immune system acts against the body's own tissues), kidney disease, diabetes, and sarcoidosis*.

□ □ □

□ Angiogram

WHAT IT IS AND WHY IT'S OBTAINED

An angiogram is an **X-ray contrast study** designed to visualize blood vessels and nearby organs. Although the prefix angio- means "blood vessel," the term angiogram is usually synonymous with the term arteriogram, which refers to the study of arteries as opposed to veins. The X-ray contrast study of veins is called a **venogram.** Thus, an arm angiogram or arteriogram is used to evaluate the arteries in the arm. Commonly ordered tests include the carotid angiogram, cerebral angiogram, and coronary angiogram. The circulation of any area of the body may be studied.

HOW IT WORKS

The general principle of the angiogram is to thread a catheter into an artery and inject an X-ray contrast agent into it while taking **X rays** of the area of interest. The usual approach is through the femoral artery in the groin, from which most of the major organs can be reached. Alternatively, the brachial artery in the arm may be used. Angiograms are usually carried out in a special procedure room with surgical and X-ray equipment. For some studies you will receive a mild sedative. Your vital signs (pulse, blood pressure, respiration, and temperature) will first be taken and an intravenous fluid line will be started in your arm. You will be lying flat on the examining table, the skin over the artery will be cleansed with an antiseptic and an injection with local anesthetic will be made. This will sting or burn slightly. Next, a needle or small catheter will be introduced into the artery and the contrast dye will be injected. You may feel warmth or flushing and a salty or metallic taste in your mouth and you may feel nauseated, but the sensations should be transient. The X rays will then be taken. It is important, as in all imaging tests, to try to remain as still as possible.

BEFORE THE TEST

Preparation varies according to the test and the laboratory protocol. Some doctors prefer an overnight fast, whereas others allow a clear liquid diet. Follow instructions carefully.

AFTER THE TEST

You will be kept on bed rest for a number of hours and your vital signs will be taken frequently. It is important not to move your leg on the side of the puncture to prevent bleeding. The site of the puncture will be checked at intervals for bleeding and your pulses will be palpated to make certain there has been no interruption of blood flow. Allergic reactions to the contrast dye are possible, ranging from mild skin rashes to severe breathing difficulties. These often occur in those with a history of allergy to iodine. The symptoms are transient but if uncomfortable may be treated with antihistamines or steroids. Although uncommon, kidney failure has occurred in those who are dehydrated or who have kidney disease.

SIGNIFICANCE OF RESULTS

Many abnormalities may be discovered by angiography, including blood clots, fistulas, injuries, arteriosclerosis, tumors, aneurysms, and inflammation. A less invasive angiogram using a **radionuclide scan** provides similar information but the images are not so detailed.

SYNONYMS AND INCLUDED TESTS

Arteriogram.

◻ ◻ ◻

☐ Angiotensin converting enzyme

WHAT IT IS AND WHY IT'S OBTAINED

Angiotensin converting enzyme (ACE) is an enzyme which is mostly found in the lungs. Blood levels are used to monitor the activity and treatment of sarcoidosis*, a disease of unknown origin which can affect almost any organ in the body but which often causes lung damage.

HOW IT WORKS

You will be asked to provide a **venous blood sample** from which serum* will be separated. Several methods may be used in the laboratory analysis.

BEFORE THE TEST

No special preparation is required although some laboratories request an overnight fast.

AFTER THE TEST

Follow **venous blood sample** aftercare.

SIGNIFICANCE OF RESULTS

Increased ACE is found in active sarcoidosis* and roughly parallels disease activity, especially if the lungs are involved. It decreases if treatment is successful. ACE is also increased in Gaucher's disease and leprosy and is sometimes used to assist in the diagnosis of these diseases. ACE levels, however, may also be increased in diabetes*, hyperthyroidism*, and liver disease. ACE blood levels are decreased if you are taking the blood pressure medications known as "ACE inhibitors" such as captopril, enalapril, and lisinopril.

☐ ☐ ☐

❏ Anion gap

WHAT IT IS AND WHY IT'S OBTAINED

Anions are negatively charged ions. The anion gap is a calculation based upon **electrolytes** which is used to evaluate acid-base balance*, most commonly metabolic acidosis*.

HOW IT WORKS

You will be asked to provide a **venous blood sample** from which serum* will be separated and electrolytes determined. The anion gap is the difference between the major positive ion, **sodium,** and the two major negative ions, **chloride** and **bicarbonate.**

BEFORE THE TEST

No special preparation is required.

AFTER THE TEST

Follow **venous blood sample** aftercare.

SIGNIFICANCE OF RESULTS

A normal anion gap is found in the metabolic acidosis caused by the kidney disease called renal tubular acidosis, some drugs, and severe diarrhea. A high anion gap is found in lactic acidosis (from many causes), starvation, diabetic acidosis, alcoholic acidosis, and poisoning with salicylates (aspirin), methanol (wood alcohol), and ethylene glycol (antifreeze). A low anion gap usually means laboratory error.

❏ ❏ ❏

❏ Anoscopy

WHAT IT IS AND WHY IT'S OBTAINED

Anoscopy is a technique for directly examining the lower part of the rectum and anus. It is used to evaluate a variety of symptoms, including rectal bleeding, growths, and rectal pain.

HOW IT WORKS

The procedure may be carried out in a special treatment room in a hospital or clinic or in a private doctor's office. You will be asked to disrobe from the waist down and to put on an examination gown. Most often you will be asked to lie on your left side with your right leg drawn up to your abdomen or chest. The anoscope is a plastic or metal tube about two to three inches long. It will be lubricated and inserted gently into your anus and advanced into the lower portion of your rectum. You will feel some pressure but no real pain unless you have some disease causing abnormal tenderness in the area. As the instrument is slowly withdrawn, the walls of the rectum and anus are examined. Biopsies or cauterization may be performed if indicated.

BEFORE THE TEST

No special preparation is required.

AFTER THE TEST

No special aftercare is needed if no surgical treatment was performed. If it was, follow your doctor's instructions.

SIGNIFICANCE OF RESULTS

Possible diseases which may be uncovered include hemorrhoids, abscesses, tumors, polyps, foreign bodies, ulcers, fistulas, and fissures. Deeper views of the intestine can be obtained with **sigmoidoscopy** and **colonoscopy.**

SYNONYMS AND INCLUDED TESTS

Proctoscopy.

□ □ □

☐ Anti-DNA

WHAT IT IS AND WHY IT'S OBTAINED

Deoxyribonucleic acid (DNA) is the genetic material present in the nucleus of a cell. Antibodies (blood proteins which are an important part of the immune system) to it are used to diagnose and monitor treatment of systemic lupus erythematosus (SLE), the most well-known autoimmune disease (where the immune system acts against the body's own tissues), particularly with regard to kidney disease.

HOW IT WORKS

You will be asked to provide a **venous blood sample** from which serum* will be separated. Immunoassay* is used for the laboratory analysis.

BEFORE THE TEST

No special preparation is required.

AFTER THE TEST

Follow **venous blood sample** aftercare.

SIGNIFICANCE OF RESULTS

A negative test means that the antibody level was within normal limits. A positive test is highly specific for SLE, but is not necessary for the diagnosis. False positives ("drug-induced lupus") may be caused by the drugs procainamide and hydralazine.

SYNONYMS AND INCLUDED TESTS

The test is sometimes referred to as anti-native DNA, which means anti-double-stranded DNA, to distinguish it from denatured, or single-stranded DNA. The anti-native DNA test is the more specific.

☐ ☐ ☐

☐ Antibacterial activity

WHAT IT IS AND WHY IT'S OBTAINED

This test is used to monitor the effectiveness of antibiotic treatment in a specific infection. It is used most often in bone and joint infections and in endocarditis (infection of the heart valves).

HOW IT WORKS

A sample of the bacteria causing your infection will have been obtained using **bacterial culture** and you will be undergoing treatment with an antibiotic, either intravenously, intramuscularly, or orally. Depending upon the antibiotic and how you are taking it, a **venous blood sample** will be obtained at some point after one dose and another blood sample before the next dose. In the laboratory the serum* from these samples will be incubated with the bacteria causing your disease to see how well it is able to kill it or inhibit its growth.

BEFORE THE TEST

No special preparation is required.

AFTER THE TEST

Follow **venous blood sample** aftercare.

SIGNIFICANCE OF RESULTS

This test is very useful in adjusting dosages and predicting cure rates for certain chronic and deep-seated infections which require prolonged antibiotic treatment. It is particularly helpful in managing bone infections (osteomyelitis).

☐ ☐ ☐

☐ Antideoxyribonuclease-B

WHAT IT IS AND WHY IT'S OBTAINED

Antideoxyribonuclease-B (AD-B) is an antibody (blood protein important to the immune system) which is present in bacterial infections due to *Streptococcus* species. Blood levels are used to diagnose such infections.

HOW IT WORKS

You will be asked to provide a **venous blood sample** from which serum* will be separated and analyzed in the laboratory.

BEFORE THE TEST

No special preparation is required.

AFTER THE TEST

Follow **venous blood sample** aftercare.

SIGNIFICANCE OF RESULTS

Elevated AD-B strongly suggests a recent streptococcal infection. This test is especially valuable if multiple tests are done and if the concentration (titer) rises over time. It can be used in conjuction with the **antistreptolysin O** and **antihyaluronidase** for increased sensitivity.

SYNONYMS AND INCLUDED TESTS

Antistreptococcal DNase-B.

☐ ☐ ☐

☐ Antihyaluronidase

WHAT IT IS AND WHY IT'S OBTAINED

Antihyaluronidase (AH) is an antibody (a blood protein important to the immune system) produced by *Streptococcus* infections. Blood levels are used to document such infections.

HOW IT WORKS

You will be asked to provide a **venous blood sample** from which serum* will be separated. Several methods may be used for the assay.

BEFORE THE TEST

No special preparation is required.

AFTER THE TEST

Follow **venous blood sample** aftercare.

SIGNIFICANCE OF RESULTS

A significant increase in AH strongly suggests a recent streptococcal infection, especially if multiple tests are used. This test can be used with the **antistreptolysin O** and **antideoxyribonuclease-B** for increased accuracy.

SYNONYMS AND INCLUDED TESTS

Antistreptococcal hyaluronidase.

☐ ☐ ☐

☐ Antimitochondrial antibody

WHAT IT IS AND WHY IT'S OBTAINED

Antimitochondrial antibody (AMA) is used to aid in the diagnosis of liver disease, particularly to confirm primary biliary cirrhosis, an uncommon disease predominantly of middle-aged women.

HOW IT WORKS

You will be asked to provide a **venous blood sample** from which serum* will be separated. Immunoassay* is used for the laboratory analysis.

BEFORE THE TEST

No special preparation is required.

AFTER THE TEST

Follow **venous blood sample** aftercare.

SIGNIFICANCE OF RESULTS

A positive AMA is highly suggestive of primary biliary cirrhosis, but it may be present in other liver diseases and some autoimmune diseases (in which the immune system reacts against the body's own tissues). This test must be interpreted along with other **liver function tests.**

☐ ☐ ☐

☐ Antineutrophil antibody

WHAT IT IS AND WHY IT'S OBTAINED

Neutrophils are a type of white blood cell which are crucial to the immune system. Blood antibodies* to them are used to investigate the cause of a low **white blood cell count.**

HOW IT WORKS

You will be asked to provide a **venous blood sample** from which serum* will be separated. Immunoassay* is used for the laboratory analysis.

BEFORE THE TEST

No special preparation is required.

AFTER THE TEST

Follow **venous blood sample** aftercare.

SIGNIFICANCE OF RESULTS

A high antineutrophil antibody suggests the diagnosis of the disease known as autoimmune neutropenia.

SYNONYMS AND INCLUDED TESTS

Granulocyte antibody.

□ □ □

□ Antineutrophil cytoplasmic antibody

WHAT IT IS AND WHY IT'S OBTAINED

Blood levels of antineutrophil cytoplasmic antibody (ACA) are used to diagnose and monitor the course of Wegener's granulomatosis, a severe form of vasculitis (inflammation of blood vessels).

HOW IT WORKS

You will be asked to provide a **venous blood sample** from which serum* will be separated. Immunoassay* is used for the laboratory analysis.

BEFORE THE TEST

No special preparation is required.

AFTER THE TEST

Follow **venous blood sample** aftercare.

SIGNIFICANCE OF RESULTS

High ACA is mainly seen in Wegener's granulomatosis but other types of vasculitis, ulcerative colitis, and rheumatoid arthritis may cause increases as well.

SYNONYMS AND INCLUDED TESTS

ACPA, ANCA.

□ □ □

□ Antinuclear antibody

WHAT IT IS AND WHY IT'S OBTAINED

The nucleus of a cell is found at its center and contains DNA. Antibodies (blood proteins important to the immune system) to it are called antinuclear antibodies (ANA) and are found in diseases such as systemic lupus erythematosus (SLE). These diseases are often called autoimmune diseases and indicate that the immune system is reacting against the body's own tissues. ANA blood levels are used to screen for these diseases.

HOW IT WORKS

You will be asked to provide a **venous blood sample** from which serum* will be separated. Immunoassay* is used for the laboratory analysis.

BEFORE THE TEST

No special preparation is required.

AFTER THE TEST

Follow **venous blood sample** aftercare.

SIGNIFICANCE OF RESULTS

A positive ANA in a significant concentration (titer) is characteristic of SLE, but must be interpreted in the light of your symptoms. Low concentrations may be found in other autoimmune diseases, such as scleroderma, chronic active hepatitis, mixed connective tissue disease, and Sjögren's syndrome. Numerous drugs, including penicillin, can also produce a positive result, and a certain number of normal people have positive ANAs, especially the elderly.

Positive ANAs will often be further distinguished by a "pattern" of staining of the nucleus. A "peripheral" pattern is usually associated with SLE, a "homogenous" pattern with SLE and other autoimmune disorders, a "nucleolar" pattern with scleroderma, and a "speckled" pattern with mixed connective tissue disease.

A positive ANA will almost always be followed by other tests designed to further investigate your problem. Among these are **anti-DNA, scleroderma antibody, rheumatoid factor,** and **complement.**

□ □ □

□ Antiphospholipid antibody

WHAT IT IS AND WHY IT'S OBTAINED

Blood levels of antiphospholipid antibody (APA) are used to investigate symptoms suggestive of autoimmune diseases (in which the immune system acts against the body's own tissues). These symptoms may include recurrent blood clots, miscarriages, and neurological symptoms, or abnormal blood tests such as a long **partial thromboplastin time** or a positive **serologic test for syphilis.**

HOW IT WORKS

You will be asked to provide a **venous blood sample** from which serum* will be separated. Immunoassay* is used for the laboratory analysis.

BEFORE THE TEST

No special preparation is required.

Follow **venous blood sample** aftercare.

SIGNIFICANCE OF RESULTS

The APA must be interpreted along with other tests since it can be associated with many abnormalities. An isolated, elevated APA along with the symptoms listed above is sometimes called the "antiphospholipid antibody syndrome."

SYNONYMS AND INCLUDED TESTS

Anticardiolipin antibody, lupus anticoagulant.

□ □ □

□ Antistreptolysin O

WHAT IT IS AND WHY IT'S OBTAINED

Antistreptolysin O (ASO) is an antibody (a blood protein important to the immune system) against streptolysin, a substance produced by *Streptococcus* bacteria. Blood levels are used to diagnose recent streptococcal infections.

HOW IT WORKS

You will be asked to provide a **venous blood sample** from which serum* will be separated. Immunoassay* is used for the laboratory analysis.

BEFORE THE TEST

No special preparation is required.

AFTER THE TEST

Follow **venous blood sample** aftercare.

SIGNIFICANCE OF RESULTS

An elevated ASO, especially if rising, strongly suggests a recent streptococcal infection, especially "strep throat." This is important because streptococcal infections can give rise to rheumatic fever and kidney disease after the actual infection has subsided. The ASO test is relatively insensitive to streptococcal infections of the skin and may be falsely elevated in liver disease. Accuracy may be increased by obtaining **antideoxyribonuclease-B** and **antihyaluronidase** tests.

SYNONYMS AND INCLUDED TESTS

ASLO.

□ ⊏ □

□ Apolipoprotein A and B

WHAT IT IS AND WHY IT'S OBTAINED

An apolipoprotein (Apo) is the **protein** part of a fat (lipid)–protein complex. Apo A is the protein part of high-density lipoprotein (HDL) and Apo B of low-density lipoprotein (LDL). HDL is associated with "good cholesterol" and LDL with "bad cholesterol." Blood levels of Apo A and B are used to predict coronary artery disease. Because of difficulties in performing these tests in the laboratory, however, **cholesterol** and the **lipid profile** are more widely used.

HOW IT WORKS

You will be asked to provide a **venous blood sample** from which serum* will be separated. Immunoassay* is used for the laboratory analysis.

BEFORE THE TEST

You should fast overnight.

Follow **venous blood sample** aftercare.

SIGNIFICANCE OF RESULTS

The ratio of Apo B to Apo A is reported as a profile. Low figures signify a low risk of coronary artery disease, high figures signify a high risk.

□ □ □

□ Apolipoprotein E

WHAT IT IS AND WHY IT'S OBTAINED

An apolipoprotein (Apo) is the **protein** part of a fat (lipid)-protein complex. Certain types of Apo E have been linked to Alzheimer's disease.

HOW IT WORKS

You will be asked to provide a **venous blood sample**. A **polymerase chain reaction** is used to test the sample.

BEFORE THE TEST

No special preparation is required.

AFTER THE TEST

Follow **venous blood sample** aftercare.

SIGNIFICANCE OF RESULTS

Although studies have shown that there is a statistical link between the presence of certain genetic types of Apo E and an increased risk of Alzheimer's disease, this test is not accurate enough to be relied upon at this time.

□ □ □

☐ Apt test

WHAT IT IS AND WHY IT'S OBTAINED

The Apt test is used to determine whether a given sample of blood is from a mother or baby. It may be performed on any source of blood, such as amniotic fluid, mucus, or blood found on a diaper. The distinction may be important in certain circumstances, such as if amniotic fluid obtained during an **amniocentesis** is bloody, or if blood is found in an infant's mouth but its source cannot be determined.

HOW IT WORKS

The specimen, from whatever source, is dissolved in water and treated with sodium hydroxide. A mother's blood will appear yellow-brown; the infant's blood remains pink.

BEFORE THE TEST

No special preparation is required.

AFTER THE TEST

No special aftercare is needed.

SIGNIFICANCE OF RESULTS

If the source of blood in or on an infant is found to be the mother there is no need for an extensive evaluation of the infant.

☐ ☐ ☐

☐ Arterial blood sample

WHAT IT IS AND WHY IT'S OBTAINED

Arterial blood is used for **blood gas** determinations. As such it is much more rarely used than a **venous blood sample,** and is almost always performed in the hospital.

48

HOW IT WORKS

You will be asked to lie or sit comfortably, usually in a hospital bed. The radial artery, located over the thumb side of your wrist where the pulse is taken, is most often used. Alternative sites are the brachial artery, located just above the crook of the elbow, or the femoral artery, in the groin. If the radial artery is selected, the "Allen's test" will be performed to make certain there is sufficient circulation to your hand. This is done by the examiner's compressing both your radial and ulnar arteries (located on the other side of your wrist) to cut off circulation to your hand completely. This will cause your skin to become pale, but it is not painful. The compression over the ulnar artery will then be released. If circulation is adequate, your hand will turn pink again. If circulation is adequate, you may receive local anesthesia. If so, it will sting or burn slightly as it is injected into your skin. Then a needle will be introduced into the skin over the radial artery and advanced until bright red blood pulsates into the syringe. The syringe will be capped with a rubber stopper, packed in ice, and rushed to the laboratory for immediate analysis. Puncturing an artery is considerably more difficult than puncturing a vein, and it is not unusual for even an experienced doctor to have difficulty with it. More than one try is frequently needed.

BEFORE THE TEST

No special preparation is required.

AFTER THE TEST

Firm pressure to prevent bleeding after an arterial puncture is crucial, and it should be applied by a nurse or technician, with your arm elevated, for at least ten minutes. If you are taking a blood thinner (anticoagulant), fifteen minutes of pressure is required. You should report any symptoms of swelling, bleeding, numbness, tingling, or discoloration of your hand. Although rare, gangrene has occurred after this procedure.

SIGNIFICANCE OF RESULTS

Arterial blood samples are mainly obtained for blood gas determination. Depending upon the circumstances, **anion gap, calcium, electrolytes, carboxyhemoglobin,** and **methemoglobin** may also be measured.

□ □ □

□ Arthrogram

WHAT IT IS AND WHY IT'S OBTAINED

The arthrogram is an **X-ray contrast study** designed to visualize the joints. Any joint may be tested, such as the ankle, knee, hip, shoulder, elbow, or wrist, as well as the temperomandibular joint in the jaw.

HOW IT WORKS

The test is performed in a special room with X-ray equipment. The skin over the joint to be X-rayed will be cleansed with an antiseptic. A small amount of local anesthetic will sting or burn slightly as it is injected into your skin. A needle and syringe will then be guided into the joint space, often with the aid of fluoroscopy—a type of X ray which produces an image on a screen rather than on film. Joint fluid, if present, may be removed as in a **joint tap** and may be sent for **joint fluid analysis.** The X-ray contrast dye and air will then be injected into the joint space. You will feel pressure but no real pain. You will then be asked to move the joint in order to disperse the fluid. X rays will be taken from various angles.

BEFORE THE TEST

No special preparation is required.

AFTER THE TEST

Follow instructions with regard to activity, since this depends upon your underlying condition. Most joints should be wrapped with an elastic bandage for a few days.

SIGNIFICANCE OF RESULTS

Many abnormalities may be detected by arthrography, including diseases and tears in the cartilage, ligaments, and joint capsule.

SYNONYMS AND INCLUDED TESTS

Joint study.

□ □ □

□ Arthroscopy

WHAT IT IS AND WHY IT'S OBTAINED

Arthroscopy is a technique for looking into the interior of joints, most commonly the knee. It is used to evaluate joint symptoms, to investigate abnormalities found on **X ray** or **arthrogram,** and to monitor the progress of joint diseases. It has become popular because it is accurate and allows many surgical procedures to be carried out at the same time.

HOW IT WORKS

Arthroscopy for diagnosis is most often performed under local anesthesia as an outpatient, but spinal or general anesthesia may be used when surgery is anticipated. Discuss the options with your doctor. If you are particularly anxious you also may receive a mild tranquilizer. There are several techniques, depending upon the preference of the orthopedic surgeon. The following is typical for a knee. You will be asked to lie on a table and the skin of your leg will be shaved and cleansed with an antiseptic. Next, an inflatable tourniquet will be placed around your thigh and a sterile tubular cloth will be applied around your knee. Your leg will then be elevated and an elastic bandage will be wrapped around it from foot to thigh. The tourniquet will be inflated, the elastic bandage removed, and your leg lowered to a comfortable angle. Some of the tubular cloth will then be cut away and a local anesthetic will be injected. This will sting or burn slightly. A small incision with a scalpel will be made at a site depending upon the area to be studied, and the arthroscope will be inserted. You may feel a "thud" as the arthroscope is advanced but you should feel no real pain. Your leg may be moved about in order to examine different parts of the joint or another incision and insertion may be made, depending upon what the surgeon finds. After the examination is completed your knee joint will be flushed with sterile saline solution.

BEFORE THE TEST

Follow instructions carefully, since requirements often differ. In general you should fast overnight for a morning examination and avoid aspirin for at least a week and ibuprofen, ketoprofen, or naproxen for one day.

AFTER THE TEST

Follow instructions regarding activity, although in general you will be allowed to walk immediately. Also follow instructions regarding wound care of the incision, which is usually closed with a sterile tape. Report any fever or undue pain or swelling.

SIGNIFICANCE OF RESULTS

Findings may reveal damage to a meniscus, ligament, bone, or synovial membrane. Cysts, arthritis, or changes associated with gout may also be identified. If a **biopsy** was taken, several days may elapse before the results are known.

□ □ □

□ Aspartate aminotransferase

WHAT IT IS AND WHY IT'S OBTAINED

Aspartate aminotransferase (AST) is an enzyme found in the liver. Blood levels are used as **liver function tests.**

HOW IT WORKS

You will be asked to provide a **venous blood sample** from which serum* will be separated. Several methods are available for the laboratory assay.

BEFORE THE TEST

No special preparation is required.

AFTER THE TEST

Follow **venous blood sample** aftercare.

SIGNIFICANCE OF RESULTS

High AST is seen in many liver diseases, including all forms of hepatitis and cirrhosis. AST is also high after heart attacks. As with all liver tests, a battery of results must be interpreted together.

SYNONYMS AND INCLUDED TESTS

Serum glutamic oxaloacetic transaminase, SGOT.

□ □ □

□ Aspiration

WHAT IT IS AND WHY IT'S OBTAINED

Aspiration refers to the removal of fluid or tissue by means of suction from a tumor, cyst, abscess, or other mass. Aspiration may be performed in a variety of circumstances, but the common denominator is that there is a mass or lump which can be felt and which by its characteristics is presumed to contain a fluid or a semifluid substance. The more common indications are for cysts of the breast, skin, lymph nodes, thyroid gland, neck, and mouth.

HOW IT WORKS

The skin over the mass will be felt by the doctor and held firm. Local anesthesia is usually not used since it distorts the tissue and makes the procedure less reliable. A needle on a syringe will then be introduced through your skin while suction is applied on the syringe. This should be only mildly uncomfortable. When the needle enters the mass it is sometimes moved back and forth and rotated in order to free up the tissue and provide a representative sample from several areas. The samples are sent to the laboratory and may be analyzed by **cytology, bacterial culture, fungal culture,** or other methods. On occasion imaging techniques such as **ultrasound** or fluoroscopy (a type of X ray in which the image is produced on a screen rather than on film) may be used during the procedure to guide the needle.

BEFORE THE TEST

No special preparation is required. Avoid aspirin for at least a week and ibuprofen, ketoprofen, or naproxen for one day.

AFTER THE TEST

Pressure should be applied for at least five minutes to stop bleeding. There may be mild soreness at the site of the aspiration but it should not last long.

SIGNIFICANCE OF RESULTS

Aspiration is often helpful in the diagnosis of masses but repeat aspirations or further surgery may be needed. The main question to be answered is whether the mass is benign or malignant, or, if infected, what germ is responsible.

SYNONYMS AND INCLUDED TESTS

Fine needle aspiration, FNA.

□ □ □

☐ Autohemolysis test

The autohemolysis test is used to evaluate anemia, particularly the type called congenital spherocytosis, in which red blood cells are shaped like spheres rather than like disks.

HOW IT WORKS

You will be asked to provide a **venous blood sample** which will be mixed with glass beads to remove fibrin. The sample is divided into three parts, incubated with and without additives, and the percent of hemolysis—disruption of the red blood cell membranes—measured.

BEFORE THE TEST

No special preparation is required.

AFTER THE TEST

Follow **venous blood sample** aftercare.

SIGNIFICANCE OF RESULTS

An abnormal pattern of hemolysis in the three divided blood samples suggests the diagnosis of spherocytosis.

☐ ☐ ☐

☐ Bacterial antibodies

WHAT IT IS AND WHY IT'S OBTAINED

Bacterial antibodies (blood proteins important to the immune system) are used to diagnose bacterial infections. Many diseases may be tested for in this way, including whooping cough, diphtheria, chlamydia, Legionnaires' disease, or "virus" pneumonia (primary atypical pneumonia). Bacterial antibody testing is performed when direct methods of diagnosis, such as **bacterial culture,** are not feasible.

HOW IT WORKS

You will be asked to provide a **venous blood sample** from which serum* will be separated. Various methods of immunoassay* are available. Multiple determinations over time are best.

BEFORE THE TEST

No special preparation is required.

AFTER THE TEST

Follow **venous blood sample** aftercare.

SIGNIFICANCE OF RESULTS

An elevated level of antibody to a specific bacterium is indirect evidence of infection with that bacterium, but multiple tests which show a rise in concentration (titer) are more specific. In many cases both **immunoglobulin M** (indicating recent infection) and **immunoglobulin G** (indicating more remote infection) antibodies can be distinguished. Many antibodies, however, are not specific, and positive tests should be confirmed by bacterial culture if possible. There are certain cases, however, such as *Mycoplasma pneumoniae,* pneumonia ("virus" pneumonia) in which the organism is very hard to culture, and antibody tests are relied upon for diagnosis. In some cases, such as chlamydia, there are many people who have antibodies but are free of disease. Positive tests may shed light on the situation, but sometimes provoke needless worry. Positive or negative antibody tests should be interpreted in the light of symptoms, signs, and the results of other tests.

SYNONYMS AND INCLUDED TESTS

Bacterial serology.

□ □ □

☐ Bacterial antigens

WHAT IT IS AND WHY IT'S OBTAINED

An antigen is any substance to which the immune system reacts. Bacterial antigen tests are used to help determine the specific organism causing an infection. They are most useful in meningitis when no organisms have been found in the fluid (cerebrospinal fluid or CSF) obtained from a **spinal tap.**

HOW IT WORKS

Either CSF, urine, or blood may be tested. If CSF is used, you will have undergone a **spinal tap.** For urine, a random urine sample will be used. For blood, you will be asked to provide a **venous blood sample** from which serum* will be separated. The specimen may be tested for *Pneumococcus, Meningococcus, Haemophilus influenzae,* or *Streptococcus* by immunoassay*.

BEFORE THE TEST

No special preparation is required.

AFTER THE TEST

For CSF, follow **spinal tap** aftercare; for blood, follow **venous blood sample** aftercare.

SIGNIFICANCE OF RESULTS

A positive test points to the specific organism causing the infection in question, particularly in meningitis caused by bacteria. A negative result only means that the bacterial antigens were not detected and does not rule out bacterial meningitis. The definitive way of diagnosing bacterial infections is the **bacterial culture.**

☐ ☐ ☐

☐ **Bacterial culture**

WHAT IT IS AND WHY IT'S OBTAINED

Bacterial culture is used to identify the organism or organisms causing a suspected infection. It should be noted that a culture is not a **biopsy,** which is the microscopic examination of tissue. Bacterial culture should be distinguished also from **viral culture** and **fungal culture,** both of which test for different classes of organism.

HOW IT WORKS

Any source of biological specimen or fluid may be used: blood, fluid from a spinal tap (cerebrospinal fluid), pus, urine, mucus, drainage, exudate, bone marrow, throat swabbings, stool, or tissue. The specimen is placed in a nutrient in a shallow glass or plastic container (Petri dish) and incubated. Growth on the nutrient is noted and subjected to various tests to determine the specific germ.

BEFORE THE TEST

No special preparation is required. Be certain to tell your doctor if you have taken any antibiotics.

AFTER THE TEST

No special aftercare is needed.

SIGNIFICANCE OF RESULTS

Although culture of a specific germ is usually proof of infection with that germ, contamination must always be kept in mind, and the symptoms and signs must be taken into consideration if something doesn't make sense. The main reason for positive bacterial identification is to allow proper antibiotic treatment by coupling it with **bacterial sensitivity.** Antibiotics, however, will often have been started by the time the culture results are known. The chosen antibiotic may have been correct (a good guess) or incorrect. In the latter case, if the infection seems to be clearing, common practice is to continue the first antibiotic rather than switch to a new one.

□ □ □

□ Bacterial sensitivity

WHAT IT IS AND WHY IT'S OBTAINED

This test is coupled with **bacterial culture** to determine how well antibiotics kill or inhibit the growth of specific bacteria. The two tests are almost always ordered together as a "C & S."

HOW IT WORKS

A **bacterial culture** of the germ causing your infection will have been growing in the laboratory in the nutrient. The culture will be treated with different antibiotics and any change in growth will be noted and recorded. A few specialized laboratories also test multiple antibiotic sensitivities to determine if two of them have a greater effect than the simple additive effects of each (synergy).

BEFORE THE TEST

No special preparation is required.

AFTER THE TEST

No special aftercare is needed.

SIGNIFICANCE OF RESULTS

The sensitivity of an organism to a given antibiotic is usually reported as follows: susceptible, intermediate, or resistant. The most intelligent antibiotic selection, clearly, is the safest, least expensive one which falls in the first category. At times, such as in tuberculosis, repeat bacterial sensitivity testing may be indicated in order to detect resistant organisms which may be developing during treatment.

□ □ □

□ Barium enema

WHAT IT IS AND WHY IT'S OBTAINED

The barium enema is an **X-ray contrast study** used to detect diseases of the colon and rectum. It is indicated in the investigation of abdominal pain, changed bowel habits, diarrhea, constipation, or blood or mucus in the stool.

HOW IT WORKS

The procedure is performed in the X-ray department of a hospital or clinic, or in a private radiologist's office. You will be asked to undress, to put on a hospital gown, and to lie on your side. A lubricated soft rubber tube will then be inserted into your anus. Barium sulfate, the contrast agent, will be introduced slowly and you may experience some cramping and the urge to defecate. Try to retain the barium as long as possible. Sometimes a rectal tube with a balloon is used to make this easier. During the time the **X rays** are taken you will be asked to assume different positions. If a "double contrast" enema was requested, air will be instilled into your colon and multiple films will be obtained in various positions. When the complete series of X rays has been taken you will be moved to a nearby toilet to expel the material.

BEFORE THE TEST

Adequate preparation is crucial to a good test and you should follow instructions given to you carefully. There are several ways to clean the bowel, all involving a period of about twenty-four hours of taking in clear liquids along with a laxative. Then, shortly before the test, multiple enemas may be taken until they are clear. GoLYTELY is a popular product which does not require enemas. It is taken by mouth and produces a rapid diarrhea. Modifications may be necessary if you cannot drink large amounts of fluid.

AFTER THE TEST

If no further X rays are to be taken, no special aftercare is needed. If you are to have a **barium meal,** however, you must cleanse your bowel of residual barium. Follow instructions regarding laxatives and enemas.

SIGNIFICANCE OF RESULTS

Many abnormalities can be revealed by the barium enema, such as tumors, diverticulitis, ulcerative colitis, polyps, and other diseases of the colon. The barium enema is used along with other tests such as **ultrasound, colonoscopy, computed tomography,** or **magnetic resonance imaging** to evaluate diseases of the lower gastrointestinal tract. All these tests provide a different type of visualization. The advantage of the barium enema over colonoscopy is that more of the colon can be seen with it. Its main disadvantage is that disease cannot be observed directly, nor can biopsies be taken.

SYNONYMS AND INCLUDED TESTS

Lower gastrointestinal X rays, lower GI, colon X ray.

❑ ❑ ❑

❑ Barium meal

WHAT IT IS AND WHY IT'S OBTAINED

The barium meal is an **X-ray contrast study** designed to visualize the esophagus, stomach, and small intestine. It is used to evaluate digestive symptoms such as abdominal pain, difficulty swallowing, heartburn, diarrhea, intestinal bleeding, and weight loss.

HOW IT WORKS

This test is usually performed in the **X-ray** department of a hospital or clinic or in a radiologist's private office. You will be asked to undress from the waist up and will be placed behind a screen used for fluoroscopy (a type of X ray in which the image appears on a screen rather than on film). You will then be asked to drink a thick, chalky liquid solution of barium sulfate, the contrast agent. A good study requires your drinking the volume as directed. The movement of the agent down your esophagus and into your stomach will be observed by fluoroscopy and recorded on film. The examiner will compress your abdomen in order to get the barium to coat the lining of your stomach better, and you may be asked to sip barium through a perforated straw in order to get a some air into your stomach or you may be asked to swallow some pills or powder which will form some gas. This is called a "double contrast" technique, which permits better outlining of the stomach walls. The X-ray table will be moved and tilted in various positions and your abdomen will be compressed by the examiner's hand as the barium moves through your bowel. Depending upon your symptoms and the speed with which the barium moves, you may have X rays repeated every hour or so for several hours.

BEFORE THE TEST

You should fast overnight. Follow carefully any instructions from the laboratory regarding medications. Some doctors prefer you to be on a low-residue diet for several days.

AFTER THE TEST

You may be given a laxative to help clear the barium from your intestines. Your stool will be light-colored for several days. Tell your doctor if you become constipated, since barium may harden if you do not eliminate it promptly.

SIGNIFICANCE OF RESULTS

Abnormal findings of a barium meal may include tumors, ulcers, strictures, foreign bodies, inflammation, fistulas, or a hiatus hernia. Biopsy or visualization by means of **upper gastrointestinal endoscopy** may be indicated. Abdominal **computed tomography, ultrasound,** or **magnetic resonance imaging** may be performed *before* the barium meal.

Upper gastrointestinal series, small bowel series, upper GI.

□ □ □

□ Barium swallow

WHAT IT IS AND WHY IT'S OBTAINED

The barium swallow is an **X-ray contrast study** designed to visualize the throat (pharynx) and esophagus. It is used to evaluate symptoms such as difficulty swallowing, heartburn, and intestinal bleeding. It can also be used to locate foreign bodies which have been swallowed.

HOW IT WORKS

This test is usually performed as part of a **barium meal** in the **X ray** department of a hospital or clinic or in a private radiologist's office. You will be asked to undress from the waist up and will be placed behind a screen used for fluoroscopy*. The fluoroscope will be turned on so that the radiologist can observe your chest and abdomen. You will then be asked to drink a thick, chalky liquid solution of barium sulfate, the contrast agent. A good study requires your drinking the volume as directed. The action of its movement down your throat and esophagus will be filmed and observed. This will be repeated, sometimes with a "barium marshmallow," a piece of bread which has been soaked in barium. The X-ray table may be tilted in various positions as the test is performed. Sometimes you may be asked to swallow some pills or powder that will form a gas to better outline the walls of the esophagus.

BEFORE THE TEST

You should fast overnight. On the morning of the test you may rinse your mouth with water but do not swallow it.

AFTER THE TEST

You may be given a laxative to help clear the barium from your intestines. Your stool will be light-colored for several days. Tell your doctor if you become constipated, since barium may harden if you do not eliminate it promptly.

SIGNIFICANCE OF RESULTS

A barium swallow may help detect growths, strictures, polyps, foreign bodies, ulcers, inflammation, fistulas, hiatus hernia, outpouchings (diverticulae), and enlarged veins (varices). Biopsy or visualization by means of **upper gastro-intestinal endoscopy** may be indicated. If abnormal movement of the barium has been discovered **esophageal motility** studies may be helpful.

SYNONYMS AND INCLUDED TESTS

Esophagram.

□ □ □

□ Bernstein test

WHAT IT IS AND WHY IT'S OBTAINED

The Bernstein test is used to evaluate chest pain, specifically, to find out if it is being caused by too much acid in the stomach or esophagus.

HOW IT WORKS

The test is carried out in a procedure room. You will be asked either to sit upright or to lie on your back. A lubricated flexible tube will be inserted into one of your nostrils and down your throat into your esophagus. This is only mildly uncomfortable. Follow directions, particularly with regard to swallowing, since you can often "swallow" the tube without gagging. If you don't fight the tube, it will pass much easier. The tube will be connected to a saline solution drip and you will be asked to report your sensations. This will continue for about fifteen minutes and then switched, without your knowing it, to a dilute hydrochloric acid solution. A positive test is considered to be a reproduction of the symptoms which brought you to the doctor. The switch may be performed several times to determine if the original findings were valid.

BEFORE THE TEST

You should fast overnight. Follow your doctor's instructions regarding antacids and stomach medications.

AFTER THE TEST

You will be given an antacid before you leave the laboratory. No special aftercare is needed.

SIGNIFICANCE OF RESULTS

A positive test is good evidence that your symptoms are due to excess acidity in the lower esophagus. This usually means reflux esophagitis—backward movement of acid from the stomach into the esophagus. False positives, however, can occur with other diseases of the stomach, such as gastritis, and the test is not always positive even in known cases of reflux esophagitis. **Esophageal motility,** the **acid reflux test,** and the **esophageal pH study** are designed to evaluate similar symptoms.

SYNONYMS AND INCLUDED TESTS

Acid infusion test, acid perfusion test.

□ □ □

□ Beta₂-microglobulin

WHAT IT IS AND WHY IT'S OBTAINED

Beta₂-microglobulin is a substance which is released into the circulation in a variety of serious diseases such as AIDS,

65

lymphoma (lymphatic cancer), and kidney disease. Blood levels are used to monitor the course of those diseases.

HOW IT WORKS

You will be asked to provide a **venous blood sample** from which serum* will be separated. Immunoassay* is used for the laboratory analysis.

BEFORE THE TEST

No special preparation is required.

AFTER THE TEST

Follow **venous blood sample** aftercare.

SIGNIFICANCE OF RESULTS

Elevated beta$_2$-microglobulin tends to correspond with the seriousness of certain diseases, rising if the outlook is poor, falling if there is response to treatment.

◻ ◻ ◻

◻ Bicarbonate

WHAT IT IS AND WHY IT'S OBTAINED

Bicarbonate (HCO_3) is one of the major negatively charged ions in the body and is crucial in maintaining the proper pH* of the blood. The chemical name for a substance of this type is a buffer. Blood levels are used to evaluate problems related to acid-base balance*.

HOW IT WORKS

You will be asked to provide either a **venous blood sample** or an **arterial blood sample**. Measurement of pH and **carbon dioxide** will allow HCO_3 to be calculated. Direct measurement is also possible.

BEFORE THE TEST

No special preparation is required.

AFTER THE TEST

Follow **venous blood sample** or **arterial blood sample** after-care.

SIGNIFICANCE OF RESULTS

Bicarbonate is high in metabolic alkalosis* and low in metabolic acidosis*. Its significance is generally the same as for **carbon dioxide** and should be interpreted along with **blood gas** and **electrolytes**.

□ □ □

□ Bilirubin

WHAT IT IS AND WHY IT'S OBTAINED

Bilirubin is a waste product of normal red blood cell breakdown and is the major constituent of bile produced in the liver and stored in the gall bladder. There are two types of bilirubin, one which is formed before it is processed by the liver (indirect or unconjugated bilirubin) and that which is formed after it is processed by the liver (direct or conjugated bilirubin). Blood levels of either type serve mainly as **liver function tests.**

HOW IT WORKS

You will be asked to provide a **venous blood sample** from which serum* will be separated. For infants a **heelstick blood sample** is obtained. Spectrophotometry* and other methods are used in the laboratory for the actual measurement.

BEFORE THE TEST

No special preparation is required.

AFTER THE TEST

Follow **venous blood sample** aftercare.

SIGNIFICANCE OF RESULTS

High *indirect* bilirubin usually signifies that the liver has been so damaged that it can no longer process bilirubin, such as in severe hepatitis, alcoholic cirrhosis, and cancer involving the liver. A high *direct* bilirubin usually means that there is a blockage to the normal outflow of bile, such as occurs with gallstones. Many drugs, including birth control pills, erythromycin, penicillin, and steroids, can produce elevated bilirubin and other abnormal liver function tests.

□ □ □

□ Biopsy

WHAT IT IS AND WHY IT'S OBTAINED

A biopsy is a form of surgery performed to remove tissue for laboratory examination. A sample of any organ can be taken, the limiting factor being difficulty of access and potential problems because of the location. A **skin biopsy** is done in an office and is simple, fast, and poses few risks. A **bone biopsy** is more involved, and heart or brain biopsies require strict preparation, much experience, and a hospital stay. Most biopsies are done to rule out cancer.

HOW IT WORKS

The details and technique depend entirely upon the organ being biopsied. Mild or strong sedation may be used before local or general anesthesia. Minor biopsies may be performed in examining or procedure rooms whereas those which are more involved require operating rooms.

BEFORE THE TEST

This depends upon the organ being biopsied. Avoid aspirin for at least a week and ibuprofen, ketoprofen, or naproxen for one day.

AFTER THE TEST

This also depends upon the organ being biopsied. Follow instructions carefully.

SIGNIFICANCE OF RESULTS

A biopsy is interpreted by a pathologist. Most of the time a diagnosis can be made but there are instances of border-line results or insufficient tissue for examination. Occasionally a report is delayed while consultation is sought or further testing on the tissue specimen is performed, such as special staining or electron microscopy. The pathologist will on occasion call for another biopsy or recommend surgical removal of the entire lesion to be on the safe side.

□ □ □

□ Bleeding time

WHAT IT IS AND WHY IT'S OBTAINED

The bleeding time is a screening test for symptoms such as easy bruisability, spontaneous bleeding, or prolonged bleeding.

HOW IT WORKS

There have been several attempts at standardizing this test, and different doctors and laboratories use different techniques. In one method a blood pressure cuff will be placed on your upper arm and inflated. A site on the underside of your forearm free of veins will then be selected and cleansed with an antiseptic. Two or three small incisions or punctures will then be made in this area, a stopwatch will be started, and blood will be removed with gauze or filter paper at intervals. The time it takes for each cut to stop bleeding is noted and averaged to get the result. Variations arise in the type, length, and depth of the incision or puncture. Commercial kits with disposable equipment may also be used. Although no anesthetic is used, this test is only mildly uncomfortable.

BEFORE THE TEST

Avoid aspirin for at least a week and ibuprofen, ketoprofen, or naproxen for one day.

AFTER THE TEST

Apply a small amount of antibiotic ointment such as bacitracin to the cuts and cover with a Band-Aid or sterile gauze for a day or two.

SIGNIFICANCE OF RESULTS

Prolonged bleeding times occur in a variety of bleeding disorders, such as low or dysfunctional platelets, capillary weakness, and coagulation factor deficiencies. Recent intake of aspirin or ibuprofen, ketoprofen, or naproxen will also prolong the bleeding time. This test is evaluated with other tests for bleeding disorders such as the **platelet count, prothrombin time,** and **partial thromboplastin time.** A variant of this test is called the "aspirin tolerance test" and is performed before and after taking aspirin. This is mainly used to detect aspirin "hyperresponders" who have abnormally long bleeding times after they take small amounts of aspirin.

□ □ □

◻ Blood culture

WHAT IT IS AND WHY IT'S OBTAINED

A blood culture is a type of **bacterial culture** which is used to investigate unexplained fevers and suspected cases of heart valve infection (endocarditis).

HOW IT WORKS

You will be asked to provide a **venous blood sample** which will be carefully obtained in order to avoid contamination. Multiple specimens will probably be needed on different days because bacteria cannot always be recovered from the blood, even when they are there. The specimens will immediately be inoculated into a nutrient, incubated, and observed for signs of bacterial growth.

BEFORE THE TEST

No special preparation is required.

AFTER THE TEST

Follow **venous blood sample** aftercare.

SIGNIFICANCE OF RESULTS

Blood is sterile. Any organisms obtained by culture are due to either disease or contamination during collection. A positive result is highly significant. A negative result means that no organisms were recovered but does not rule out the presence of bacteria in the bloodstream.

☐ Blood gas

WHAT IT IS AND WHY IT'S OBTAINED

The main gases present in the blood are oxygen and **carbon dioxide.** Finding out how much of each is present is used to evaluate how well the lungs and heart are able to transfer oxygen into the blood and carbon dioxide out of the blood. Lung diseases such as asthma and emphysema, and heart diseases such as congestive heart failure and heart attacks may require blood gas determinations. Because of the time, expense, and risks of the procedure it is generally confined to more serious conditions and it is almost always performed in the hospital.

HOW IT WORKS

You will be asked to provide an **arterial blood sample** if you are an adult. A **heelstick blood sample** is used in infants. Great care will be taken to transport the specimen to the laboratory immediately. Besides oxygen and carbon dioxide, which are measured as "partial pressures" and which are reported as "pO_2" and "pCO_2," the pH of the blood and **hematocrit** are also measured.

BEFORE THE TEST

No special preparation is required.

AFTER THE TEST

Follow **arterial blood sample** aftercare. In infants, follow **heelstick blood sample** aftercare.

SIGNIFICANCE OF RESULTS

Low oxygen or high carbon dioxide in the blood indicates some problem in either the heart, the lungs, or both. The degree of abnormality is highly significant and those sick enough to warrant these studies often require further monitoring and treatment, such as a change in oxygen administration, respirator setting, or administration of medications, along with repeat blood gases, until the problem resolves.

SYNONYMS AND INCLUDED TESTS

Arterial blood gases.

□ □ □

□ Blood loss localization

WHAT IT IS AND WHY IT'S OBTAINED

This test is a type of **radionuclide scan** designed to detect the site of hidden bleeding in the intestines, particularly the colon. It is obtained when tests such as **colonoscopy** or **barium enema** have not been helpful.

HOW IT WORKS

The test is carried out in the nuclear medicine laboratory of a hospital, clinic, or private physician's office, sometimes as part of a radiology facility. You will receive an injection of a very small amount of a radioactive isotope, called a tracer, designed for this test. The vein puncture is usually only mildly uncomfortable. The images are taken with a gamma camera, a computerized device which may stand still or may move over your abdomen. You should try to remain as still as possible; this portion of the procedure is painless. Because intestinal hemorrhage can be intermittent, repeat tests may be indicated.

BEFORE THE TEST

No special preparation is required.

AFTER THE TEST

No special aftercare is needed. Although safe, this test does involve the injection of a radioactive compound.

73

SIGNIFICANCE OF RESULTS

Abnormal results are followed up by tests such as **X-ray contrast studies, laparoscopy,** or **colonoscopy.** The main value of the blood loss localization study is to focus attention on a specific area for definitive testing.

SYNONYMS AND INCLUDED TESTS

Gastrointestinal bleed localization study, lower GI blood loss scan.

□ □ □

□ Blood typing

WHAT IT IS AND WHY IT'S OBTAINED

Blood typing is a method of classifying blood according to antigens—substances which stimulate the immune system—on the surface of the red blood cells. The most well known are the "ABO" and the "Rh" classification systems. In the ABO system the antigens are classified as either A or B. A given cell may have only A, only B, both A and B, or neither. In the Rh system, the antigen is either present or absent. Blood typing is used to determine compatibility for blood transfusions.

HOW IT WORKS

You will be asked to provide a **venous blood sample** from which serum* and red blood cells will be separated. Your red cells will be mixed with antibodies (proteins which react with antigens) to antigen A and antibodies to antigen B. Clumping signifies the presence of antigens. The test will then be verified by mixing your serum with known group A and group B red blood cells. A similar test will be performed to determine your Rh status. Your serum will also usually be tested for antibodies to red cells. This is termed an "antibody screen." A "crossmatch" is the mixing of a blood

74

donor's red blood cells with the recipient's serum for incompatibility.

BEFORE THE TEST

No special preparation is required.

AFTER THE TEST

Follow **venous blood sample** aftercare.

SIGNIFICANCE OF RESULTS

Blood typing is reported as A, B, AB, or O. Type A blood has the A antigen; type B the B antigen; type AB, both antigens, and type O, neither antigen. The suffix "positive" or "negative" refers to whether the Rh antigen is present or absent. Although O negative blood is considered the universal donor and AB positive the universal recipient, typing and crossmatching for complete compatibility is the best way to insure that a transfusion reaction will not occur. There is little practical value in knowing your blood type; if you need a transfusion, even as an emergency, your blood will be typed and crossmatched before you receive the blood.

□ □ □

□ Blood urea nitrogen

WHAT IT IS AND WHY IT'S OBTAINED

Urea is the main waste product of protein metabolism. Blood levels of it are referred to as blood urea nitrogen (BUN) and are used to evaluate kidney disease.

HOW IT WORKS

You will be asked to provide a **venous blood sample** from which serum* will be separated. Several methods are available for assay.

BEFORE THE TEST

No special preparation is required.

AFTER THE TEST

Follow **venous blood sample** aftercare.

SIGNIFICANCE OF RESULTS

A high BUN is the hallmark of kidney disease. It is also high in heart failure, increased protein breakdown, diabetic acidosis, dehydration, intestinal bleeding, and muscle degeneration. Certain drugs cause an elevated BUN, as will a recent meal heavy in protein. Low BUN is associated with excess fluid intake, malnutrition, liver disease, and pregnancy. **Creatinine** and **creatinine clearance** are used to further evaluate kidney disease. Frequent monitoring of kidney disease is essential and is often obtained by means of **kidney function tests.**

SYNONYMS AND INCLUDED TESTS

Urea nitrogen.

□ □ □

□ **Blood viscosity**

WHAT IT IS AND WHY IT'S OBTAINED

Blood viscosity measures how easily blood flows. It is used primarily to evaluate poor circulation in newborn infants.

HOW IT WORKS

A **heelstick blood sample** is usually obtained and a microviscometer used for the analysis. The viscosity of serum* or plasma* may be measured separately from that of whole blood. If you are an adult you will be asked to provide a **venous blood sample.**

BEFORE THE TEST

No special preparation is required.

AFTER THE TEST

Follow **venous blood sample** or **heelstick blood sample** aftercare.

SIGNIFICANCE OF RESULTS

Increased viscosity of the blood may be due to polycythemia (in which there are increased numbers of red blood cells), leukemia, abnormal red blood cells, or increased blood **protein.** The viscosity of blood is not the same as its ability to clot, which can be measured by the **activated clotting time.**

□ □ □

□ Blood volume

WHAT IT IS AND WHY IT'S OBTAINED

As its name implies, blood volume is an estimate of how much blood your body contains. It is used to diagnose polycythemia, a disease in which there are large numbers of red blood cells.

HOW IT WORKS

You will be asked to provide a **venous blood sample.** The **protein** or red blood cells or both will then be incubated with a radioactive substance and reinjected intravenously. After a period of time another blood sample will be taken. The amount of radioactivity in this sample will be measured and the blood volume calculated from the degree of dilution which has taken place.

BEFORE THE TEST

No special preparation is required.

AFTER THE TEST

Follow **venous blood sample** aftercare. Although safe, this test does involve the injection of a radioactive compound.

SIGNIFICANCE OF RESULTS

Polycythemia is first suspected when there is an increase in the **red cell count, hematocrit,** and **hemoglobin.** But this may not reflect a *total* increase in red blood cells, because the same result may occur when the blood is concentrated, such as in dehydration or burns. A *normal* or *increased* blood volume under these circumstances, therefore, suggests polycythemia.

□ □ □

□ Bone biopsy

WHAT IT IS AND WHY IT'S OBTAINED

This procedure is used to obtain a tissue sample for microscopic analysis after an **X ray, computed tomography** (CT), or **magnetic resonance imaging** has detected a localized abnormality in a bone. It should be distinguished from a **bone marrow** examination.

HOW IT WORKS

A bone biopsy is usually performed in the X-ray department of a hospital. You will probably be given a mild sedative. The skin over the bone to be biopsied will be first be cleansed with an antiseptic and a small amount of local anesthetic will be injected into your skin and the deeper tissue. This will sting or burn slightly. Next, a small incision will be made and through it a special needle will be introduced. The needle is guided by fluoroscopy (an X ray in which the image appears on a screen rather than on film) or CT until it touches the bone abnormality. The needle will be rotated first one way, then back again to remove a core of bone. This is painful, but the pain lasts only a few seconds. There is no way, unfortunately, to anesthetize the bone. The specimen will be sent to the laboratory for analysis. Bone may also be obtained by a surgeon in an operating room using general anesthesia.

BEFORE THE TEST

Avoid aspirin for at least a week and ibuprofen, ketoprofen, or naproxen for one day.

AFTER THE TEST

If the biopsy requires general anesthesia or is done on your spine, hospitalization will usually be required. Bone biopsy is generally safe but bleeding and infection may occur. It is normal for the biopsy site to be tender for several days but you should report any significant pain, redness, or drainage of pus.

SIGNIFICANCE OF RESULTS

Bone biopsy is most often performed to differentiate benign from malignant tumors. The pathologist is usually able to make this distinction and a report is generated in a matter of days.

□ □ □

□ Bone marrow

WHAT IT IS AND WHY IT'S OBTAINED

The term bone marrow (BM) actually refers to two different procedures, *bone marrow aspiration* and *bone marrow biopsy*. BM in the minds of many implies a painful and serious procedure, but there are many reasons for obtaining these tests since they provide information which can be obtained in no other way. Of the two, BM aspiration is the more common, but some hematologists routinely perform both procedures on all patients in which either study is indicated. BM is used to evaluate a wide range of disorders but mainly those of the blood. It is also of value in determining the extent or spread of infections such as tuberculosis.

HOW IT WORKS

BM aspiration refers to the sampling of the bone marrow itself, whereas BM biopsy is the removal of a complete core of the bone and marrow. If both are being done at the same time, opinions differ as to which should come first. If you are not told, you should ask, since it helps to prepare for the procedure if you know what to expect. For BM *aspiration* several sites are possible. Although the breast bone, spine, or rib may be used, the best site is the pelvic bone, specifically the "posterior superior iliac crest," one of the two bony prominences located just above your buttocks near the lower spine. The *anterior* superior iliac crest—the prominence on your side above your hip—may also be used. In children the best site is the leg, specifically the upper portion of the shin. If the test is being done on your pelvic bone, you will be asked to lie on your side. The skin will be cleansed with an antiseptic and anesthetized with a local anesthetic, which stings or burns mildly. Once the superficial area is numb, more anesthetic will be injected deeper. A small incision will then be made and a special needle introduced through it down to the bone and into the marrow cavity. When it is in the cavity a syringe is attached and negative pressure is applied. You will be warned just before this is done because it is the point at which you will feel the most discomfort. The specimen is checked immediately to see if it is adequate. If so, and if only an aspiration was planned, the procedure ends here. If the specimen is not adequate, what is called a "dry tap," it will be repeated. If the test is to include a BM *biopsy,* a nearby but different site will be used. Another small incision will be made and a different type of needle will be introduced and rotated into the bone and marrow. The sensation is one of "drilling" and is usually more uncomfortable than the aspiration, although on occasion it is less. The removal of the core of bone marrow also takes longer than the aspiration, but it is only a matter of seconds. Again the specimen is examined for adequacy and is transported to the laboratory for microscopic examination.

BEFORE THE TEST

No special preparation is required.

AFTER THE TEST

Pressure will be applied to the site for several minutes (longer if you are having trouble with bleeding). If the back of the pelvis was used you should lie on your back for at least thirty minutes. Complications of BM are few, particularly from the pelvic bone. Although rare, perforation of the chest and heart has occurred in cases of BM *aspiration* from the breast bone. This bone is never used for a BM *biopsy*.

SIGNIFICANCE OF RESULTS

The slides of the material obtained are interpreted by a pathologist. Results may confirm a clinical suspicion, indicate the direction for further testing, or offer a specific diagnosis. BM is interpreted in conjunction with a wide range of other tests. In cases of suspected infection a portion of the specimen may be sent for **bacterial culture** or **fungal culture.**

□ □ □

□ **Bone scan**

WHAT IT IS AND WHY IT'S OBTAINED

The bone scan is a type of **radionuclide scan** used to visualize the skeleton. It is obtained to detect cancer in bones, to monitor bone diseases, to assess the progress of bone grafts, to diagnose bone infections, to detect fractures, and to evaluate unexplained bone pain. It is a common study in the field of nuclear medicine and is valuable because it can detect bone disorders much earlier than conventional X rays. Sometimes a **gallium scan** is done at the same time.

HOW IT WORKS

The test takes several hours, of which about an hour is spent "under the camera." It is carried out in the nuclear medicine department of a hospital, clinic, or private physician's office, sometimes as part of a radiology facility. You will receive an injection of a very small amount of a radioactive isotope ("tracer") designed for this test. The vein puncture is usually only mildly uncomfortable. You will then be asked to wait for two to three hours for the tracer to disperse while you drink four to six glasses of water. Just before the actual scan you should empty your bladder. The images are taken with a gamma camera, a computerized device which will move over your body to produce pictures. Some studies may be performed with you sitting, standing, or lying down, but the whole body scan is best done as you lie flat on the table. You will be asked to remain still as the actual scanning takes place. It is painless.

BEFORE THE TEST

Do not drink large quantities of water or other liquids *before* the injection of the tracer.

AFTER THE TEST

Follow **venous blood sample** aftercare. Although safe, this test does involve the injection of a radioactive compound.

SIGNIFICANCE OF RESULTS

The tracer will concentrate at varying levels depending on the metabolism of the bone in question; diseased bone exhibits increased metabolism which shows up as a "hot spot." Tumors or fractures show up particularly well, the bone scan being the most sensitive test to reveal either. Questionable areas may then be further studied with **X ray, computed tomography,** or **bone biopsy.**

SYNONYMS AND INCLUDED TESTS

Whole body bone scan, bone scintigram.

□ □ □

□ Brain scan

WHAT IT IS AND WHY IT'S OBTAINED

The brain scan is a type of **radionuclide scan** which is used to visualize the brain to evaluate symptoms such as paralysis, seizures, dementia, or certain types of severe headaches.

HOW IT WORKS

The test takes about forty-five minutes. It is carried out in the nuclear medicine department of a hospital, clinic, or private physician's office, sometimes as part of a radiology facility. You will receive an injection of a very small amount of a radioactive isotope ("tracer") designed for this test. The vein puncture is usually only mildly uncomfortable. The images are taken with a gamma camera, a computerized device which will rotate very close to your head and shoulders. You should remain absolutely still during the scanning, which is painless and takes about three minutes. Thirty minutes to two hours later another scan, taking about thirty minutes, will be performed, and again you will be asked to lie still.

BEFORE THE TEST

No special preparation is required.

AFTER THE TEST

Follow **venous blood sample** aftercare at the injection site.

Although safe, this test does involve the injection of a radioactive compound.

SIGNIFICANCE OF RESULTS

In strokes, the brain scan often becomes abnormal before other tests such as **computed tomography** or **magnetic resonance imaging.** Brain tumors, aneurysms, or Alzheimer's disease may show characteristic patterns.

SYNONYMS AND INCLUDED TESTS

Brain scintigram, SPECT scan.

□ □ □

□ Brain stem auditory evoked responses

WHAT IT IS AND WHY IT'S OBTAINED

Brain stem auditory evoked responses (BAER) are used to investigate symptoms related to the function of the hearing (acoustic) nerve. It can be helpful in diagnosing brain tumors, strokes, and degenerative diseases of the nerves and brain. It is also sometimes used to confirm brain death.

HOW IT WORKS

Electrodes will be placed on your scalp and on the ear lobule of the ear being tested. You will then be asked to wear headphones or insert earphones. When the test starts you will hear clicks of varying loudness. The total number of clicks per ear is between 500 and 2,000, and is closer to the latter. The electrodes pick up your brain waves produced by the sound, and these waves are amplified, sent to a computer, averaged, and recorded. The test is painless and you don't have to respond. The analysis of what is going on inside your brain is performed automatically by the computer.

No special preparation is required.

AFTER THE TEST

No special aftercare is needed.

SIGNIFICANCE OF RESULTS

The BAER is interpreted by a neurologist, ear, nose, and throat specialist, or neurophysiologist. Abnormalities can suggest the location of a problem anywhere in the pathway from the ear to the areas of the brain which receive nerve impulses from the ear. Characteristic findings are found in acoustic neuroma, multiple sclerosis, elevated pressure in the skull, and damage to the inner ear. More accurate interpretation is possible when the results of a hearing test are available.

SYNONYMS AND INCLUDED TESTS

Brain stem auditory evoked potentials.

□ □ □

□ Breast biopsy

WHAT IT IS AND WHY IT'S OBTAINED

A breast **biopsy** is the removal of a portion of the breast for laboratory examination. It is used to evaluate breast masses, abnormalities discovered by **mammography** which cannot be felt, or discharge or bleeding from the nipple. If a lump appears to be a cyst it may be diagnosed by **aspiration**. A nipple discharge may first be evaluated by **cytology**.

HOW IT WORKS

A breast biopsy may be performed under local or general anesthesia, in an outpatient surgical facility or hospital operating room. You should discuss the options with your doctor. For a biopsy performed under local anesthesia the skin over the area of concern will be cleansed with an antiseptic and a small amount of local anesthetic will be injected into your skin. This will sting or burn slightly. A cut will be made into the skin of your breast, the tissue separated and dissected, and the lump identified and removed. If it is small, the entire mass will probably be removed; if larger, only a part will be taken out. The skin will be closed with stitches. If the lesion was detected by mammography and could not be felt by your doctor, you will first go the X-ray department, where a needle will be placed within the area in question. The needle may be used to inject a colored dye into the suspicious area or it may be left in place. You will then go to the operating room, where your surgeon will either remove the tissue surrounding the tip of the needle or the tissue colored by the dye. Breast biopsy by needle is also possible. Discuss this option with your doctor. Advantages of it include decreased scarring, discomfort, and cost, but less tissue is available for analysis.

BEFORE THE TEST

Avoid aspirin for at least a week and ibuprofen, ketoprofen, or naproxen for one day. If you are to receive general anesthesia you should fast overnight.

AFTER THE TEST

If you received a general anesthetic you will be placed in a recovery area and your vital signs (pulse, blood pressure, respiration, and temperature) will be taken until the anesthetic has worn off. Follow instructions regarding wound care and report any undue pain, bleeding, or abnormal discharge. Return for removal of stitches in about a week.

SIGNIFICANCE OF RESULTS

A variety of tumors, both benign and malignant, may be identified by biopsy. If malignant, the type of cancer is important in determining the best treatment. Besides its appearance under the microscope, a cancer will usually be tested for its response to hormones. There are many types of breast cancer and grades of malignancy within those types. Some cancers almost never spread; others do so at an early stage. The issue of outlook is complicated and depends not only upon a tumor's characteristics but upon its size, location, spread to other organs, and your general health.

□ □ □

□ Bronchography

WHAT IT IS AND WHY IT'S OBTAINED

Bronchography is an **X-ray contrast study** used to visualize the bronchial tubes. Because of complications and complexity it has largely been replaced by **computed tomography** and **bronchoscopy.** *Localized* bronchography is rarely used to document localized bronchiectasis, an uncommon disease in which a pocket of infection occurs within the lung. It is better tolerated than complete bronchography.

HOW IT WORKS

The general procedure is similar to that of **bronchoscopy,** with an X-ray contrast material being instilled as part of that procedure. **X rays** of your chest will then be taken.

BEFORE THE TEST

You should fast overnight.

AFTER THE TEST

You will be encouraged to cough in order to eliminate the contrast medium. Fever is fairly common after bronchography, as is mild transient difficulty in breathing which clears in a day or two. You will be allowed to eat and drink when your gag reflex returns. Allergic reactions to the contrast agent are possible. If you develop a rash, wheezing, difficulty in breathing, or any other symptom which is unusual for you, contact your doctor.

SIGNIFICANCE OF RESULTS

Abnormalities may include tumors, obstructions from foreign bodies, or cavities.

SYNONYMS AND INCLUDED TESTS

Bronchogram.

□ □ □

□ Bronchoscopy

WHAT IT IS AND WHY IT'S OBTAINED

Bronchoscopy is used to look inside the trachea, larynx, vocal cords, and bronchial tubes in order to evaluate abnormalities found on chest X ray, unexplained persistent cough, or bloody sputum.

HOW IT WORKS

Bronchoscopy is performed in a special room in a hospital or clinic, either as an inpatient or outpatient. You will receive a tranquilizer, painkiller, or both, and will be asked to gargle with a local anesthetic. The procedure may be performed as you lie on your back or sit. The bronchoscope, which is a flexible tube with fiberoptic illumination and multiple channels, will be inserted slowly into your nose or mouth, and additional local anesthetic will be sprayed through it to suppress your tendency to gag. There is some discomfort associated with this but no real pain. You will not choke because oxygen will be provided through the tube. Try to relax and breathe normally. You will remain conscious but groggy and your recollection of the event will be hazy. Depending upon the findings, biopsies, cultures, or brushings may be taken using instruments passed through the bronchoscope. The entire procedure takes about an hour.

BEFORE THE TEST

You should fast overnight. Follow your doctor's instructions regarding medications. Usually, medications (especially asthma medications) may be taken with a small amount of water.

AFTER THE TEST

You will be kept in the hospital or outpatient facility for several hours until the local anesthetic wears off and your gag reflex returns. During this time your vital signs (pulse, blood pressure, respiration, and temperature) will be monitored. If a biopsy was taken you will be told to refrain from clearing your throat and coughing. Try to spit out saliva rather than swallow it. You will have a sore throat for day or so and be hoarse and it is possible to lose your voice temporarily. Bronchoscopy is generally safe, although perforation of the airway leading to a collapsed lung (pneumothorax), spasm of the bronchial tubes, or hemorrhage may rarely occur.

SIGNIFICANCE OF RESULTS

Abnormal findings on bronchoscopy may include inflammation, infection, tumors, foreign bodies, cavities, sites of hemorrhage, and ulcers. If specimens were taken for biopsy, **bacterial culture** or **fungal culture** reports may take days or weeks to be returned.

□ □ □

□ Buccal smear for sex chromatin

WHAT IT IS AND WHY IT'S OBTAINED

This test is used to determine sex.

HOW IT WORKS

You will be asked to open your mouth. Tongue depressors will be used to scrape the inside of both of your cheeks. The superficial skin cells will be transferred to glass slides, stained, and examined under a microscope for "Barr bodies" (sex chromatin), which indicates the female pattern.

BEFORE THE TEST

No special preparation is required.

AFTER THE TEST

No special aftercare is needed.

SIGNIFICANCE OF RESULTS

This is a screening test which is in general accurate in determining whether a person is genetically male (XY) or female (XX). Definitive results can be obtained with a **chromosome analysis.**

□ □ □

□ Buffy coat bacteremia detection

WHAT IT IS AND WHY IT'S OBTAINED

The buffy coat is a white layer which appears between the red blood cells and the serum when blood is centrifuged (spun down). It consists of white blood cells. Bacteremia refers to bacteria in the blood. Buffy coat bacteremia detection is used to detect bacteria in the bloodstream.

HOW IT WORKS

You will be asked to provide a **venous blood sample.** This will be centrifuged and the buffy coat will be smeared on a glass slide, stained, and examined under a microscope.

BEFORE THE TEST

No special preparation is required.

AFTER THE TEST

Follow **venous blood sample** aftercare.

SIGNIFICANCE OF RESULTS

The presence of bacteria in the buffy coat is highly suggestive of bacteria in the bloodstream (bacteremia), which is a serious condition. **Blood culture,** however, is a more specific test.

□ □ □

□ BUN/creatinine ratio

WHAT IT IS AND WHY IT'S OBTAINED

The BUN/creatinine ratio is a calculation derived from two other tests, the **blood urea nitrogen (BUN),** and **creatinine.** It is helpful in assessing kidney function.

HOW IT WORKS

You will be asked to provide a **venous blood sample** from which serum* will be separated. The BUN and creatinine are measured and the ratio between them calculated.

BEFORE THE TEST

No special preparation is required.

AFTER THE TEST

Follow **venous blood sample** aftercare.

High BUN/creatinine ratios occur in inadequate blood supply to the kidney, shock, dehydration, gastrointestinal bleeding, and a high protein diet. Low ratios are found in malnutrition (particularly protein deprivation), pregnancy, liver disease, prolonged intravenous fluid therapy, kidney dialysis, and with certain drugs, such as tetracycline, cimetidine, and trimethoprim.

□ □ □

□ C-peptide

WHAT IT IS AND WHY IT'S OBTAINED

C-peptide is produced in the pancreas along with **insulin.** Blood levels are used to evaluate low blood sugar (hypoglycemia) and diabetes.

HOW IT WORKS

You will be asked to provide a **venous blood sample** from which serum* will be separated. Immunoassay* is used for the laboratory analysis.

BEFORE THE TEST

You should fast overnight.

AFTER THE TEST

Follow **venous blood sample** aftercare.

SIGNIFICANCE OF RESULTS

In hypoglycemia, a high C-peptide usually indicates an insulin-secreting tumor in the pancreas. A low C-peptide along with elevated insulin signifies that the individual is taking insulin by injection. In diabetes, the C-peptide level corresponds to how much functioning pancreas tissue remains and may assist in deciding the best treatment.

SYNONYMS AND INCLUDED TESTS

Connecting peptide insulin.

□ □ □

□ C-reactive protein

WHAT IT IS AND WHY IT'S OBTAINED

C-reactive protein (CRP) is a substance which increases in response to inflammation and infection. Blood levels are most often used to detect the presence of hidden bacterial infection.

HOW IT WORKS

You will be asked to provide a **venous blood sample** from which serum* will be separated. Several methods of immunoassay* are available.

BEFORE THE TEST

No special preparation is required.

AFTER THE TEST

Follow **venous blood sample** aftercare.

SIGNIFICANCE OF RESULTS

High CRP is found in bacterial infections, injuries, appendicitis, heart attacks, rheumatoid arthritis, Crohn's disease, cancer, and immediately following surgery. Viral infections may cause increases but they are typically less than those found in bacterial infections. Low or normal CRP is found in ulcerative colitis and lupus erythematosus*, which may be of use in differentiating these diseases from Crohn's disease and rheumatoid arthritis, respectively. CRP is often used after surgery or in leukemia to detect bacterial infections. Similar findings are seen in the **erythrocyte sedimentation rate,** but CRP tends to rise more quickly in the presence of disease.

SYNONYMS AND INCLUDED TESTS

Acute phase reactant.

□ □ □

□ C1 esterase inhibitor

WHAT IT IS AND WHY IT'S OBTAINED

Blood levels of C1 esterase inhibitor are used to diagnose hereditary angioneurotic edema, an uncommon disease characterized by recurrent swelling of the face and other areas.

HOW IT WORKS

You will be asked to provide a **venous blood sample** from which serum* will be separated. Immunoassay* is used for the laboratory analysis.

BEFORE THE TEST

No special preparation is required.

AFTER THE TEST

Follow **venous blood sample** aftercare.

SIGNIFICANCE OF RESULTS

Decreased levels of C1 esterase inhibitor indicate hereditary angioneurotic edema.

□ □ □

☐ CA 125

WHAT IT IS AND WHY IT'S OBTAINED

CA 125 is a blood test used to monitor the progress and treatment of cancer, particularly cancer of the ovary.

HOW IT WORKS

You will be asked to provide a **venous blood sample** from which serum* will be separated. Immunoassay* is used for the laboratory analysis.

BEFORE THE TEST

No special preparation is required.

AFTER THE TEST

Follow **venous blood sample** aftercare.

SIGNIFICANCE OF RESULTS

Many benign conditions may cause a rise in CA 125, including menstruation, pregnancy, and pelvic inflammatory disease. It is most helpful when repeated measurements are made at intervals along with other tests to detect cancer recurrence.

SYNONYMS AND INCLUDED TESTS

Cancer antigen 125.

☐ ☐ ☐

☐ CA 15-3

WHAT IT IS AND WHY IT'S OBTAINED

CA 15-3 is a blood test used to test for recurrence and spread of breast cancer.

HOW IT WORKS

You will be asked to provide a **venous blood sample** from which serum* will be separated. Immunoassay* is used for the laboratory analysis.

BEFORE THE TEST

No special preparation is required.

AFTER THE TEST

Follow **venous blood sample** aftercare.

SIGNIFICANCE OF RESULTS

An elevated CA 15-3 suggests spread or recurrence of breast cancer. This test is often used along with **carcinoembryonic antigen** and **CA 125**. The TAG 72 test works in a similar way. It is not used to screen for breast cancer.

SYNONYMS AND INCLUDED TESTS

Carbohydrate antigen 15-3.

□ □ □

□ CA 19-9

WHAT IT IS AND WHY IT'S OBTAINED

CA 19-9 is a blood test which is used to monitor the progress and treatment of cancer, particularly cancer of the pancreas.

HOW IT WORKS

You will be asked to provide a **venous blood sample** from which serum* will be separated. Immunoassay* is used for the laboratory analysis.

BEFORE THE TEST

No special preparation is required.

AFTER THE TEST

Follow **venous blood sample** aftercare.

SIGNIFICANCE OF RESULTS

The CA 19-9 is most useful when several measurements are made at intervals along with other tests to detect recurrence or spread of the cancer in question. An elevated level is not specific for cancer and should not be used as a screening test.

SYNONYMS AND INCLUDED TESTS

Carbohydrate antigen 19-9.

□ □ □

□ Calcitonin

WHAT IT IS AND WHY IT'S OBTAINED

Calcitonin is a hormone produced in the thyroid gland which acts to stabilize the level of **calcium** in the blood. Blood levels are used to evaluate thyroid enlargement and to screen family members of those with certain thyroid tumors.

HOW IT WORKS

You will be asked to provide a **venous blood sample** from which serum* will be separated. Immunoassay* is used for the laboratory analysis.

BEFORE THE TEST

You should fast overnight.

AFTER THE TEST

Follow **venous blood sample** aftercare.

SIGNIFICANCE OF RESULTS

A high calcitonin is very suggestive of "medullary carcinoma" of the thyroid. Although uncommon, it is important to detect this cancer early, since it may be cured by surgery. Calcitonin may also be elevated in an early stage of medullary carcinoma of the thyroid, which is called "C cell hyperplasia." If the results of this test are inconclusive, calcitonin stimulation with intravenous calcium or pentagastrin is performed. In these cases, an elevated calcitonin is considered a positive test.

SYNONYMS AND INCLUDED TESTS

Thyrocalcitonin.

□ □ □

□ Calcium

WHAT IT IS AND WHY IT'S OBTAINED

Calcium is crucial to health and is the major component of bone. Its blood level is kept within strict limits by the body. High or low levels can lead to critical situations, including coma and death. Blood levels of calcium are routinely obtained to evaluate general health, acid-base balance, irregularities of the heartbeat (arrhythmias), blood clotting diseases, diseases of the endocrine glands, and diseases of bones. Urine levels are used to evaluate bone disease, kidney stones, parathyroid gland disease, and calcium intake.

HOW IT WORKS

For blood testing you will be asked to provide a **venous blood sample** from which serum* will be separated. For

urine you will be asked to provide a **24-hour urine sample.**
In either case cresophthalein complexone is used to measure the amount of calcium present.

BEFORE THE TEST

You should fast overnight. For urine testing try to stay on your normal diet and activity levels for as long as possible before and during the test.

AFTER THE TEST

Follow **venous blood sample** aftercare.

SIGNIFICANCE OF RESULTS

The most common causes of increased *blood* calcium are primary hyperparathyroidism, cancer, various medications and drugs, Paget's disease, sarcoidosis, and increased intake of vitamin A, vitamin D, or calcium itself. Dehydration will give the appearance of a slight elevation. Low *blood* calcium levels are found with low **protein,** kidney disease, hypoparathyroidism, vitamin D deficiency, and certain drugs, such as anticonvulsants, steroids, and insulin. *Urine* calcium is high in hyperparathyroidism, sarcoidosis, prolonged bed rest, Paget's disease, steroid use, diabetes, hyperthyroidism, cancer, and increased intake of vitamin A, vitamin D, and calcium. It is low with hypoparathyroidism, kidney disease, vitamin D deficiency, and in those taking certain diuretics.

□ □ □

□ Capillary fragility test

WHAT IT IS AND WHY IT'S OBTAINED

The capillary fragility test evaluates the smallest blood vessels, the capillaries, and is used to investigate bleeding disorders.

HOW IT WORKS

There are several ways to perform this test. In one, a circle will be drawn on your forearm, your blood pressure will be taken, and the blood pressure cuff will be reinflated to a pressure midway between the systolic (high number) and diastolic (low number) readings. The cuff will be kept in place for five minutes, deflated, and the number of petechiae (flat, tiny, and round red-purple spots signifying hemorrhage in the skin) within the circle will be recorded. In another variant, a suction device will be applied to your forearm until at least one petechia forms. The amount of pressure required to produce this result is then noted. The suction device produces only mild discomfort.

BEFORE THE TEST

No special preparation is required.

AFTER THE TEST

Open and close your hand a few times to restore blood flow to your arm.

SIGNIFICANCE OF RESULTS

Positive tests are seen in a wide variety of bleeding disorders, including low platelets (thrombocytopenia) and disseminated intravascular coagulation*, and must always be interpreted in the light of other tests for bleeding disorders, such as the **platelet count, prothrombin time,** and **partial thromboplastin time.** False positives often occur in women, particularly around menstruation. Although inexpensive, this test is nonspecific.

SYNONYMS AND INCLUDED TESTS

Rumpel-Leede test, tourniquet test.

□ □ □

☐ Carbon dioxide

WHAT IT IS AND WHY IT'S OBTAINED

Carbon dioxide (CO_2) is the major waste product of normal metabolism. Blood levels are used to evaluate acid-base balance, particularly in those with breathing problems.

HOW IT WORKS

You will be asked to provide a **venous blood sample.** Either serum* or whole blood may be used. There are several laboratory methods for measurement.

BEFORE THE TEST

No special preparation is required.

AFTER THE TEST

Follow **venous blood sample** aftercare.

SIGNIFICANCE OF RESULTS

The level of CO_2 in the blood should be interpreted along with other **electrolytes,** blood pH, and, on occasion, with **blood gas** determination. Since the main route of excretion of CO_2 is through the lungs, high levels are found in those with breathing difficulties such as pneumonia or emphysema. High CO_2 is also seen when there has been a loss of acid from the body, such as in prolonged vomiting. Low CO_2 may be seen when there is increased respiration, as in hyperventilation, and when there is an accumulation of acid in the blood (acidosis).

☐ ☐ ☐

☐ Carboxyhemoglobin

WHAT IT IS AND WHY IT'S OBTAINED

Carboxyhemoglobin is the substance formed when carbon monoxide combines with **hemoglobin.** Blood levels, therefore, are used to detect and determine the extent of carbon monoxide poisoning. This test is indicated when there has been smoke inhalation or when there is unexplained headache, irritability, nausea, vomiting, dizziness, or coma. It can also be used to determine the harmful effects of cigarette smoking.

HOW IT WORKS

You will be asked to provide either a **venous blood sample** or an **arterial blood sample,** the latter often when **blood gas** is being tested. Spectrophotometry* and other methods are available for analysis.

BEFORE THE TEST

No special preparation is required.

AFTER THE TEST

Follow **venous blood sample** or **arterial blood sample** aftercare.

SIGNIFICANCE OF RESULTS

Carboxyhemoglobin levels are given as a percent of normal hemoglobin. The table reveals the usual interpretation:

Carboxyhemoglobin level	Situation
Less than 2%	Nonsmokers
4–5%	1–2 packs of cigarettes per day
8–9%	More than 2 packs of cigarettes per day

10–30%	Disturbed judgment, headache, dizziness
50–60%	Coma
60–80%	Death

SYNONYMS AND INCLUDED TESTS

Carbon monoxide.

□ □ □

□ Carcinoembryonic antigen

WHAT IT IS AND WHY IT'S OBTAINED

Carcinoembryonic antigen (CEA) is a substance which is released into the bloodstream in a number of diseases. Blood levels are used to monitor the progress and treatment of cancer, particularly cancer of the colon and rectum.

HOW IT WORKS

You will be asked to provide a **venous blood sample** from which serum* will be separated. Immunoassay* is used for the laboratory analysis.

BEFORE THE TEST

No special preparation is required.

AFTER THE TEST

Follow **venous blood sample** aftercare.

SIGNIFICANCE OF RESULTS

An elevated CEA is not specific to cancer and should not be used as a screening test. High CEA may be seen in liver disease, inflammation of the bowel, hypothyroidism, and cigarette smoking. To detect recurrence or spread of cancer it is most useful when multiple measurements are made over time along with other diagnostic tests.

□ □ □

□ Cardiac catheterization

WHAT IT IS AND WHY IT'S OBTAINED

Cardiac catheterization entails the passing of a flexible tube into the heart in order to evaluate the coronary blood vessels, heart valves, heart muscle, and heart architecture. Although invasive, it has become common because of the extent of coronary artery disease and because of the popularity of coronary bypass surgery. It provides details about the heart which are available in no other way.

HOW IT WORKS

Procedures vary according to the laboratory and doctor but are always performed in a special room devoted to the purpose. Usually the preliminaries will be performed in one room and you will then be wheeled on a gurney into the cardiac catheterization laboratory. In general, you will be asked to disrobe, to put on a hospital gown, and to lie flat. If the blood vessels in your groin are to be used you will be shaved in that area. At some point your vital signs (pulse, blood pressure, respiration, and temperature) will be taken, an intravenous fluid drip will be started, you will be given a sedative, and electrodes, as for an **electrocardiogram,** will be placed on your chest and extremities. Either your arm or your groin veins and arteries may be used for the actual procedure, depending upon the doctor's preference. If the right side of your heart is to be catheterized, a vein is used; for the left side, an artery. In either case the skin over the proposed site will be injected with a local anesthetic, which causes slight stinging or burning. Next, either a puncture or an incision is made, again depending upon the preference of the doctor. The catheter will next be introduced into the desired blood vessel and directed into your heart using fluoroscopy (in which X-ray images are formed on a screen rather than on film). You may feel some unusual pressure during this phase but no pain. Next, a series of tests will be conducted depending upon the information being sought. Pressure readings cause no discomfort but the injection of X-ray contrast dye may produce a hot flush or nausea. These sensations pass quickly. Follow any instructions you may be given about breathing or coughing. If you experience chest pain during the procedure you may be given medications to alleviate it.

BEFORE THE TEST

Follow your doctor's instructions carefully regarding medications, food, and fluid intake. In general, if the catheterization is to be done in the morning, do not eat breakfast; if in the afternoon, do not eat lunch and have only liquids such as juice and coffee for breakfast. You may drink water.

AFTER THE TEST

You will be kept on bed rest and your vital signs will be monitored until they are stable. The wound site will be checked for bleeding. If a groin artery was used you will be kept on bed rest for a period of time with a pressure on the site. Stitches, if any, can be removed in about a week. Cardiac catheterization is generally a safe procedure. Complications, though uncommon, include bleeding from the catheterization site, infection, blood clot formation, or the precipitation of a heart attack.

SIGNIFICANCE OF RESULTS

The interpretation of a cardiac catheterization will be performed by the cardiologist and cardiac surgeon, if one is involved. The decisions on medical or surgical treatment, the type of surgery, risks, and benefits, will be reviewed with you.

□ □ □

☐ Cardiac enzymes

WHAT IT IS AND WHY IT'S OBTAINED

Cardiac enzymes are blood tests which are often bundled together to assist in the diagnosis and progress of a heart attack. The panel usually includes **creatine kinase, lactic dehydrogenase,** and often **aspartate aminotransferase.**

HOW IT WORKS

You will be asked to provide a **venous blood sample** from which serum* will be separated. Various laboratory methods of analysis are in use.

BEFORE THE TEST

No special preparation is required.

AFTER THE TEST

Follow **venous blood sample** aftercare.

SIGNIFICANCE OF RESULTS

See the individual entries for interpretation. The **electrocardiogram** is also essential in diagnosing and monitoring a heart attack.

☐ ☐ ☐

☐ Carotene

WHAT IT IS AND WHY IT'S OBTAINED

Carotene is a precursor of vitamin A. Blood levels are mainly used to diagnose carotenemia, in which the skin turns orange-yellow, and in screening for abnormal fat excretion in the feces (steatorrhea) and diseases in which there are problems with absorption of nutrients by the intestines (intestinal malabsorption).

HOW IT WORKS

You will be asked to provide a **venous blood sample** from which serum* will be separated. Chromatography* is used in the laboratory analysis.

BEFORE THE TEST

You should fast overnight.

AFTER THE TEST

Follow **venous blood sample** aftercare.

SIGNIFICANCE OF RESULTS

High levels of carotene are seen in carotenemia, a benign condition caused by excessive intake of vegetables containing carotene, such as carrots. Low levels are found in smokers and in those taking birth control pills. This test is of questionable value because blood carotene varies greatly. A high level of carotene is sometimes interpreted as ruling out steatorrhea, but a better test is **fecal fat**.

SYNONYMS AND INCLUDED TESTS

Beta-carotene.

□ □ □

□ Catecholamines

WHAT IT IS AND WHY IT'S OBTAINED

Catecholamines are a group of hormones which affect virtually every part of the body. Two of the most important, epinephrine (adrenalin) and norepinephrine, are produced by the adrenal gland as part of the "flight or fight" response to stress. In certain tumors, most notably pheochromocytoma, abnormal amounts of catecholamines are released into the bloodstream and cause high blood pressure. Testing for catecholamines, therefore, is used to evaluate high blood pressure.

HOW IT WORKS

Either blood or urine may be tested. For blood, you will be asked to provide a **venous blood sample** from which serum* will be separated. For urine, you will be asked to provide a **24-hour urine sample** which should be refrigerated during collection. Chromatography* and other methods are used in the laboratory analysis.

BEFORE THE TEST

Avoid stress, exercise, smoking, pain, extremes of cold or heat, or low blood sugar, as they all influence catecholamines. Many drugs interfere with this test, including caffeine, certain nosedrops, and some cough medicines. Obtain a complete list from your doctor or the laboratory. An overnight fast is recommended for the blood test.

AFTER THE TEST

Follow **venous blood sample** aftercare for the blood test. Resume normal diet and activity.

SIGNIFICANCE OF RESULTS

This test is usually obtained as part of a battery of tests designed to evaluate high blood pressure and must be interpreted accordingly. In general, a high level of catecholamines is associated with pheochromocytoma. Many false positives, however, can occur with the blood test; fewer are seen with the urine test. **Metanephrines** is a better test to screen for pheochromocytoma.

☐ ☐ ☐

□ Centromere/kinetochore antibody

WHAT IT IS AND WHY IT'S OBTAINED

Blood levels of this antibody are used to aid in the diagnosis of a certain variant of scleroderma, a systemic disease in which the skin becomes hard and inelastic.

HOW IT WORKS

You will be asked to provide a **venous blood sample** from which serum* will be separated. Immunoassay* is used for the laboratory analysis.

BEFORE THE TEST

No special preparation is required.

AFTER THE TEST

Follow **venous blood sample** aftercare.

SIGNIFICANCE OF RESULTS

Elevated levels of the centromere/kinetochore antibody are found in a majority of people with the CREST (calcinosis, Raynaud's phenomenon, esophageal dysfunction, sclerodactyly, and telangiectasia) variety of scleroderma and in few of those with other types of scleroderma.

□ □ □

□ Ceruloplasmin

WHAT IT IS AND WHY IT'S OBTAINED

Ceruloplasmin is a **protein** which is involved in copper and iron metabolism. Blood levels are used to evaluate liver disease, neurological symptoms, nutritional status, and, in infants, failure to develop normally.

HOW IT WORKS

You will be asked to provide a **venous blood sample** from which serum* will be separated. Several laboratory methods are available for analysis.

BEFORE THE TEST

No special preparation is required.

AFTER THE TEST

Follow **venous blood sample** aftercare.

SIGNIFICANCE OF RESULTS

Low ceruloplasmin levels are seen in Menkes' kinky hair syndrome, Wilson's disease, and protein loss. High levels are found in certain cancers, autoimmune diseases (in which the immune system reacts against the body's own tissues), pregnancy, copper toxicity, and in those taking birth control pills. Blood **copper** is usually obtained at the same time as ceruloplasmin in order to provide a comparison. Wilson's disease is best diagnosed by injecting radioactive copper intravenously and then measuring its incorporation into ceruloplasmin.

□ □ □

□ Cervical punch biopsy

WHAT IT IS AND WHY IT'S OBTAINED

Cervical punch biopsy is the surgical removal of tissue from the cervix of the uterus. It is usually obtained if the **Pap smear** is abnormal or a suspicious lesion is found on pelvic examination.

HOW IT WORKS

The procedure is performed about a week after your menstrual period, when the cervix contains the least amount of blood. You will be asked to lie on your back in the usual position for a pelvic examination and the procedure followed as for **colposcopy**. The punch biopsy instrument is introduced into the vagina after a speculum has been inserted. The actual biopsy is only mildly uncomfortable since the cervix has few nerve endings. Anesthesia is not needed.

BEFORE THE TEST

No special preparation is required.

AFTER THE TEST

Avoid strenuous exercise for a day and intercourse for forty-eight hours. A gray-green discharge with a bad odor is possible, and may persist for a week. Report any bleeding that is heavier than your normal menstrual flow.

SIGNIFICANCE OF RESULTS

A negative result means that the tissue was normal. A positive result may be reported as dysplasia, superficial ("intraepithelial") cancer, or invasive cancer. If the specimen was either dysplastic or superficial, a more extensive biopsy, such as a cone biopsy, is usually indicated.

□ □ □

□ Chloride

WHAT IT IS AND WHY IT'S OBTAINED

Chloride is one of the two major **electrolytes** in the blood, the other being **sodium.** The two together constitute sodium chloride (salt). Chloride levels in blood are routinely used to evaluate acid-base balance and water balance.

HOW IT WORKS

You will be asked to provide a **venous blood sample** from which serum* will be separated. Several methods are available for the assay. Urine may also be tested.

BEFORE THE TEST

No special preparation is required.

AFTER THE TEST

Follow **venous blood sample** aftercare.

SIGNIFICANCE OF RESULTS

High blood chloride is seen in dehydration, ammonium chloride ingestion, metabolic acidosis (due to excess acid or loss of base), and hyperparathyroidism. Low chloride is associated with congestive heart failure, excess fluid intake, the syndrome of inappropriate secretion of antidiuretic hormone, Addison's disease (underactive adrenal gland), kidney disease, burns, metabolic alkalosis (due to excess base or loss of acid, as in prolonged vomiting), and with use of some types of diuretics ("water pills").

□ □ □

□ Cholecystogram

WHAT IT IS AND WHY IT'S OBTAINED

The cholecystogram is an **X-ray contrast study** designed to visualize the gallbladder. It is obtained to evaluate symptoms suggestive of gallbladder disease, such as abdominal or right shoulder pain, jaundice (yellow color of the skin), or fatty food intolerance.

HOW IT WORKS

You will be given a contrast dye in pill form to be taken orally the evening before the examination. In the X-ray department the next day a series of **X rays** of your abdomen will be taken.

BEFORE THE TEST

You should fast overnight. Some doctors recommend a high-fat lunch the day before.

AFTER THE TEST

No special aftercare is needed.

SIGNIFICANCE OF RESULTS

The test will be interpreted by a radiologist. Abnormalities may suggest the presence of inflammation (cholecystitis), gallstones, or tumors. In general, gallbladder **ultrasound** is a better test and has largely replaced the oral cholecysto-gram.

SYNONYMS AND INCLUDED TESTS

Gallbladder X ray.

◻ ◻ ◻

◻ **Cholesterol**

WHAT IT IS AND WHY IT'S OBTAINED

Cholesterol is present throughout the body and is essential to health. The popularity of blood levels for its stems from the close link between cholesterol and coronary artery disease (CAD). Cholesterol is carried in the blood in several forms, including high-density lipoprotein (HDL), low-density lipoprotein (LDL), and very–low density lipo-protein (VLDL). Importantly, each of these can be mea-sured independently, for, in general, high levels of HDL are associated with a *low* incidence of CAD, whereas high levels of LDL are associated with a *high* incidence of CAD.

113

HOW IT WORKS

You will be asked to provide a **venous blood sample** from which serum* will be separated. Several methods are available for analysis.

BEFORE THE TEST

For the most accurate cholesterol level, your diet should not have changed for three weeks, your body weight should be stable, you should be fasting for twelve hours, and you should not have consumed alcohol for three days.

AFTER THE TEST

Follow **venous blood sample** aftercare.

SIGNIFICANCE OF RESULTS

In general a desirable blood cholesterol is below 200 (mg/dL). If the level is 200 to 239 and if you have two or more risk factors for CAD (male sex, family history of premature CAD, smoke more than ten cigarettes per day, high blood pressure, low HDL cholesterol, diabetes, history of stroke or vascular disease, or are severely obese) then a **lipid profile** should be obtained. All cases in which the level is over 240 should have a **lipid profile.** The best correlation with risk of CAD is the ratio of HDL cholesterol to total cholesterol. The desired ratio is 4:1 or less. The greater it is above 5, the higher the risk, and the less it is below 4, the lower the risk. High cholesterol is seen in hypercholesterolemia, kidney disease, hypothyroidism, primary biliary cirrhosis, and diabetes. Low levels are associated with poor nutrition, intestinal malabsorption, hyperthyroidism, some cancers, and some very rare diseases. There are several medications which will interfere with this test, including, most obviously, drugs which lower cholesterol. Steroids, estrogens, and certain diuretics may also change cholesterol levels.

□ □ □

☐ Cholinesterase

WHAT IT IS AND WHY IT'S OBTAINED

Acetylcholine is a substance which helps transmit impulses across nerve junctions. Cholinesterase is an enzyme which breaks down the acetylcholine and prevents it from accumulating and causing paralysis. There are two instances where obtaining blood levels of cholinesterase are important. The first is to diagnose and monitor recovery from poisoning and the second is to screen before general anesthesia using certain muscle relaxants which inactivate cholinesterase. Industrial workers who may be at risk from toxic exposure to chemicals such as pesticides or military nerve gases often have baseline levels of cholinesterase taken before starting work and at intervals thereafter.

HOW IT WORKS

You will be asked to provide a **venous blood sample.** Cholinesterase may be measured in serum* (also called pseudocholinesterase) or red blood cells (also called true cholinesterase), the former for acute poisoning, the latter for chronic poisoning. There are several laboratory systems which may be used to measure the level of the enzyme.

BEFORE THE TEST

No special preparation is required.

AFTER THE TEST

Follow **venous blood sample** aftercare.

SIGNIFICANCE OF RESULTS

Low levels of cholinesterase are found in insecticide (parathion, malathion, diazinon, or carbamyl) or nerve gas poisonings and are often due to industrial exposure. Low levels of cholinesterase may also be found in liver disease and may be inherited. Anyone with a congenitally low level of cholinesterase will be particularly sensitive to the effects of succinylcholine (suxamethonium), a muscle relaxant used in surgery. Low levels may be further investigated using the **dibucaine number.**

SYNONYMS AND INCLUDED TESTS

Acetylcholinesterase, pseudocholinesterase.

□ □ □

□ Chromium

WHAT IT IS AND WHY IT'S OBTAINED

Chromium is a chemical element which is present in very small amounts in the body, but it is important in sugar **(glucose)** and **insulin** metabolism. Blood and urine levels are obtained to evaluate chromium deficiency and toxicity. Inadequate chromium causes sugar imbalance, whereas excessive amounts can cause breathing difficulties and lung cancer. Extremely high levels may produce kidney disease, liver disease, and convulsions.

HOW IT WORKS

You will be asked to provide a **venous blood sample** from which serum* will be separated. Special metal-free equipment will be used. If urine is being tested, a **24-hour urine sample** is required. Laboratory measurement is very difficult because of the small amounts of chromium normally present.

BEFORE THE TEST

You should fast overnight for a blood sample.

Follow **venous blood sample** aftercare.

SIGNIFICANCE OF RESULTS

Low chromium is uncommon except in extremely malnourished infants. High chromium is seen with industrial exposure.

◻ ◻ ◻

◻ Chromosome analysis

WHAT IT IS AND WHY IT'S OBTAINED

There are forty-six human chromosomes, composed of DNA, which carry the genetic material which make us unique individuals. Chromosome analysis, a field which continues to become more and more sophisticated, analyzes these chromosomes for defects which either produce disease themselves or which might lead to genetic disease in future generations.

HOW IT WORKS

Many sources of sampling material may be used, the most common of which are amniotic fluid obtained during **amniocentesis,** a **venous blood sample,** or **bone marrow.** The technique is to culture cells, to stimulate their growth, to arrest their growth, to stain the cells, and to photograph them under a microscope. The individual chromosomes can be identified by differences in their shapes and sizes.

BEFORE THE TEST

No special preparation is required.

AFTER THE TEST

Aftercare depends upon the source of the specimen.

SIGNIFICANCE OF RESULTS

A number of diseases may be identified through abnormal chromosome patterns. Among these are ataxia telangiectasia, Bloom's syndrome, chronic myelogenous leukemia, cri du chat syndrome, Down's syndrome, Edward's syndrome, Fanconi's anemia, the fragile X syndrome, Klinefelter's syndrome, Miller-Dieker syndrome, Prader-Willi syndrome, retinoblastoma, Wiedemann-Beckwith syndrome, Wilm's tumor, and the XXX syndrome.

□ □ □

□ Clomiphene test

WHAT IT IS AND WHY IT'S OBTAINED

Clomiphene is a steroid which blocks the effects of estrogen. Estrogen, among many other effects, normally suppresses the secretion of **follicle stimulating hormone** (FSH) and **luteinizing hormone** (LH) by the pituitary gland. Clomiphene, therefore, *stimulates* FSH and LH under normal conditions. The clomiphene test is used to evaluate women who are not ovulating but who otherwise have normal ovaries.

HOW IT WORKS

You will be asked to record four weeks of basal body temperatures after which a **pregnancy test** will be obtained. If you are not pregnant you will be asked to take 50 mg of clomiphene orally for five days beginning on the fifth day of your menstrual cycle. About a week after the last dose a **venous blood sample** is obtained for LH and FSH. Two weeks after the last dose a blood **progesterone** may be ordered to see if you ovulated.

BEFORE THE TEST

No special preparation is required.

AFTER THE TEST

Continue to obtain basal body temperature. One side effect of clomiphene is to induce ovulation, thereby facilitating conception, which may be multiple (twins or more).

SIGNIFICANCE OF RESULTS

A normal test means that FSH and LH both increased with clomiphene. If they did not, an abnormality in the way the brain (hypothalamus), pituitary gland, and ovaries are working is indicated.

SYNONYMS AND INCLUDED TESTS

Clomid test.

□ □ □

□ Clot lysis time

WHAT IT IS AND WHY IT'S OBTAINED

The normal blood clotting system involves both the formation and the dissolving of blood clots. Without the ability to dissolve blood clots, the circulation would eventually turn to sludge. The clot lysis time (CLT) measures the ability of the body to break down blood clots and is used to monitor treatment with clot dissolving (thrombolytic) medications.

HOW IT WORKS

You will be asked to provide a **venous blood sample.** There are several variants of the actual measurement but all involve allowing the blood to clot after chemical treatment. The time it takes for the clot to dissolve is then recorded.

BEFORE THE TEST

No special preparation is required.

AFTER THE TEST

Follow **venous blood sample** aftercare.

SIGNIFICANCE OF RESULTS

A short CLT in the absence of treatment with thrombolytic medications usually indicates that there is excessive stimulation of natural anticoagulants (blood thinners).

SYNONYMS AND INCLUDED TESTS

Whole blood clot lysis, diluted whole blood clot lysis, euglobulin clot lysis time, fibrinolysis time.

□ □ □

□ Coagulation factor screen

WHAT IT IS AND WHY IT'S OBTAINED

There are twelve substances, called factors, which are important to the development of a normal blood clot. Deficiency of any may cause bleeding or abnormal screening tests for blood clotting such as the **prothrombin time** (PT) or **partial thromboplastin time** (PTT). The best known and most common bleeding disorder is hemophilia, which is due to factor VIII deficiency. Symptoms of factor problems range from none, such as factor XII deficiency, to incompatible with life, such as absence of factor II. The others produce a variety of diseases, such as prolonged bleeding from cuts or scrapes, bleeding into joints or the skin, or severe hemorrhage. Nine factors may be tested: II, V, VII, VIII, IX, X, XI, XII, and XIII (see table).

Coagulation factors and synonyms	
Factor	**Synonym**
I	Fibrinogen
II	Prothrombin

Factor	Synonym
III	Tissue thromboplastin
IV	Calcium
V	Proaccelerin
VII	Proconvertin
VIII	Antihemophiliac factor
IX	Christmas factor
X	Stuart-Prower factor
XI	Plasma thromboplastin antecedent
XII	Hageman factor
XIII	Fibrin stabilizing factor

HOW IT WORKS

You will be asked to provide a **venous blood sample** from which plasma* is separated. For all factors except XIII the plasma is mixed with another plasma known to be deficient in the one factor being tested. If the PT and PTT are abnormal for this mixture, the test sample is presumed to be deficient in the factor. For factor XIII a clotted blood sample is incubated with urea and observed for twenty-four hours, at which time the clot should still be intact.

BEFORE THE TEST

No special preparation is required.

AFTER THE TEST

Follow **venous blood sample** aftercare.

SIGNIFICANCE OF RESULTS

Interpretation of these results is done under the supervision of a hematologist. In many cases within each class of factor deficiency there are subclasses which can range widely in severity. Blood thinners can interfere with results of any of these tests. Birth control pills may increase factors II, VII, IX, and X.

SYNONYMS AND INCLUDED TESTS

Factor assay.

□ □ □

☐ Cold agglutinins

WHAT IT IS AND WHY IT'S OBTAINED

Cold agglutinins are antibodies (proteins important to the immune system) which cause red blood cells to clump in the cold. Blood levels of these antibodies are mainly used to support the diagnosis of certain cases of pneumonia (primary atypical pneumonia, or "virus" pneumonia). Symptoms may be cough, fever, sore throat, and nasal congestion, but tend to be less severe than pneumonia caused by bacteria.

HOW IT WORKS

You will be asked to provide a **venous blood sample** from which serum* will be separated. Immunoassay* is used for the laboratory analysis.

BEFORE THE TEST

No special preparation is required.

AFTER THE TEST

Follow **venous blood sample** aftercare.

SIGNIFICANCE OF RESULTS

Cold agglutinins are found to some extent in most people, but a high concentration of them is evidence for infection with *Mycoplasma pneumoniae,* especially if the level rises over time. Smaller elevations may occur following infectious mononucleosis ("mono"). **Bacterial antibodies** are also helpful in diagnosing "virus" pneumonia.

□ □ □

□ Colonoscopy

WHAT IT IS AND WHY IT'S OBTAINED

Colonoscopy is used to examine the colon (large intestine) by means of an instrument called a colonoscope, a flexible tube several feet long and about a half an inch wide. It is performed to evaluate rectal bleeding, diarrhea, abdominal pain, abnormalities found on **barium enema** or **stool for occult blood** and the extent of bowel diseases such as ulcerative colitis. It is also used to check for spread or recurrence of colon cancer.

HOW IT WORKS

Colonoscopies are performed either by gastroenterologists, who are internal medical subspecialists, or by surgeons and may be done without anesthesia, under intravenous sedation, or under general anesthesia. You should discuss options with your doctor, but the best way is with intravenous sedation, which creates partial amnesia. You will be asked to get undressed and to put on a hospital gown. If the intravenous sedation option is selected, an intravenous fluid line will be started and a mild sedative injected. You will be asked to lie on your left side and to bring your right leg up to your chest. The doctor will first perform a digital rectal examination after which the colonoscope will be inserted into your anus. This produces a cold sensation but minimal discomfort. As the colonoscope is introduced farther into the rectum you will feel pressure and cramping. During the procedure air is introduced to distend the intestine and this will cause further cramping and a feeling that you have to

123

expel gas. Don't fight the feeling. Suction to remove secretion or feces is noisy but painless. Biopsies, if taken, are also painless. The procedure may last up to an hour, but because of the sedation your recollection will be that it took less time.

BEFORE THE TEST

Preparation for the test is crucial. Follow any instructions you have been given carefully, the idea being to clear the intestine as completely as you can. One regimen is to have a clear liquid diet for two days and to take several warm tap water enemas the day before along with a laxative. GoLYTELY is a popular product which does not require enemas. If your bowel is not cleansed properly colonoscopy will take longer and be more uncomfortable.

AFTER THE TEST

After the procedure you will feel groggy until the anesthesia or sedative wears off. You will also feel some cramping and extra gas. A small amount of blood in your stool is normal if a biopsy was taken. Severe pain, pronounced rectal bleeding, or fever should be reported to your doctor. Although rare, perforation of the intestine sometimes occurs and may require surgery for repair.

SIGNIFICANCE OF RESULTS

A negative result means that nothing suspicious was found. Positive results are reported according to the findings. If the test was done to investigate bloody diarrhea, for example, evidence of ulcerative colitis may be evident immediately. If polyps, growths, or other lesions were biopsied it may take a week or longer for the definitive results to be returned.

□ □ □

☐ Color vision testing

WHAT IT IS AND WHY IT'S OBTAINED

Color vision testing is used to evaluate color blindness.

HOW IT WORKS

Several techniques are available. In the most common, using pseudoisochromatic plates, you will be shown a page containing seemingly randomly arranged colored dots and will be asked to detect numbers or certain shapes within the dotted area. In the Farnsworth-Munsell test you will be asked to arrange buttons or chips by color or increasing hue. In the Nagel test you will match a yellow hue by using mixtures of red and green.

BEFORE THE TEST

No special preparation is required.

AFTER THE TEST

No special aftercare is needed.

SIGNIFICANCE OF RESULTS

There are various kinds of color blindness which can be distinguished by color vision testing. Color blindness may not only be inherited but also acquired as a result of diseases of the retina or of the optic nerve.

SYNONYMS AND INCLUDED TESTS

Ishihara plates, Farnsworth-Munsell test, Nagel anomaloscope.

☐ ☐ ☐

☐ Colposcopy

WHAT IT IS AND WHY IT'S OBTAINED

Colposcopy is a technique for obtaining a magnified image of the cervix and is mainly used to evaluate an abnormal **Pap smear.**

HOW IT WORKS

You will be asked to lie on your back in the usual position for a pelvic examination. The colposcope, a type of telescope with lights, will be inserted into your vagina and the surface of your cervix examined. A **cervical punch biopsy** or other procedure may be performed at this time.

BEFORE THE TEST

No special preparation is required.

AFTER THE TEST

If a procedure was performed, follow instructions carefully.

SIGNIFICANCE OF RESULTS

Abnormalities may include visible signs of infection, inflammation, tumors, erosions, or atrophy.

☐ ☐ ☐

☐ Complement

WHAT IT IS AND WHY IT'S OBTAINED

The term complement refers to a group of proteins which play an important part in the immune system. Blood levels are used to evaluate and monitor the treatment of autoimmune diseases (in which the immune system reacts against the body's own tissues) and to detect hereditary complement deficiencies.

HOW IT WORKS

You will be asked to provide a **venous blood sample** from which serum* will be separated. Several methods are available for the assay, which may be of total complement or of the more important complement components.

BEFORE THE TEST

No special preparation is required.

AFTER THE TEST

Follow **venous blood sample** aftercare.

SIGNIFICANCE OF RESULTS

Interpretation of the total complement and component levels should take into account your symptoms and diagnosis because a change in the complement level doesn't indicate any one disease. In general a low level is more significant than a high level because it means either that there is congenital deficiency of complement, or, more likely, that complement is being used up by an immune reaction in the body, which is the case in many autoimmune diseases. If multiple determinations are made over time, a falling level of complement may predict flare-ups in these diseases.

□ □ □

□ Complete blood count

WHAT IT IS AND WHY IT'S OBTAINED

The complete blood count and differential (CBC) is the most commonly ordered blood test and is the standard way of evaluating blood cells. It normally consists of the **white blood cell count, white blood cell differential, red blood cell count, hemoglobin, hematocrit,** and **platelet count.** Abnormalities are seen in a wide variety of conditions such as anemia, autoimmune diseases (in which the immune system reacts against the body's own tissues), allergic reactions, bleeding disorders, cancer, and infections. The CBC is used extensively both to diagnose and monitor the progress of disease.

HOW IT WORKS

You will be asked to provide a **venous blood sample**. Analysis is by machine.

BEFORE THE TEST

No special preparation is required.

AFTER THE TEST

Follow **venous blood sample** aftercare.

SIGNIFICANCE OF RESULTS

A CBC may be abnormal in many different ways. See individual listing of the components for interpretation.

SYNONYMS AND INCLUDED TESTS

Complete blood count and differential.

□ □ □

□ Computed tomography

WHAT IT IS AND WHY IT'S OBTAINED

Computed tomography (CT) is an **X-ray** imaging technique for internal organs in which cross sectional images are constructed from multiple radiation readings. Any part of the body may be scanned, such as the abdomen, joints, bones, head, larynx, eye sockets, sinuses, pelvis, spine, and chest. It is particularly valuable for brain tumors and other diseases within the skull, and for evaluating chest and abdominal cancer and injuries. It is also used to guide instruments for taking a **biopsy,** to plan surgery, and to detect complications after surgery. CT is usually obtained *after* conventional X rays or **ultrasound** of the area to be examined.

HOW IT WORKS

CT relies upon the ability of a computer to translate hundreds of thousands of X-ray readings into multiple cross sectional images. You will be placed face up on a table which is then rolled into the CT scanner. The scanner revolves around the table, taking multiple X rays. You will hear the clicking and whirring of the machine. Depending upon the study this may take an hour or less. CT scans are sometimes performed with contrast agents to increase the ability to visualize organs. If contrast medium is used the table will be slid out of the scanner and the medium will be injected intravenously. You may feel flushed, dizzy, have a headache, and be nauseated. This is a normal reaction. If the scan is of the abdominal cavity you may be given a contrast agent (barium sulfate) orally or rectally. If the scan is of the pelvis, women may have a vaginal tampon implanted in order to increase visualization. The table will then be rolled back into the scanner and the test repeated. In the variant called "ultrafast" CT, the scanner takes pictures in one tenth of a second, whereas normally about two seconds are needed. The ultrafast method is used for heart CT, in which clear images between heartbeats can be obtained.

BEFORE THE TEST

If contrast media is used you should take nothing by mouth for four hours before the test.

AFTER THE TEST

No special aftercare is needed if a plain CT scan has been obtained. If an injectable contrast agent has been employed, you will be observed for signs of allergy—hives, shortness of breath, or wheezing—for a period of time after the test.

SIGNIFICANCE OF RESULTS

The interpretation of CT scans is usually by a radiologist. Results are reported to the doctors who are involved with ultimate responsibility for your care, such as your internist, oncologist, or surgeon. Serial CT scans are very useful for following the course of disease.

SYNONYMS AND INCLUDED TESTS

Computed transaxial tomography, CAT scan.

□ □ □

□ Coombs' test

WHAT IT IS AND WHY IT'S OBTAINED

There are two types of Coombs' test, the direct and the indirect, both of which are used to investigate a particular type of anemia (hemolytic) which is characterized by disruption of the red blood cell membranes. The *direct* test detects the presence of antibodies on the surface of red blood cells, whereas the *indirect* test detects antibodies in the blood serum. The indirect test is also used before blood transfusions.

HOW IT WORKS

You will be asked to provide a **venous blood sample.** Immunoassay* is used for the laboratory analysis.

BEFORE THE TEST

No special preparation is required.

AFTER THE TEST

Follow **venous blood sample** aftercare.

SIGNIFICANCE OF RESULTS

A positive Coombs' test is helpful in evaluating autoimmune hemolytic anemia. **Cold agglutinins,** and the drugs methyldopa and mefenamic acid may cause false positives.

SYNONYMS AND INCLUDED TESTS

Antiglobulin test.

❏ ❏ ❏

❏ Copper

WHAT IT IS AND WHY IT'S OBTAINED

Although present in trace amounts, copper is critical to many chemical reactions in the body. Its functions are complex and intertwined with the metabolism of **zinc.** Too much zinc, for example, can cause copper deficiency. Blood copper levels are particularly important in the diagnosis of Wilson's disease, an inherited condition in which large amounts of copper are deposited in the liver and brain. They are also useful in malnutrition or excessive ingestion.

HOW IT WORKS

You will be asked to provide a **venous blood sample** from which serum* will be separated. As with all trace element assays, special care must be given to avoid contamination, and the type of needle and collection tube is important. The assay is performed by means of atomic absorption.

BEFORE THE TEST

No special preparation is required.

AFTER THE TEST

Follow **venous blood sample** aftercare.

SIGNIFICANCE OF RESULTS

Low copper levels are found in malnutrition, Menkes' kinky hair syndrome, Wilson's disease, kidney disease, and leukemia. High copper is seen in nutritional excess, cirrhosis, in smokers, during pregnancy, with estrogen and birth control therapy, cancer, infections, thyroid diseases, and autoimmune diseases (in which the immune system reacts against the body's own tissues).

□ □ □

□ Corneal topography

WHAT IT IS AND WHY IT'S OBTAINED

Corneal topography is used to screen for certain diseases of the cornea of the eye and to evaluate candidates for refractive surgery.

HOW IT WORKS

You will be seated in a chair and a device which projects illuminated rings or patterns of light onto the cornea is brought close to each of your eyes. The images are reflected back to a video camera and then to a monitor and computer. The computer will analyze the picture and a color map of the corneal surface will be produced.

BEFORE THE TEST

If you have contact lenses do not wear them for several days.

AFTER THE TEST

No special aftercare is needed.

SIGNIFICANCE OF RESULTS

Corneal topography may help in detecting defects or irregularities of the corneal architecture, such as astigmatism or keratoconus (in which the cornea assumes a conical shape).

◻ ◻ ◻

◻ Cortisol

WHAT IT IS AND WHY IT'S OBTAINED

Cortisol is a hormone produced by the adrenal gland which affects all tissues in the body. Lack of it produces Addison's disease, which causes weakness, low blood pressure, and skin pigmentation. Too much produces Cushing's syndrome, which is marked by obesity ("moon face" and "buffalo hump"), acne, purple stretch marks, irregular menstrual periods, abnormal hair growth, and backache. Blood levels of cortisol are used to diagnose Addison's disease in the **cosyntropin test,** whereas urine levels are used to evaluate symptoms suggestive of Cushing's syndrome.

HOW IT WORKS

For blood, you will be asked to provide a **venous blood sample** from which serum* will be separated. At least two samples must be obtained, one in the morning and one in the evening, because the level of cortisol varies greatly. For urine you will be asked to provide a **24-hour urine sample.** Follow instructions regarding refrigeration of the specimen. Immunoassay* is used for the laboratory analysis.

BEFORE THE TEST

Follow instructions given by the laboratory or your doctor regarding intake of food and drugs. Avoid excessive physical exertion and stress during the urine collection period.

AFTER THE TEST

Follow **venous blood sample** aftercare for the blood test.

SIGNIFICANCE OF RESULTS

A single *blood* cortisol level without knowing when it was taken is practically meaningless, since there is such great variation. In general, however, low blood cortisol levels are found in Addison's disease, which can be caused by several diseases which affect the adrenal glands. A low *urine* cortisol, on the other hand, does not necessarily mean inadequate production of cortisol.

High blood and urine cortisol levels are found in Cushing's syndrome due to pituitary gland tumors or adrenal gland tumors, congenital adrenal hyperplasia, some cancers (such as lung and thyroid), and in the condition called pseudo-Cushing's disease. Increased cortisol levels are also seen in pregnancy, with birth control pills, and in those under stress. Elevated urine levels are in general more significant than elevated blood levels. But if blood cortisol levels reveal loss of the normal daily rhythm, even if the values are otherwise normal, it may mean that cortisol is being produced independent of the normal inhibitions present in the endocrine system.

SYNONYMS AND INCLUDED TESTS

Hydrocortisone.

□ □ □

□ Cosyntropin test

WHAT IT IS AND WHY IT'S OBTAINED

Cosyntropin is a drug which stimulates the adrenal gland. Administration of it is used to evaluate adrenal gland function, particularly adrenal insufficiency (Addison's disease). This test is better than the "ACTH stimulation test" because it is more rapid and less prone to produce allergic reactions.

HOW IT WORKS

You will be asked to provide a **venous blood sample** in the morning. You will then receive an injection of cosyntropin, either intravenously or in a muscle. Further blood samples will be taken after thirty minutes and after sixty minutes. All blood samples are analyzed by immunoassay* for **cortisol.**

BEFORE THE TEST

You should fast overnight. Follow instructions from the laboratory or your doctor regarding medications.

AFTER THE TEST

Follow **venous blood sample** aftercare. Resume medications as directed.

SIGNIFICANCE OF RESULTS

A rise of cortisol levels in the samples taken at thirty and sixty minutes signify that the adrenal glands are functioning. At this point a **metyrapone test** may be ordered to see whether pituitary and adrenal glands are interacting properly. If the cortisol does not rise, the adrenal gland itself is at fault. This may be the result of a number of problems, such as infection, cancer, or autoimmune disease (where the immune system acts against the body's own tissues).

SYNONYMS AND INCLUDED TESTS

Rapid ACTH test.

❑ ❑ ❑

☐ Creatine kinase

WHAT IT IS AND WHY IT'S OBTAINED

Creatine kinase (CK) is an enzyme which is found mostly in muscles and the brain; damage to these tissues, therefore, releases the enzyme into the blood. There are three types of CK: CK-BB, found in the brain; CK-MB, found in heart muscle; and CK-MM, found in other muscle. Blood levels of CK are most often used to assist in the diagnosis of a heart attack but are also of value in diseases of muscle degeneration.

HOW IT WORKS

You will be asked to provide a **venous blood sample** from which serum* will be separated. Several methods of analysis are available in the laboratory.

BEFORE THE TEST

If CK is being obtained to evaluate or monitor muscle disease, avoid strenuous exercise for forty-eight hours.

AFTER THE TEST

Follow **venous blood sample** aftercare.

SIGNIFICANCE OF RESULTS

High total CK is seen in diseases of muscle degeneration, such as muscular dystrophy and dermatomyositis, and after heart attacks, surgery, and strenuous exercise. Small elevations occur after intramuscular injections or other muscle injuries. When assessing heart attacks multiple CK determinations are necessary, because values are usually normal at the onset of the attack, increase to a peak after about eighteen hours, then gradually return to normal. With heart attacks it is also important that CK be used in conjunction with other tests, such as the **electrocardiogram** and **lactic dehydrogenase.** In cases of doubt as to the source of the elevated CK the different fractions may be analyzed.

SYNONYMS AND INCLUDED TESTS

Creatine phosphokinase.

□ □ □

□ **Creatinine**

WHAT IT IS AND WHY IT'S OBTAINED

Creatinine is a waste product of normal metabolism. Blood levels—along with **blood urea nitrogen**—are the most common **kidney function tests.**

HOW IT WORKS

You will be asked to provide a **venous blood sample** from which serum* will be separated. The Jaffé reaction (picric acid in an alkaline solution producing a red color) is generally used in the laboratory.

BEFORE THE TEST

You should fast overnight.

AFTER THE TEST

Follow **venous blood sample** aftercare.

SIGNIFICANCE OF RESULTS

High creatinine is associated with any of a number of kidney diseases, but provides only a rough approximation of the extent of disease and does not identify its cause. High levels can also be due to decreased blood supply to the kidney, as occurs in shock. Diseases such as hyperthyroidism and muscle disorders may also increase creatinine, as will several ingested substances, including meats, vitamin

C, cimetidine (Tagamet), and some antibiotics. Low creatinine is seen in debilitation and some severe liver diseases. More accurate information about kidney function can be obtained with **creatinine clearance.**

□ □ □

□ Creatinine clearance

WHAT IT IS AND WHY IT'S OBTAINED

Creatinine clearance is a very good test for kidney function. It is obtained when more common **kidney function tests,** such as **blood urea nitrogen** and **creatinine,** are abnormal and when more detailed information is needed. It is also used to follow the course of kidney disease and to adjust the dosage of certain medications which depend upon the kidneys for excretion.

HOW IT WORKS

You will be asked to provide a **24-hour urine sample,** although two-, four-, six-, or twelve-hour specimens are sometimes used. Keep the specimen bottle refrigerated during collection period. At some time during the collection a **venous blood sample** will be obtained and analyzed for blood creatinine. A formula taking into consideration the volume of urine, the concentration of creatinine in blood and urine, and the body surface area is then used to calculate the creatinine clearance number.

BEFORE THE TEST

Avoid nonessential medications before the collection begins. Drink plenty of liquids before and during collection.

AFTER THE TEST

Follow **venous blood sample** aftercare.

SIGNIFICANCE OF RESULTS

A low creatinine clearance suggests the presence of kidney disease or low blood flow to the kidneys, such as occurs in shock or heart failure. Certain drugs, especially cephalosporin antibiotics, may reduce creatinine clearance. A high creatinine clearance is not significant and normally occurs after exercise or during pregnancy.

□ □ □

□ Cryoglobulin

WHAT IT IS AND WHY IT'S OBTAINED

Cryoglobulins are abnormal proteins which precipitate out of the blood at low temperatures. Blood levels are used to evaluate symptoms such as coldness and discoloration of the fingers and toes (Raynaud's phenomenon) and bleeding beneath the skin (purpura).

HOW IT WORKS

You will be asked to provide a **venous blood sample** from which serum* will be separated and chilled. A cloudy precipitate signifies the presence of cryoglobulins.

BEFORE THE TEST

No special preparation is required.

AFTER THE TEST

Follow **venous blood sample** aftercare.

SIGNIFICANCE OF RESULTS

A negative test means that no cryoglobulins were found. Cryoglobulins are relatively nonspecific and may occur in a variety of diseases such as leukemia, Waldenstrom's macro-globulinemia, multiple myeloma, lupus erythematosus, and viral infections.

□ □ □

□ Cyclic AMP

WHAT IT IS AND WHY IT'S OBTAINED

Although cyclic AMP is important to the functioning of many hormones, blood levels are used to evaluate parathyroid hormone function, especially to evaluate cases of increased blood **calcium** (hypercalcemia).

HOW IT WORKS

Both blood and urine should be studied. For blood, you will be asked to provide a **venous blood sample** from which serum* will be separated. For urine, a **24-hour urine specimen** is used, although lesser quantities can be analyzed. Urine should be frozen during collection. Immunoassay* is used for the laboratory analysis.

BEFORE THE TEST

No special preparation is required.

AFTER THE TEST

Follow **venous blood sample** aftercare.

SIGNIFICANCE OF RESULTS

A high cyclic AMP signifies increased activity of the parathyroid gland (hyperparathyroidism) but may also be caused by cancer or vitamin D deficiency. Low cyclic AMP signifies underactivity of the parathyroid gland (hypoparathyroidism). A normal cyclic AMP is seen in both pseudohypoparathroidism and pseudo-pseudohypoparathyroidism. Interpretation of cyclic AMP should take into account blood **parathyroid hormone, calcium, phosphorus,** and **creatinine.**

SYNONYMS AND INCLUDED TESTS

Cyclic adenosine monophosphate.

□ □ □

□ **Cystogram**

WHAT IT IS AND WHY IT'S OBTAINED

The cystogram is an **X-ray contrast study** used to visualize and diagnose diseases of the urinary bladder and urethra.

HOW IT WORKS

The test is done in the **X-ray** department of a hospital or clinic or in a private radiologist's office. You will be asked to undress, put on a hospital gown, and lie on your back on the examining table. A soft, flexible, lubricated tube (catheter) will be inserted into your urinary opening (urethra) and then into your bladder. This is only mildly uncomfortable. A fluid that shows up on the X ray (contrast dye) will then be allowed to drip into your bladder until it is full. A series of X rays will then be taken as you are asked to assume different positions. In the variant known as the voiding cystourethrogram, the catheter will be removed and you will be asked to urinate while an X-ray videotape is taken.

BEFORE THE TEST

No special preparation is required.

AFTER THE TEST

No special aftercare is needed.

SIGNIFICANCE OF RESULTS

Many abnormalities of the urinary bladder and urethra may be demonstrated using the cystogram, including tumors, stones, bladder rupture, and outpouchings called diverticulae. The voiding cystourethrogram can show dynamically the reasons for difficulty in urination, as well as abnormal backflow of urine from the bladder to the kidneys.

SYNONYMS AND INCLUDED TESTS

Voiding cystourethrogram.

□ □ □

□ Cystometry

WHAT IT IS AND WHY IT'S OBTAINED

Cystometry is a test of urinary bladder function which is used to evaluate urinary incontinence, urinary frequency or urgency, or urinary retention.

HOW IT WORKS

The term cystometry actually refers to a number of tests of varying complexity, ranging from simple methods which can be performed by nurses to more sophisticated procedures done in a special urodynamic laboratory. All rely upon the principle of instilling water, saline, or sometimes carbon dioxide gas into the bladder and measuring volumes and pressures as you perform various maneuvers and report your sensations. A typical scenario is as follows. The test begins with your voiding as completely as you can. Then a lubricated flexible tube (catheter) will be inserted into your bladder through your urinary opening (urethra). This is only mildly uncomfortable. Any residual urine is drained and its volume measured. Next, sterile water at room temperature will be dripped through the catheter into your bladder and you will be asked to report your sensations:

when you first feel the desire to void, then when you feel the need to void. At this point the test will stop. You may also be asked exert maximum force to empty your bladder. All the while pressures and volumes are being recorded on a strip of paper. Many variations of this test are possible. Sometimes a pressure-sensing device will be inserted into your rectum, and you may be given drugs to increase or decrease the muscle tone of your bladder, or be asked to sit or stand while the test goes on.

BEFORE THE TEST

Discontinue all nonessential medications and others as directed by your doctor, particularly those which may interfere with bladder function, such as antihistamines. Ask about the specifics of the test you will be having.

AFTER THE TEST

No special aftercare is needed. Resume medications as directed.

SIGNIFICANCE OF RESULTS

A urologist will interpret the results of this test, taking into consideration your symptoms and the results of other bladder tests, such as a cystourethrogram or **cystoscopy.** Many diseases may be responsible for abnormal bladder function, including a number of nerve disorders such as strokes, spinal cord injuries, Parkinson's disease, diabetes, or multiple sclerosis. Diseases of the bladder itself, injury (for example after prostate surgery), or obstruction to urinary flow by a large prostate are also possibilities.

SYNONYMS AND INCLUDED TESTS

Cystometrogram, urodynamic testing of bladder function.

□ □ □

□ Cystoscopy

WHAT IT IS AND WHY IT'S OBTAINED

Cystoscopy is used to examine the bladder and urethra. It is done to evaluate symptoms related to the urinary tract, such as difficulty voiding or blood in the urine, and to evaluate urinary tract abnormalities detected by **X ray, ultrasound,** or **cystogram.**

HOW IT WORKS

This procedure may be performed in a special room in a urologist's office, clinic, or hospital. It is usually done under local anesthesia, although spinal or general anesthesia may be used if an additional surgical procedure is contemplated. Discuss these options with your doctor. If you are having this test under local anesthesia you will be asked to undress from the waist down and to lie on your back with your legs spread. Your genital skin will be cleansed with an antiseptic solution and a tube which has been lubricated with a local anesthetic will be gently guided into your urinary opening (urethra) and then into your bladder. There is some discomfort associated with this, but no real pain. Your bladder will next be irrigated with a solution. This will give you the feeling that you have to urinate. Do not fight the sensation. The urologist will examine the lining of the bladder and urethra and may perform a **biopsy** or other surgical procedure through the tube.

BEFORE THE TEST

If you are to receive spinal or general anesthesia you should fast overnight.

AFTER THE TEST

If you received a general or spinal anesthetic you will be taken to a recovery area where your vital signs (pulse, blood pressure, respiration, and temperature) will be taken until the anesthetic wears off. Drink plenty of fluids as directed.

You might experience mild burning upon urination and frequency of urination and may or may not have blood in your urine, depending upon whether a biopsy was taken. Follow instructions carefully. Tell your doctor if you do not void in eight hours, if you experience persistent blood in your urine, or if you develop fever, chills, or back pain. Although generally very safe, infections and hemorrhage occasionally occur.

SIGNIFICANCE OF RESULTS

A variety of abnormalities may be seen, including bladder stones, tumors, fistulas, ulcers, and abnormalities of the openings which lead to the kidneys (ureters). Enlargement of the prostate can be seen in men. If a biopsy was taken, several days may elapse before the results are known.

SYNONYMS AND INCLUDED TESTS

Cystourethroscopy.

□ □ □

□ Cytology

WHAT IT IS AND WHY IT'S OBTAINED

Cytology is the microscopic study of cells. Mostly it is used to detect cancer, but other diseases may be diagnosed as well. The best example and the most well known is the **Pap smear,** but virtually any body fluid can be tested, such as urine or that obtained during a **thoracentesis, spinal tap,** or **bronchoscopy.** The general principle is the same, that of examining the specimen for cells which appear abnormal.

HOW IT WORKS

An aspiration, smear, or brushing from the organ in question is obtained and placed on a slide or into a container. In the laboratory the specimen is examined under a microscope.

Preparation depends upon the organ being studied.

AFTER THE TEST

Aftercare depends upon the way in which the specimen was obtained.

SIGNIFICANCE OF RESULTS

Negative results mean that the cells in question appeared normal. Positive results almost always need confirmation by a repeat test or some other study, such as a **biopsy.**

SYNONYMS AND INCLUDED TESTS

Cytopathology.

□ □ □

□ Darkfield examination

WHAT IT IS AND WHY IT'S OBTAINED

The term "darkfield" refers to a way of indirectly providing light to a microscope. This test is mainly used to diagnose early (primary or secondary) syphilis.

HOW IT WORKS

A specimen of drainage will be taken from the sore, growth, or rash in question either by suctioning with a small glass tube or by rubbing with a piece of gauze and pressing a glass slide directly on to your skin. The slide will be examined immediately under a special microscope.

BEFORE THE TEST

No special preparation is required.

AFTER THE TEST

No special aftercare is needed.

SIGNIFICANCE OF RESULTS

Treponema pallidum, the organism which causes syphilis, can often be identified by this method, particularly in early lesions of syphilis (chancres) on the genitals. A negative test, however, does not rule out its presence and repeat tests may be necessary. A **serologic test for syphilis** should be obtained also and repeated in about six weeks. Some specialized laboratories use immunoassay* for directly examining smears of suspected syphilis.

□ □ □

□ Dehydroepiandosterone

WHAT IT IS AND WHY IT'S OBTAINED

Dehydroepiandosterone (DHEA) is a hormone produced by the adrenal gland which causes the formation of male features. Blood levels are used to evaluate infertility, menstrual abnormalities, and virilization (the appearance of male characteristics) in women. It is also used to monitor treatment with drugs that reduce DHEA levels.

HOW IT WORKS

You will be asked to provide a **venous blood sample** from which serum* will be separated. Immunoassay* is used for the laboratory analysis.

BEFORE THE TEST

No special preparation is required.

AFTER THE TEST

Follow **venous blood sample** aftercare.

SIGNIFICANCE OF RESULTS

High DHEA is found with increased adrenal gland function, which may be due to congenital adrenal hyperplasia, Cushing's disease, or cancer of the adrenal. It is sometimes elevated, however, in the absence of other identifiable diseases. It is also high in those taking DHEA. It is best interpreted with other hormone tests, such as **testosterone, androstenedione,** and, sometimes, **17-ketosteroids.**

□ □ □

□ Delta aminolevulinic acid

WHAT IT IS AND WHY IT'S OBTAINED

Delta aminolevulinic acid is a substance which is important in the manufacture of **hemoglobin.** Urine levels are used to diagnose certain types of porphyria, a group of uncommon diseases with a range of symptoms.

HOW IT WORKS

You will be asked to provide a **24-hour urine sample.** Keep the specimen refrigerated. Several methods may be used for the laboratory assay.

BEFORE THE TEST

No special preparation is required.

AFTER THE TEST

No special aftercare is needed.

SIGNIFICANCE OF RESULTS

Elevated urine delta aminolevulinic acid indicates one of the following porphyrias: acute intermittent porphyria, hereditary coproporphyria, and porphyria variegata. It is also high in lead poisoning.

□ □ □

☐ Dexamethasone suppression test

WHAT IT IS AND WHY IT'S OBTAINED

Dexamethasone is a synthetic steroid which will normally suppress the production of **adrenocorticotropic hormone** (ACTH) by the pituitary gland, which in turn suppresses the production of **cortisol** by the adrenal gland. The dexamethasone suppression test (DST) is used to evaluate the causes of increased cortisol production.

HOW IT WORKS

You will be asked to provide a **venous blood sample** from which serum* will be separated. You will then be given dexamethasone to be taken before you go to sleep at night. The following day more blood samples will be taken, usually in the late afternoon and at night. All samples will be analyzed for cortisol. The test may be repeated with higher doses of dexamethasone if the first ones do not lower your cortisol.

BEFORE THE TEST

You should fast overnight.

AFTER THE TEST

Follow **venous blood sample** aftercare.

SIGNIFICANCE OF RESULTS

The DST must be interpreted with other hormone tests, including ACTH. Positive results (no cortisol suppression) with *low* doses of dexamethasone can occur as a result of Cushing's syndrome from pituitary gland or adrenal gland disease, psychiatric illness (particularly depression), alcoholism, stress, and many drugs. Suppression only with *high* doses of dexamethasone tends to rule out pituitary causes of Cushing's syndrome.

☐ ☐ ☐

◻ Dibucaine number

WHAT IT IS AND WHY IT'S OBTAINED

The dibucaine number is used to evaluate low levels of **cholinesterase.**

HOW IT WORKS

You will be asked to provide a **venous blood sample** from which serum* will be separated. The amount of cholinesterase inhibition by dibucaine and fluoride is measured by a chemical reaction at different temperatures.

BEFORE THE TEST

Muscle relaxants should not have been administered for twenty-four hours before the test.

AFTER THE TEST

Follow **venous blood sample** aftercare.

SIGNIFICANCE OF RESULTS

There are several genetic variants of cholinesterase deficiency which may be detected by this method, each having a distinct sensitivity to the muscle relaxant succinylcholine, a muscle relaxant which is used in general anesthesia.

◻ ◻ ◻

◻ DNA identification testing

WHAT IT IS AND WHY IT'S OBTAINED

The DNA in each of us is unique, unless one is an identical twin. It is possible, therefore, if the exact structure of this molecule is known, to identify us positively. As it is, there are some parts of the DNA molecule that most of us share and other parts which show great variation from one person to another. It is the latter areas of the DNA which are analyzed for identification. DNA identification testing is used to establish paternity or other family relationships such as in cases where infants have been switched at birth. It is also used in identification of the dead, in rape cases, and in many types of legal and criminal investigations.

HOW IT WORKS

Many specimen sources are possible, including blood, semen, hair, tissue, or cultured cells. To establish an identity between two family members, both members must submit a sample, the most common of which is a **venous blood sample.** Southern blot* is used for the analysis.

BEFORE THE TEST

If blood is used, you should have received no transfusions for ninety days.

AFTER THE TEST

If blood is used, follow **venous blood sample** aftercare.

SIGNIFICANCE OF RESULTS

The interpretation of DNA for medical or legal purposes is a subject of much dispute. Since the entire structure of DNA is not analyzed, but only parts of it, results are reported in terms of probability. Thus, in cases of paternity testing, one can be 99.99 percent certain that a given person is not the father of a given child. Some might think this is virtual certainty, whereas others say that all you need is 10,000 tests to get a false positive. The other major cause for controversy is in the collection of the sample. This is a valid concern, since it is easy to contaminate the specimen with foreign DNA. As more sites on the DNA molecule are capable of being analyzed the specificity will improve and one day will be able to provide indisputable evidence of identity.

DNA fingerprinting, paternity testing, RFLP analysis for parentage.

□ □ □

□ DNA probe testing

WHAT IT IS AND WHY IT'S OBTAINED

DNA probe testing presently is used mainly to identify DNA from germs, such as bacteria, viruses, and parasites. Tests for gonorrhea, chlamydia, papillomavirus, and mycoplasma are currently in use, and others are being developed.

HOW IT WORKS

Any source of DNA can be used, such as blood, body fluids, or tissue. The DNA is extracted from the specimen, denatured, and incubated with a specific radioactive DNA "probe" which is then analyzed using electrophoresis* and photography.

BEFORE THE TEST

This depends upon the source of the specimen.

AFTER THE TEST

Depends upon the source of the specimen.

SIGNIFICANCE OF RESULTS

A positive DNA probe test virtually proves the presence of the DNA being sought. If the DNA is from a germ, further testing should be performed, since the identification of DNA from bacteria, for example, tells us nothing about how the body is responding to the infection via the immune system. For this, **bacterial antibodies** should be obtained. In addition, a positive DNA bacterial test does not substitute for a **bacterial culture** which also usually includes **bacterial sensitivity,** information which can be crucial in proper treatment. Some DNA tests, unfortunately, are not good enough to be used routinely. This is the case with the wart virus (papillomavirus) DNA tests. The reason for this is that there are over fifty types of this virus, and the DNA test detects only seven of them. A negative test, therefore, is virtually meaningless, and although certain types of papillomavirus are associated with a higher risk of developing cervical cancer, the relationship is not at all clear. The main advantage of DNA probe tests is they are fast.

□ □ □

□ Drug testing

WHAT IT IS AND WHY IT'S OBTAINED

Although drug testing is commonly associated with detecting substance abuse, there are valid medical reasons for finding out about a drug or drugs in the body. It is fairly common, for instance, that someone suffering a drug overdose is unwilling or unable to divulge the name of the drug. Another indication is what is termed "therapeutic drug monitoring." Some medications, such as antibiotics, heart medications, anticonvulsants, and psychiatric medications, work best if a certain blood level can be maintained. In these cases blood levels may be obtained and dosage adjusted.

HOW IT WORKS

For *therapeutic drug monitoring* you will be asked to provide a **venous blood sample** from which serum* will be separated. The timing of taking this specimen varies with the drug being analyzed. For some drugs, two determinations are made, to measure the highest and lowest levels. Many methods may be used for the laboratory analysis.

For *detecting drug abuse* you will be asked to provide a urine sample. Urine is used because it is easier to collect and because concentrations of drugs are usually greater in urine than in blood. There are many machines which will perform these analyses and screen for hundreds of drugs. If you are submitting a urine sample for drug analysis, certain precautions (short of having someone watching you void) are taken to prevent you from switching samples or diluting your urine with water. Only cold water, for example, is available in the collection room, and the toilet water is dyed. The color and temperature of your urine will be noted shortly after you submit it, as well as its specific gravity and **creatinine** content, to see if it was diluted.

BEFORE THE TEST

No special preparation is required.

AFTER THE TEST

Follow **venous blood sample** aftercare if a blood sample was taken.

SIGNIFICANCE OF RESULTS

For therapeutic drug monitoring the concentration of the drug in your blood will be compared to known effective levels. Your doctor will take into account your age, weight, the disease being treated, and other medications you are taking which may influence the effectiveness of the drug being tested. For drug abuse testing, a positive or negative result will be given for each drug. A negative result may not mean that there was *no* drug present but only that the amount of drug did not meet the threshold for reporting a positive. Further testing may be done to quantify drugs found to be present. The most commonly abused drugs are alcohol, amphetamines, barbiturates, benzodiazepines, marijuana, cocaine, heroin, morphine and other opiates, phencyclidine (PCP), methaqualone, and propoxyphene. These are often included in a drug abuse or pre-employment screen.

The following is a list of only some of the many substances and classes of substances which may be detected through testing:

Acetominophen
Alcohol
Amiodarone
Amitriptyline
Amoxapine
Amphetamines
Amphotericin B
Antibiotics
Anticonvulsants
Antidepressants
Antipsychotics
Arsenic
Aspirin and other
    salicylates
Barbiturates
Benzodiazepines (Valium,
    Librium, Halcion, and
    others)
Cadmium
Caffeine
Carbamazepine (Tegretol)
Chloramphenicol
    (Chloromycetin)
Chlorpromazine
Clonazepam
Cocaine
Codeine
Cyanide
Cyclosporine
Diazepam
Digoxin
Disopyramide
Doxepin
Encainide (Enkaid)
Ethchlorvynol

Ethosuximide
Ethotoin
Ethylene glycol
Felbamate
Flecainide
Flucytosine
Fluoride
Fluoxetine
Fluphenazine
Flurazepam
Gentamicin
Glutethimide
Gold
Haloperidol
Heroin
Imipramine
Itraconazole
Ketoconazole
Lead
Lidocaine
Lithium
Maprotiline
Marijuana and other
    cannabinoids
Meperidine
Mephenytoin
Meprobamate
Mercury
Methadone
Methaqualone
Methotrexate
Mexiletine
Morphine
Nortriptyline
Opiates

Oxazepam
Phenacemide
Phencyclidine
Phenothiazines
Phenytoin (Dilantin)
Primidone
Procainamide
Propoxyphene
Propranolol
Quinidine

Thallium
Theophylline
Thiocyanate
Tocainide
Trazodone
Valproic acid
Verapamil
Warfarin
Zidovudine

□ □ □

□ Echocardiogram

WHAT IT IS AND WHY IT'S OBTAINED

The echocardiogram is a type of **ultrasound** of the heart. Echocardiography is an excellent noninvasive test which produces a picture of the heart as it beats. It is used to evaluate diseases of the heart muscle, valves, and blood vessels.

HOW IT WORKS

You will be asked to disrobe from the waist up and to put on a hospital gown. Three electrodes for an **electrocardiogram** will be attached and a clear jelly applied to your chest. As you lie on your left side a transducer will be moved across your skin while the doctor watches the image on a screen. The procedure is completely safe and painless and takes forty-five minutes to an hour. There are a number of technical variations which give different views, such as two-dimensional, M-mode, and Doppler, all of which can be performed at the same time. A phonocardiogram, which records heart sounds as they are heard through a stethoscope, may also be obtained.

BEFORE THE TEST

No special preparation is required.

AFTER THE TEST

No special aftercare is needed.

SIGNIFICANCE OF RESULTS

Interpretation of this test is performed by a cardiologist. Many abnormalities may be detected, such as heart valve dysfunction, septal defects ("holes" in the heart), fluid collections around the heart (pericardial effusion), cardiac enlargement, tumors of the heart, and disease of the heart muscle (cardiomyopathy).

SYNONYMS AND INCLUDED TESTS

Doppler echo, 2-D echo, M-mode echo, color Doppler.

□ □ □

□ Electrocardiogram

WHAT IT IS AND WHY IT'S OBTAINED

The electrocardiogram (ECG) records the electrical activity of the heart and is the most common test of heart function. It is used in a variety of circumstances both by itself and as a basis for other tests, such as the **stress test** and **Holter monitor,** to evaluate chest pain, shortness of breath, palpitations, and other symptoms.

HOW IT WORKS

You will be asked to disrobe from the waist up. For the full "12-lead" recording, electrode paste will be applied to your ankles and wrists and to sites on the left side of your chest. The technician will switch between the various electrodes to obtain different views and the results are recorded on a paper strip. The ECG measures electrical activity of the heart as it is transmitted throughout the body.

BEFORE THE TEST

No special preparation is required.

AFTER THE TEST

No special aftercare is needed. There are no complications.

SIGNIFICANCE OF RESULTS

The interpretation of the ECG is a science in itself. Generally, the basis of the ECG is that the electrical activity of the heart can be recorded as a characteristic pattern which changes with heart disease. A normal result is good evidence that you do not have heart disease but does not rule it out completely. Characteristic patterns can be seen in recent and ongoing heart attacks, old heart attacks, heart enlargement, pericarditis, ventricular aneurysms, conduction defects, and the effects of drugs and **electrolytes.**

SYNONYMS AND INCLUDED TESTS

EKG.

□ □ □

□ Electroencephalogram

WHAT IT IS AND WHY IT'S OBTAINED

The electroencephalogram (EEG) records the electrical activity of the brain and is used to evaluate epilepsy, meningitis, encephalitis, head injuries, strokes, brain abscesses, and brain tumors. It is also used to distinguish between psychological disorders and mental retardation.

HOW IT WORKS

The test is usually performed in a special procedure room or laboratory. You will be asked to sit in a chair or upright recliner, or to lie flat on a bed or examining table. Electrodes will then be placed on your scalp and forehead. The electrodes are usually flat, but occasionally small needle electrodes are used. In the latter case there will be slight discomfort. Wires attach these electrodes to the electroencephalograph, which amplifies the signals received through them and translates them into wave forms which are recorded on a long paper strip. You will usually be observed through a window in an adjoining room and will be given certain instructions regarding positioning and breathing. If the test is being used to evaluate epilepsy a strobe light may be flashed in front of your eyes or you may be asked to overbreathe (hyperventilate).

BEFORE THE TEST

Check with your doctor concerning medications and foods to be stopped before the test. Do not skip the meal before the test. Shampoo thoroughly the night before the test and do not apply hair sprays or other cosmetics to your hair. On occasion you may be asked to stay up all night before the test for a sleep-deprived EEG. In some studies you may be asked to take a hypnotic medication, since sometimes the EEG is only abnormal during sleep.

AFTER THE TEST

Resume medications which may have been discontinued or withheld before the test. If you have epilepsy a seizure may have been induced by one or more of the stimuli employed during the EEG, such as the strobe light. Medical personnel are trained to observe carefully for this complication.

SIGNIFICANCE OF RESULTS

The EEG is interpreted by studying the recorded wave forms. There are four basic patterns: alpha, beta, theta, and delta. Characteristic abnormalities are found in the various types of epilepsy, dementia due to organic brain disease, encephalitis, brain tumors, and severe head injuries. The EEG tends to be normal in psychiatric illnesses and Alzheimer's disease. **Computed tomography** and **magnetic resonance imaging** of the head often provide crucial additional information about the brain.

□ □ □

□ Electrolytes

WHAT IT IS AND WHY IT'S OBTAINED

Electrolytes are substances which exist as ions (charged particles) in the blood and which have many important functions, including that of keeping the pH of the blood stable. This test commonly includes **sodium, chloride, potassium,** and **carbon dioxide. Anion gap** is sometimes included as well. Electrolytes are used to evaluate dehydration, vomiting, diarrhea, severe illnesses, and acid-base balance.

HOW IT WORKS

You will be asked to provide a **venous blood sample** from which serum* will be separated. Various laboratory methods are used to analyze the different ions. Urine may also be analyzed.

BEFORE THE TEST

No special preparation is required.

AFTER THE TEST

Follow **venous blood sample** aftercare.

SIGNIFICANCE OF RESULTS

For interpretation, see the individual components.

□ □ □

☐ Electromyogram

WHAT IT IS AND WHY IT'S OBTAINED

The electromyogram (EMG) records electrical activity within muscles. It is used mainly to tell the difference between muscle diseases and nerve diseases that may cause similar symptoms, such as weakness, twitching, or poor coordination.

HOW IT WORKS

The procedure is performed in a special procedure room or laboratory. In most cases you will be asked to lie on your back on an examining table but if your back muscles are to be tested you will be asked to lie face down. The basic procedure is for the examiner to cleanse your skin and insert a needle into the muscle to be tested. The needle is attached to an amplifier which translates the impulses into sounds and waves. Unfortunately, no anesthesia or sedation can be used, and the testing tends to be uncomfortable. As the test proceeds you will hear the loudspeaker crackle. As a needle is inserted there will be a burst of electrical activity, which is called insertional activity. After this subsides you will be asked to relax the muscle, then flex it a little, then again, as hard as you can. All of these activities are measured and the patterns recorded. It is usually neither necessary nor desirable to test every muscle, just representative samples.

BEFORE THE TEST

Check with your doctor regarding medications to avoid.

AFTER THE TEST

No special aftercare is needed. You may have some transient tenderness in the muscles tested.

SIGNIFICANCE OF RESULTS

The EMG is interpreted by a neurologist or physiatrist (physical medicine specialist). Different diseases produce different electrical patterns during needle insertion, rest, or contraction, and all patterns are taken into consideration. In nerve diseases it is usually possible to distinguish between the two basic types, called upper motor neuron disease, such as tumors of the spinal cord, and lower motor neuron disease, such as amyotrophic lateral sclerosis (Lou Gehrig's disease) or polio. Primary muscle diseases can also usually be distinguished, such as muscular dystrophy, myotonia, dermatomyositis, and the muscle wasting which occurs in alcoholics. The EMG is often performed in conjunction with **nerve conduction studies.**

□ □ □

□ Electrophysiologic eye testing

WHAT IT IS AND WHY IT'S OBTAINED

The two major electrophysiologic eye tests are the electrooculogram and the electroretinogram. Both measure electrical impulses generated by the eyes and are used to evaluate severe visual impairment such as occurs in blindness or degenerative eye diseases. These tests are not designed for routine eye examinations.

HOW IT WORKS

The tests are conducted in a special laboratory. You will be asked to sit in a chair. For the electrooculogram drops to dilate your pupils will be instilled and electrodes will be placed on the skin at the corners of your eyes and your forehead. The room will be darkened and you will be asked to repeatedly glance at an object to the left and then at an object to the right. The same procedure will be conducted with the lights on. For the electroretinogram anesthetic eye drops will be instilled and a contact lens containing an embedded electrode will be placed on your eye. Light sources of different intensities will then be shined into your eyes, again both in the dark and in the light. The electrical responses of your retina to these stimuli will be recorded on a paper strip.

BEFORE THE TEST

No special preparation is required.

AFTER THE TEST

No special aftercare is needed.

SIGNIFICANCE OF RESULTS

In total blindness, no electrical response is noted. If the test is abnormal only in the dark, the rods of the retina are impaired; if the test is abnormal only in the light, the cones are at fault. Varying degrees of visual impairment are suggestive of a number of hereditary and degenerative diseases of the retina.

SYNONYMS AND INCLUDED TESTS

Electrooculogram, EOG, electroretinogram, ERG.

□ □ □

□ Endomysial antibodies

WHAT IT IS AND WHY IT'S OBTAINED

Endomysin is a protein found in muscle. Antibodies to it are formed in diseases which are triggered by wheat protein (gluten) sensitivity. Blood levels of endomysial antibodies are used to diagnose these diseases.

HOW IT WORKS

You will be asked to provide a **venous blood sample** from which serum* will be separated. Immunoassay* is used for the laboratory analysis.

BEFORE THE TEST

No special preparation is required.

AFTER THE TEST

Follow **venous blood sample** aftercare.

SIGNIFICANCE OF RESULTS

Elevated endomysial antibodies are seen in dermatitis herpetiformis, an itchy skin disease, and gluten-sensitive enteropathy, an intestinal disease characterized by diarrhea and intestinal malabsorption. A gluten-free diet will often alleviate symptoms.

□ □ □

□ Endoscopic retrograde cholangiopancreatography

WHAT IT IS AND WHY IT'S OBTAINED

Endoscopic retrograde cholangiopancreatography (ERCP) is a method for examining the ducts which lead from the pancreas and gallbladder into the intestine. It is used to evaluate jaundice where obstruction of the flow of bile (the digestive aid formed in the liver and stored in the gallbladder) is suspected and to investigate diseases of the pancreas such as pancreatitis or suspected pancreatic cancer. It is a type of **X-ray contrast study.**

HOW IT WORKS

ERCP takes place in a special room with X-ray equipment. You will have your vital signs (pulse, blood pressure, respiration, and temperature) taken and the blood pressure cuff will remain on your arm. You will have an intravenous fluid drip started and will be given a mild sedative and a painkiller. This will make you feel drowsy and groggy but you will still be conscious. You will be asked to lie on your left side, although other positions are possible, and will be given a plastic mouthpiece to protect your teeth. A local anesthetic will next be sprayed onto the back of your throat. At this point you will be unable to swallow your saliva and will be instructed to let it drain out of the side of your mouth into a basin. The doctor will then guide a lubricated flexible tube into your mouth with the aid of his finger. Follow instructions with regard to swallowing and head position carefully. The sensation is unusual but not painful. You will not choke on the tube. After a time you will not swallow at all as the doctor slowly advances the tube. At times you will feel pressure, fullness, or other sensations in your chest or belly but no real pain. Although the main purpose of this test is to visualize a portion of the gastrointestinal tract with a contrast dye, there are multiple small channels in the endoscope which allow for surgical procedures such as a **biopsy.**

BEFORE THE TEST

Follow instructions carefully with regard to food and medications. It is usual to fast overnight for an early morning test and to be without food for eight hours in any event. Antacids interfere with this test and should be discontinued as directed.

AFTER THE TEST

Your vital signs will be monitored in a recovery area depending upon your physical condition. After about an hour your gag reflex will be tested by a nurse or technician touching the back of your throat with a tongue depressor. After the reflex has returned you will be allowed clear liquids. This procedure is usually *not* performed as an outpatient, but if it is, have someone drive you home since you will be groggy for twelve hours or more. Although generally safe, ERCP can produce complications such as perforation of the esophagus or stomach, acute pancreatitis, heartbeat irregularities (arrhythmias), and infection. Report any abnormal pain, palpitations, difficulty breathing, fever, chills, black stool, or vomiting blood.

SIGNIFICANCE OF RESULTS

A normal test means that the pancreatic ducts and bile ducts appeared normal. ERCP may reveal stones, strictures, inflammation, tumors, and cysts. It may take a week for results of biopsy specimens to be reported. Abdominal **ultrasound, computed tomography, liver and spleen scan,** and **magnetic resonance imaging** are also helpful in visualizing this area.

□ □ □

□ Endothelial photography

WHAT IT IS AND WHY IT'S OBTAINED

This test is used to evaluate the cornea before eye surgery or to detect the presence of certain corneal diseases.

HOW IT WORKS

You will be asked to sit in a chair and anesthetic drops will be used to numb your eyes. A photographic microscope will then be advanced gently until it touches the surface of your eye and photographs will be taken of the cornea. The photographs are analyzed for the size, shape, and number of cells lining the back surface of the cornea.

BEFORE THE TEST

No special preparation is required.

AFTER THE TEST

No special aftercare is needed.

SIGNIFICANCE OF RESULTS

A lower than normal cell count suggests to the surgeon that special precautions may need to be taken at the time of corneal surgery.

SYNONYMS AND INCLUDED TESTS

Endothelial cell count, preoperative corneal evaluation, specular microscopy.

◻ ◻ ◻

◻ Eosinophil count

WHAT IT IS AND WHY IT'S OBTAINED

Eosinophils are a type of white blood cell which are involved in allergies. The eosinophil count is usually a part of the **complete blood count** but may be ordered separately to evaluate allergic diseases, diseases caused by parasites, endocrine (hormonal) diseases, cancer, and autoimmune diseases (in which the immune system reacts against the body's own tissues).

HOW IT WORKS

You will be asked to provide a **venous blood sample** or **fingerstick blood sample** which will be smeared on a slide and stained. The eosinophils, which show up with red granules, are counted manually or by machine.

BEFORE THE TEST

No special preparation is required.

AFTER THE TEST

Follow **venous blood sample** or **fingerstick blood sample** aftercare.

SIGNIFICANCE OF RESULTS

An increase in eosinophils occurs in allergies, drug reactions, infestations with intestinal parasites, autoimmune diseases, Hodgkin's disease, certain leukemias, the hypereosinophilic syndrome, eosinophilic gastroenteritis, eosinophilia myalgia syndrome, sarcoidosis, and other diseases. An increase in the eosinophil count, in and of itself, is not sufficient to diagnose any disease in particular. A decrease in eosinophils occurs in Cushing's disease (caused by an overactive adrenal gland).

□ □ □

□ Eosinophil smear

WHAT IT IS AND WHY IT'S OBTAINED

Eosinophils are a type of white blood cell which are involved in allergies. Smears for eosinophils are used to diagnose hay fever, asthma, and intestinal parasites.

HOW IT WORKS

The procedure depends upon the specimen in question. For nasal secretions, the doctor or technician will insert a cotton swab into your nostrils and transfer the material to a slide. For sputum you will be given a plastic container in which to place sputum which you cough up. Sputum should be from a *deep* cough. For feces you will be given a container in which to place the specimen.

BEFORE THE TEST

No special preparation is required.

AFTER THE TEST

No special aftercare is needed.

An increased number of eosinophils in nasal mucus is found in hay fever (allergic rhinitis). In sputum, eosinophils are increased in asthma and chronic bronchitis. In feces, eosinophils are increased in intestinal parasites.

□ □ □

□ Erythropoietin

WHAT IT IS AND WHY IT'S OBTAINED

Erythropoietin is a substance produced by the kidney which stimulates the production of red blood cells. Blood levels are used to evaluate anemia or polycythemia (a disease caused by overproduction of red blood cells).

HOW IT WORKS

You will be asked to provide a **venous blood sample** from which serum* will be separated. Immunoassay* is used for the laboratory analysis.

BEFORE THE TEST

No special preparation is required.

AFTER THE TEST

Follow **venous blood sample** aftercare.

SIGNIFICANCE OF RESULTS

Erythropoietin is increased in the presence of certain tumors, such as brain tumors or liver cancer, pregnancy, iron deficiency anemia, in those taking androgenic steroids, and in athletes who inject themselves to increase their red blood cells. It is decreased in those taking estrogens, in kidney disease, and after surgical removal of the kidneys.

□ □ □

☐ Esophageal motility

WHAT IT IS AND WHY IT'S OBTAINED

This test is used to evaluate the function of the esophagus and to investigate symptoms of heartburn, difficulty swallowing, or chest pain.

HOW IT WORKS

The procedure is usually performed in a special room or laboratory. Your vital signs (pulse, blood pressure, respiration, and temperature) will be taken and the blood pressure cuff kept in pace. An intravenous fluid drip may or may not be started. You will be asked to lie on your back and a sensor to detect swallowing will be placed around your neck. Then, a flexible lubricated tube will next be inserted into one of your nostrils and guided to the back of your throat. Follow instructions regarding swallowing and do not fight the tube. You may feel the urge to gag but this will pass. The tube will be advanced into the lower esophagus and halted at various positions at which point pressure readings will be taken. The pressure readings are recorded on a strip of paper. You will be asked to swallow at various points and may be given water or ice chips to swallow. You may also be given a medication (edrophonium) intravenously to stimulate the sphincter at the border of your esophagus and stomach. The **Bernstein test** may be performed after the pressure readings are taken. Esophageal motility is mildly uncomfortable but not painful.

BEFORE THE TEST

You should fast overnight or for eight hours.

AFTER THE TEST

You may have a slight sore throat for a day or two.

A number of abnormalities in the way the esophagus moves may be found. Failure of the sphincter between the esophagus and stomach to relax (achalasia), spasm of the esophagus, scleroderma, polymyositis, and the "nutcracker" esophagus produce distinctive patterns on the recording strip.

SYNONYMS AND INCLUDED TESTS

Esophageal manometry.

◻ ◻ ◻

◻ Esophageal pH study

WHAT IT IS AND WHY IT'S OBTAINED

The esophageal pH study is used to evaluate symptoms of reflux esophagitis—inflammation of the lower esophagus caused by upward leakage of acid from the stomach. The most common symptom of this is heartburn, but other forms of chest pain may occur.

HOW IT WORKS

This test is most often performed in the hospital over a twelve- or twenty-four-hour period, but it is possible to have it as an outpatient. The general idea is to have an acid-sensing electrode installed in your lower esophagus over a period of time in order to correlate symptoms with the presence of excess acid. The initial part of the test is done in order to pinpoint the location of the sphincter between the stomach and esophagus and is identical to **esophageal motility.** The tube used for the first study is withdrawn and a smaller flexible tube with the pH electrode will be inserted through one of your nostrils and guided to a point above the sphincter where it remains for the duration of the test. The electrode along with a control electrode on your arm is hooked up to an electronic device and the recording begins.

You will be given a special diet free of acidic foods. Do not smoke or drink coffee or alcohol for the duration of the test. You will also be asked to record your activities, carefully noting food intake, the position of your body, and your symptoms.

BEFORE THE TEST

No special preparation is required.

AFTER THE TEST

You may have a sore throat for a day or two.

SIGNIFICANCE OF RESULTS

The symptom of heartburn is very common and most of us have experienced mild episodes which resolve spontaneously. There are those, however, who suffer considerably, often at night when they lie flat. This is often associated with a hiatal hernia. The esophageal pH study is theoretically the best way to diagnose reflux esophagitis because it mimics daily activity. It does so, however, only for twenty-four hours, and false negatives are common. **Upper gastrointestinal endoscopy** can be helpful by documenting inflammation in the lower esophagus in cases of reflux esophagitis.

SYNONYMS AND INCLUDED TESTS

Twelve- or twenty-four-hour pH study, esophageal reflux study with intraluminal pH electrode.

□ □ □

☐ Estradiol

WHAT IT IS AND WHY IT'S OBTAINED

Estradiol is the most powerful natural **estrogen.** Blood levels are used to study infertility, menstrual irregularities, sexual precocity, and delayed puberty in females. In males, blood estradiol is indicated in evaluating feminization.

HOW IT WORKS

You will be asked to provide a **venous blood sample** from which serum* will be separated. Immunoassay* is used for the laboratory analysis.

BEFORE THE TEST

No special preparation is required.

AFTER THE TEST

Follow **venous blood sample** aftercare.

SIGNIFICANCE OF RESULTS

High estradiol is found in certain tumors of the ovary or adrenal gland, and in some liver diseases. Low levels are seen in decreased functioning of the pituitary gland or the ovaries, such as occurs in menopause.

□ □ □

□ Estriol

WHAT IT IS AND WHY IT'S OBTAINED

Estriol is the most prevalent estrogen during pregnancy. Blood levels have been used to monitor the health of the fetus, but its value for this purpose is very controversial.

HOW IT WORKS

You will be asked to provide a **venous blood sample** from which serum* will be separated. Immunoassay* or chromatography* may be used in the laboratory analysis.

BEFORE THE TEST

No special preparation is required.

AFTER THE TEST

Follow **venous blood sample** aftercare.

SIGNIFICANCE OF RESULTS

A single blood estriol determination is meaningless. A gradual decline in values over the course of pregnancy has been taken to indicate problems with the fetus or placenta, but many consider this test unreliable. Many medications may interfere with accurate results.

□ □ □

□ Estrogens

WHAT IT IS AND WHY IT'S OBTAINED

Estrogens are hormones produced in the ovaries which impart female characteristics and allow for menstruation. Blood levels are used to evaluate menstrual difficulties, particularly lack of menstrual periods (amenorrhea), infertility, and sexual precocity in women. In males, it may be ordered to to study feminization.

HOW IT WORKS

You will be asked to provide a **24-hour urine sample** which should be kept refrigerated during collection. Immunoassay* is used for the laboratory analysis.

BEFORE THE TEST

No special preparation is required.

AFTER THE TEST

No special aftercare is needed.

SIGNIFICANCE OF RESULTS

Total urinary estrogens vary during the menstrual cycle, with the peak occurring at ovulation. In general, low levels signify decreased ovarian function, which may be due either to problems with the ovaries themselves or with the pituitary gland. Increased levels are seen in various ovarian tumors, testicular tumors, increased adrenal activity, liver disease, and pregnancy.

SYNONYMS AND INCLUDED TESTS

Total urinary estrogens.

□ □ □

□ Exophthalmometry

WHAT IT IS AND WHY IT'S OBTAINED

Exophthalmometry is used to measure the degree of protrusion of the eyeball. It is indicated in evaluating conditions which cause the eyeball to be displaced forward or backward.

HOW IT WORKS

You will be seated in a chair. The examiner will hold a device with a ruler and two mirrors in front of your eyes. The device will also touch the edges of the bony part of your eye sockets. The measurement takes a minute or two and is painless.

BEFORE THE TEST

No special preparation is required.

AFTER THE TEST

No special aftercare is needed.

SIGNIFICANCE OF RESULTS

The condition of protruding eyeballs is called exophthalmos and occurs in hyperthyroidism (overactive thyroid), tumors around the eye socket, hemorrhage, swelling, and infections. The opposite condition is called enophthalmos and may result from injury, infection, or a congenital defect. Abnormal results call for further testing, such as **ultrasound, X-ray, computed tomography,** and a general medical evaluation.

□ □ □

□ Febrile agglutinins

WHAT IT IS AND WHY IT'S OBTAINED

The term "febrile" refers to fever; an "agglutinin" is a type of antibody (a blood protein important to the immune system). Febrile agglutinins is actually a series of tests which are sometimes used to diagnose diseases which cause persistent fever: tularemia, brucellosis, salmonella infections, epidemic typhus, endemic typhus, scrub typhus, and Rocky Mountain spotted fever.

HOW IT WORKS

You will be asked to provide a **venous blood sample** from which serum* will be separated. Immunoassay* is used for the laboratory analysis.

BEFORE THE TEST

No special preparation is required.

AFTER THE TEST

Follow **venous blood sample** aftercare.

SIGNIFICANCE OF RESULTS

Reports are made on four diseases: salmonellosis, brucellosis, rickettsial disease, and tularemia, but positive results must be interpreted with care, since this is a rough screening test only. Most accurate results are obtained with multiple determinations over time in which rising or falling antibody levels can be noted. A single test result is practically meaningless. This test is generally considered to be outmoded because of the availability of more sophisticated antibody and culture methods for the specific diseases.

□ □ □

□ Fecal fat

WHAT IT IS AND WHY IT'S OBTAINED

This test is used to detect the presence of high levels of fat in the stool (steatorrhea), the symptoms of which are usually diarrhea and foul-smelling stool which floats in the toilet bowl.

HOW IT WORKS

You will be asked to provide a **stool specimen.** This may either be random or a three-day collection. Do not place toilet paper or any other material in the container you are provided. Refrigerate the specimen during collection. For the random specimen a small portion of stool is stained and examined under a microscope. For the three-day collection, fat is extracted with sodium hydroxide and measured.

BEFORE THE TEST

You will be given instructions for a special diet consisting of 80 to 100 grams of fat per day. Do not take mineral oil (for constipation) during the period of collection.

AFTER THE TEST

No special aftercare is needed.

SIGNIFICANCE OF RESULTS

The presence of large quantities of fat in the stool indicates disease either of the pancreas or intestine, but this test does not differentiate between them or among the different diseases which are included in each category. Other tests for intestinal malabsorption include **stool muscle fibers, d-xylose absorption, hydrogen breath test,** and **intestinal biopsy.**

SYNONYMS AND INCLUDED TESTS

Stool fat.

□ □ □

□ Ferritin

WHAT IT IS AND WHY IT'S OBTAINED

Ferritin (composed of iron and protein) is a major storehouse for iron in the body, and blood measurement provides an accurate picture of how much iron you have available in reserve. This test is used to evaluate anemia and is the best method other than a **bone marrow** for diagnosing iron deficiency.

HOW IT WORKS

You will be asked to provide a **venous blood sample** from which serum* will be separated. Immunoassay* is used for the laboratory analysis.

BEFORE THE TEST

No special preparation is required.

Follow **venous blood sample** aftercare.

SIGNIFICANCE OF RESULTS

Low ferritin is the hallmark of iron deficiency, which is the most common cause of anemia. Ferritin is high with inflammation, infection, liver disease, iron overload, certain anemias (not iron deficient), and certain cancers, such as leukemia and lymphoma.

□ □ □

□ Fibrin split products

WHAT IT IS AND WHY IT'S OBTAINED

Fibrin is a protein which is responsible for the foundation of a blood clot. As the blood clot dissolves, the fibrin splits into fragments. These fragments are called fibrin split products (FSP) and function as natural blood thinners (anticoagulants). Blood levels of FSPs are used to evaluate the blood clotting system.

HOW IT WORKS

You will be asked to provide a **venous blood sample** and the blood will be allowed to clot. As the clot dissolves, the fibrin fragments are measured by one of several methods.

BEFORE THE TEST

No special preparation is required.

AFTER THE TEST

Follow **venous blood sample** aftercare.

SIGNIFICANCE OF RESULTS

Elevated levels of FSP are associated with disseminated intravascular coagulation, a serious disease in which the substances responsible for blood clotting—mainly **fibrinogen**—are depleted, leading to excessive bleeding from multiple sites. They are also increased in pulmonary embolism, some cancers, burns, complications of pregnancy, and kidney disease.

SYNONYMS AND INCLUDED TESTS

Fibrin breakdown products, fibrin degradation products.

□ □ □

□ Fibrinogen

WHAT IT IS AND WHY IT'S OBTAINED

Fibrinogen is the precursor of fibrin, the substance which forms the meshwork of a blood clot. Blood levels of fibrinogen are used to evaluate bleeding disorders and the risk of coronary artery disease (CAD).

HOW IT WORKS

You will be asked to provide a **venous blood sample.** Many methods are available to estimate the amount of fibrinogen but most are imperfect. Some assays employ a variation of the **thrombin time.**

BEFORE THE TEST

No special preparation is required.

AFTER THE TEST

Follow **venous blood sample** aftercare.

SIGNIFICANCE OF RESULTS

Decreased fibrinogen is found in disseminated intravascular coagulation, a serious disease in which the substances responsible for blood clotting are depleted, leading to excessive bleeding from multiple sites. It is also low in hereditary absence of fibrinogen and liver disease. Increased levels are seen in pregnancy, chronic inflammation, and those taking birth control pills. High levels are also produced by cigarette smoking and are associated with an increased risk for CAD.

□ □ □

□ Fingerstick blood sample

WHAT IT IS AND WHY IT'S OBTAINED

Although much less common than the **venous blood sample,** the fingerstick blood sample is of value when veins are scarred or hard to find. If the only blood test being done is a smear on a microscope slide, however, the fingerstick method is preferred.

HOW IT WORKS

The skin on the tip of one of your fingers will be cleansed with an antiseptic and rapidly punctured with a sharp pointed stylet*. This will hurt momentarily. The first drop of blood will be wiped away and the remainder will be collected either with a small glass tube (capillary tube) or directly on a microscope slide. The finger should not be squeezed vigorously to get blood to flow, but holding it downward will help.

BEFORE THE TEST

This depends upon the nature of the individual test.

Clean the site of the puncture with soap and water. A Band-Aid is generally not necessary.

SIGNIFICANCE OF RESULTS

See individual test listings.

SYNONYMS AND INCLUDED TESTS

Skin puncture blood collection, capillary blood collection, fingerstick blood collection.

□ □ □

□ **Fluorescein angiography**

WHAT IT IS AND WHY IT'S OBTAINED

Fluorescein angiography is used to evaluate the blood vessels of the retina of the eye. It may be indicated if **ophthalmoscopy** indicates certain types of retinal disease.

HOW IT WORKS

The test is conducted by an ophthalmologist or technician. You will be asked to sit in a chair as for a **slit-lamp examination** and will receive eyedrops to dilate your pupils. Next, a vein in your arm will be selected, the skin cleansed with an antiseptic, and fluorescein injected intravenously. Rarely, you may feel slightly nauseated. The camera will take photographs of your retina at one-second intervals using a flash and will continue for about thirty seconds. Occasionally, later photographs—up to an hour—are also taken.

BEFORE THE TEST

No special preparation is required.

AFTER THE TEST

You will have blurry vision for several hours and will notice yellowish discoloration of your urine and possibly a slightly yellowish cast to your skin for one to two days. Although complications are rare, you may experience an allergic reaction to the dye, which may include difficulty breathing, hives, and vomiting.

SIGNIFICANCE OF RESULTS

A variety of abnormal blood vessel findings are possible, including aneurysms, shunts between arteries and veins, abnormal vessels, areas of completely absent blood flow, and leakage from the vessels into the retina. Eye diseases which may be evaluated in this way include those secondary to high blood pressure, diabetes, and tumors.

□ □ □

□ Folic acid

WHAT IT IS AND WHY IT'S OBTAINED

Folic acid has many important functions, including a crucial role in the formation of DNA. Blood levels are used to evaluate nutritional status. Because **vitamin B$_{12}$** is needed for folic acid to work, blood levels of this vitamin are usually obtained at the same time.

HOW IT WORKS

You will be asked to provide a **venous blood sample** from which serum* will be separated. Immunoassay* is used for the laboratory analysis.

BEFORE THE TEST

You should fast overnight. Avoid nonessential medications or as directed by your doctor.

Follow **venous blood sample** aftercare.

SIGNIFICANCE OF RESULTS

Both red blood cell and serum folic acid should be interpreted along with vitamin B_{12}. Low folic acid is common in alcoholism, pregnancy, intestinal malabsorption, poor nutrition, and after intestinal bypass surgery. An overactive thyroid (hyperthyroidism) may cause an increased or decreased folic acid. High *serum* folic acid may be seen immediately after eating or in those taking large amounts in nutritional supplements. High *serum* folic acid but low *red blood cell* folic acid may be found in vitamin B_{12} deficiency.

SYNONYMS AND INCLUDED TESTS

Folate level.

□ □ □

□ Follicle stimulating hormone

WHAT IT IS AND WHY IT'S OBTAINED

Follicle stimulating hormone (FSH) is formed in the pituitary gland and stimulates the reproductive organs in both sexes, the ovaries in women and the testicles in men. Most often, blood levels are obtained in women, along with **luteinizing hormone** (LH), to investigate infertility and menstrual disturbances. In men the test is used to evaluate testicular insufficiency which may have been picked up by a low **testosterone.** Urine levels are used to study precocious puberty in children or to determine menstrual cycles for in vitro fertilization.

HOW IT WORKS

You will be asked to provide a **venous blood sample** from which serum* will be separated. Because FSH blood levels vary greatly some laboratories recommend a series of blood samples over several hours with analysis of the pooled blood sample. A **24-hour urine sample** may also be studied. Immunoassay* is used for the laboratory analysis.

BEFORE THE TEST

No special preparation is required. It is important for women to carefully note the time of their menstrual periods and inform the laboratory, since levels of FSH vary during the menstrual cycle.

AFTER THE TEST

Follow **venous blood sample** aftercare.

SIGNIFICANCE OF RESULTS

FSH lies within the complex web of the endocrine system. In general, FSH is low if the pituitary gland itself is not functioning well or if the hypothalamus, located in the brain, is not stimulating it enough. FSH is high (because of insufficient feedback suppression) if either the ovaries or the testes are not functioning well. Thus, FSH is normally high after menopause. FSH must be interpreted along with LH and usually also with **estrogen** and **testosterone.** Most often LH and FSH parallel each other, but if one is high and the other is low a pituitary tumor may be the cause. However, if LH is much higher than FSH (more than three times), the polycystic ovary syndrome (Stein-Leventhal syndrome) is most likely the reason.

□ □ □

☐ Food allergy tests

WHAT IT IS AND WHY IT'S OBTAINED

Food allergy is controversial because most available information about it is unscientific. Food allergy testing attempts to deal with the problem more scientifically.

HOW IT WORKS

Although techniques vary, the best procedure is to employ gelatin capsules which contain a precise amount of the suspect food. You will be asked to take these at timed intervals and will be observed for signs of allergy, such as hives, wheezing, vomiting, diarrhea, or abdominal pain. If you have not experienced any symptoms after a number of doses (usually twelve), you are considered not to be allergic to that food. The test is blind: you will not know what food you are ingesting, or even if it is a food—included among the capsules are placebos which have no effect.

BEFORE THE TEST

No special preparation is required.

AFTER THE TEST

No special aftercare is needed.

SIGNIFICANCE OF RESULTS

Consistently developing allergic symptoms to one or more foods and consistently being free from allergic symptoms with placebos is strong evidence that you are allergic to the food in question. The belief that one is allergic to certain foods is commonplace and usually based upon flimsy evidence. Keeping a diary of foods and reactions to them is unreliable. The **radioallergosorbent test** is also used to evaluate food allergy, but is also unreliable. An upset stomach after eating diary products may not be a true allergy and can be evaluated by a **lactose tolerance test.**

☐ ☐ ☐

☐ Fructosamine

WHAT IT IS AND WHY IT'S OBTAINED

Fructosamines are blood proteins which have become bound to blood sugar (**glucose**). The amount of glucose in these proteins depends upon how much blood glucose is present; the higher the concentration of glucose, the higher the fructosamine level. Blood levels of fructosamine measure the *average* level of blood glucose over two to three weeks and are used to monitor the long-term control of diabetes mellitus.

HOW IT WORKS

You will be asked to provide a **venous blood sample** from which serum* will be separated. Several laboratory methods are used for the assay.

BEFORE THE TEST

No special preparation is required.

AFTER THE TEST

Follow **venous blood sample** aftercare.

SIGNIFICANCE OF RESULTS

Fructosamine results are usually reported in terms of good, fair, and poor control of diabetes. The other test which is commonly used to assess long-term control of diabetes is **glycohemoglobin.**

SYNONYMS AND INCLUDED TESTS

Glycated albumin, protein-bound glucose.

☐ ☐ ☐

☐ FTA-ABS

WHAT IT IS AND WHY IT'S OBTAINED

The FTA-ABS is a blood test which is used to confirm the diagnosis of syphilis. It is usually obtained automatically after a positive **serologic test for syphilis.**

HOW IT WORKS

You will be asked to provide a **venous blood sample** from which serum* will be separated. Immunoassay* using killed *Treponema pallidum,* the organism which causes syphilis, is used for the analysis.

BEFORE THE TEST

No special preparation is required.

AFTER THE TEST

Follow **venous blood sample** aftercare.

SIGNIFICANCE OF RESULTS

A positive FTA-ABS, along with a positive serologic test for syphilis, is diagnostic for the disease. Although sensitive and specific, there are cases of false positives in Lyme disease, leprosy, malaria, infectious mononucleosis, auto-immune diseases, drug addiction, and pregnancy. Three infectious diseases related to syphilis, pinta, yaws, and bejel, also produce positive results. Once positive, the FTA-ABS tends to remain so for life, even after adequate treatment.

SYNONYMS AND INCLUDED TESTS

Fluorescent treponemal antibody-absorption.

☐ ☐ ☐

❏ Fungal antibodies

WHAT IT IS AND WHY IT'S OBTAINED

Fungal antibody testing is used to aid in the diagnosis of suspected fungal infections. Many fungal infections may be tested for in this way, including blastomycosis, histoplasmosis, coccidioidomycosis, aspergillosis, and candidiasis.

HOW IT WORKS

You will be asked to provide a **venous blood sample** from which serum* will be separated. Various methods of immunoassay* are available. Multiple determinations over a period of time are advisable.

BEFORE THE TEST

No special preparation is required.

AFTER THE TEST

Follow **venous blood sample** aftercare.

SIGNIFICANCE OF RESULTS

An elevated level of antibody to a specific fungus is indirect evidence of infection with that fungus, but multiple tests which show a rise in concentration (titer) are more helpful. Many antibodies, however, cross react with other antibodies, and positive antibody tests should be confirmed by **fungal culture** if possible.

SYNONYMS AND INCLUDED TESTS

Fungal serology.

❏ ❏ ❏

❏ Fungal culture

WHAT IT IS AND WHY IT'S OBTAINED

The term fungus refers to a germ which is either a yeast or mold. Culture is used to confirm the presence of those which cause disease. Fungal culture is obtained in a variety of circumstances depending upon symptoms and the results of other tests. Superficial skin infections with fungi (ringworm and athlete's foot) are extremely common, as are vaginal yeast infections, whereas fungal infections of the internal organs are seen only in certain geographic areas, such as coccidioidomycosis in California, and in certain people, such as those with impaired immune systems. It should be noted that a culture is not a **biopsy,** which is the microscopic examination of tissue. Fungal culture should be distinguished also from **bacterial culture** and **viral culture.**

HOW IT WORKS

Virtually any fluid or tissue may be cultured: sputum, blood, urine, stool, cerebrospinal fluid*, skin, nails, hair, surgical or biopsy specimens from any internal organ, or bone marrow. In general, the more tissue available, the more likely is a positive identification. The specimen is placed on a suitable culture medium, incubated, and allowed to grow. Unlike bacteria, fungi grow slowly, and it is often several weeks before a definitive report can be generated.

BEFORE THE TEST

No special preparation is required.

AFTER THE TEST

This depends upon how the specimen was obtained. In general, if an invasive method was used, follow your doctor's instructions carefully.

SIGNIFICANCE OF RESULTS

The presence of fungus in a tissue sample is significant, unless contamination has occurred. Unfortunately, it may be difficult to tell whether this has taken place. *Candida,* for example, is a common contaminant in the environment, but it can cause disease if conditions are right, such as in AIDS or diabetes. Antibiotic treatment can also predispose to fungal infections. The signs, symptoms, geographical location, site of the specimen, and the species recovered are all taken into consideration when interpreting results of a fungal culture. In certain cases, **fungal sensitivity** may be helpful in planning treatment.

□ □ □

□ Fungal sensitivity

WHAT IT IS AND WHY IT'S OBTAINED

This test is coupled with **fungal culture** to determine how well a certain antifungal medication inhibits the growth of a specific fungus. Unlike **bacterial sensitivity,** however, fungal sensitivity testing is not widely performed because it is difficult to do.

HOW IT WORKS

A culture of the fungus causing your infection will be incubated with different medications and any change in the growth rate of the organism will be observed and recorded.

BEFORE THE TEST

No special preparation is required.

AFTER THE TEST

No special aftercare is needed.

SIGNIFICANCE OF RESULTS

At the present time this test is most useful if your infection is with *Candida* or if your immune system is suppressed.

□ □ □

□ Fungal skin testing

WHAT IT IS AND WHY IT'S OBTAINED

Fungal skin testing is sometimes used as an aid in the diagnosis of certain fungal diseases, such as histoplasmosis, blastomycosis, and coccidioidomycosis.

HOW IT WORKS

The technique is identical to that used for a **tuberculin skin test** except that a preparation of one or more of the fungi in question is used and observed one, two, and three days afterward for redness and swelling.

BEFORE THE TEST

No special preparation is required.

AFTER THE TEST

After the test keep the site open; do not cover with a Band-Aid. Wash normally and pat dry. Don't scratch or manipulate the test site. If it itches put a cool plain tap water compress on it.

SIGNIFICANCE OF RESULTS

Unlike the skin test for tuberculosis, the results of these tests are practically meaningless. **Fungal antibodies** and **fungal culture** are far more useful.

□ □ □

☐ Galactosemia screening test

WHAT IT IS AND WHY IT'S OBTAINED

Galactosemia is a genetic disease which can cause liver disease, mental retardation, cataracts, poor growth, and death. Three varieties of galactosemia are recognized, each being caused by a separate enzyme deficiency. Galactosemia is important to recognize early because symptoms may be reversed by proper diet. Most states require this test on all newborns.

HOW IT WORKS

Either blood from the umbilical cord or a **heelstick blood sample** can be used. Blood is placed on a piece of filter paper. Several laboratory methods are available, the most common of which is the "Paigen" assay, which uses bacteria.

BEFORE THE TEST

No special preparation is required.

AFTER THE TEST

Follow **heelstick blood sample** aftercare.

SIGNIFICANCE OF RESULTS

A positive screening test implies galactosemia. Further testing is required to determine the type.

☐ ☐ ☐

☐ Gallium scan

WHAT IT IS AND WHY IT'S OBTAINED

The gallium scan is a type of **radionuclide scan** which is used to detect hidden disease. It is indicated in evaluating the extent of infection, inflammation, or cancer, in monitoring the treatment of cancer, or in determining the cause of nonspecific symptoms such as fever of unknown origin.

HOW IT WORKS

The test is carried out in the nuclear medicine laboratory of a hospital, clinic, or private physician's office. One to two days before the scanning procedure you will receive an intravenous injection of a radioactive isotope (gallium-67 citrate), called a tracer. This is only mildly uncomfortable. During the actual procedure a computer-driven camera will move over your body and record the images. You should try to remain as still as possible during the procedure. It is painless.

BEFORE THE TEST

No special preparation is required.

AFTER THE TEST

No special aftercare is needed. Although safe, the gallium isotope is radioactive.

SIGNIFICANCE OF RESULTS

Abnormal results of a gallium scan may indicate disorders in any part of the body. It is sensitive but relatively nonspecific, since increased amounts of gallium will accumulate in tumors of virtually any type and in sites of inflammation or infection no matter what the cause. Thus, abnormal gallium scans may be found in diseases as diverse as ulcerative colitis, pneumonia, Hodgkin's disease, and lung cancer. If the scan was performed in order to detect occult disease, further and more specific testing is necessary.

☐ ☐ ☐

☐ Gamma glutamyl transferase

WHAT IT IS AND WHY IT'S OBTAINED

Gamma glutamyl transferase (GGT) is an enzyme which is important to the excretion of bile by the liver. Blood levels are used to test liver function.

HOW IT WORKS

You will be asked to provide a **venous blood sample** from which serum* will be separated. Spectrophotometry* is used for the laboratory assay.

BEFORE THE TEST

No special preparation is required.

AFTER THE TEST

Follow **venous blood sample** aftercare.

SIGNIFICANCE OF RESULTS

GGT is a sensitive test which tends to be particularly high in liver disease caused by obstruction of the outflow of bile. It is also high in other liver diseases, in cancers of the liver or pancreas, and in pancreatitis. It may be elevated in hyperthyroidism, some cases of kidney disease, and some other cancers. Levels will also be elevated for several days after drinking even a small amount of alcohol. It should be evaluated along with other **liver function tests.**

SYNONYMS AND INCLUDED TESTS

Gamma glutamyl transpeptidase.

☐ ☐ ☐

☐ Gastric intubation

WHAT IT IS AND WHY IT'S OBTAINED

Gastric intubation is the withdrawal and analysis of stomach juices. It is used to evaluate stomach disorders such as ulcers and hyperacidity and to study pernicious anemia*.

HOW IT WORKS

The test is performed in a procedure room or laboratory. You will be asked to sit in an examining chair. A soft, flexible, lubricated tube will be inserted either into your nose or mouth. It helps to cooperate, to swallow when instructed, and to remain calm. The insertion of the tube is not painful but may stimulate a gag reflex. The tube will be gently guided through your esophagus and into your stomach. You may be asked to lie on your side or back while a suctioning device withdraws stomach fluids for approximately one and a half hours, sampling every fifteen minutes. The fluid is tested for volume and acidity.

BEFORE THE TEST

You should fast overnight and avoid smoking. For twenty-four hours before the procedure you should avoid alcohol, antacids, and ulcer medications if directed to do so.

AFTER THE TEST

You may experience a transient nosebleed and some soreness of your nose and throat.

SIGNIFICANCE OF RESULTS

High levels of gastric acidity may be found in peptic ulcers. *Very* high levels may be seen in the Zollinger-Ellison syndrome, in which a tumor stimulates massive volumes of acid. Low acidity is seen in severe chronic gastritis and pernicious anemia. Blood **gastrin** may be obtained to evaluate cases of high acidity.

Basal gastric secretion test, basal acid output.

◻ ◻ ◻

◻ Gastrin

WHAT IT IS AND WHY IT'S OBTAINED

Gastrin is a hormone produced by the stomach which stimulates digestion. Blood levels of are used to investigate ulcers.

HOW IT WORKS

You will be asked to provide a **venous blood sample** from which serum* will be separated. Laboratory measurement is by immunoassay*. One variant of this test measures gastrin levels after you receive an intravenous injection of secretin, a hormone produced in the intestine which stimulates the pancreas.

BEFORE THE TEST

You should fast overnight.

AFTER THE TEST

Follow **venous blood sample** aftercare.

SIGNIFICANCE OF RESULTS

A negative test means that blood gastrin was within normal limits. Very high blood gastrin is found in certain tumors of the digestive tract called gastrinomas. These are usually in the pancreas and stimulate, through gastrin, enormous amounts of stomach acids, which can be measured by **gastric intubation.** The resulting disease is called the Zollinger-Ellison syndrome, which includes ulcers, diarrhea, and large amounts of fat in the stool. The secretin variant of this test may help diagnose a gastrinoma if it is present. The normal response to secretin stimulation is little or no elevation of the gastrin level. In the presence of gastrinomas, however, gastrin levels rise. Abdominal **computed tomography** will help locate the tumor if present. Moderately high gastrin is seen in other stomach ulcers, kidney failure, hyperparathyroidism, stomach cancer, and pernicious anemia. Any medication which reduces gastric acid, especially omeprazole and lansoprazole, may also increase gastrin levels.

□ □ □

□ Glomerular basement membrane antibody

WHAT IT IS AND WHY IT'S OBTAINED

The glomerular basement membrane is located in the kidney. Antibodies to it mainly cause severe kidney disease, but because lung tissue is similar to kidney tissue, severe lung disease as well. Blood levels are used to evaluate kidney failure and lung hemorrhage.

HOW IT WORKS

You will be asked to provide a **venous blood sample** from which serum* will be separated. Tissue from a **kidney biopsy** or lung biopsy may also be used. Immunoassay* is used for the laboratory analysis.

BEFORE THE TEST

No special preparation is required.

AFTER THE TEST

Follow **venous blood sample** aftercare.

SIGNIFICANCE OF RESULTS

The presence of glomerular basement membrane antibody indicates Goodpasture's syndrome, a serious disease of the kidneys and lungs which can be fatal.

SYNONYMS AND INCLUDED TESTS

Goodpasture's antibody.

□ □ □

□ Glucagon

WHAT IT IS AND WHY IT'S OBTAINED

Glucagon is a hormone produced in the pancreas which is involved, with **insulin,** in sugar **(glucose)** metabolism. Blood levels are used to evaluate diabetes complicated by other symptoms, such as skin rashes and weight loss.

HOW IT WORKS

You will be asked to provide a **venous blood sample** from which serum* will be separated. Immunoassay* is used for the laboratory analysis.

BEFORE THE TEST

You should fast overnight.

AFTER THE TEST

Follow **venous blood sample** aftercare.

SIGNIFICANCE OF RESULTS

A negative result means that glucagon levels were within normal limits. Moderately high levels can be found in many disorders such as diabetic coma, stress, kidney failure, liver disease, burns, severe infections, and surgery. Very high levels are associated with glucagonomas, which are rare tumors of the pancreas. Glucagonomas tend to produce a characteristic syndrome including a skin rash (migratory necrolytic erythema), severe diabetes, weight loss, anemia, and blood clots.

❑ ❑ ❑

❑ Glucose

WHAT IT IS AND WHY IT'S OBTAINED

Glucose is the main source of energy in the body. Blood levels are used to screen for and monitor the progress and treatment of diabetes mellitus ("sugar diabetes").

HOW IT WORKS

You will be asked to provide a **venous blood sample** from which serum* will be separated. Many methods are available for the assay.

BEFORE THE TEST

You should fast overnight.

AFTER THE TEST

Follow **venous blood sample** aftercare.

SIGNIFICANCE OF RESULTS

Elevated glucose is found in diabetes, after eating, stress, injury, anesthesia, liver disease, pancreatic disease, and in those taking steroids, birth control pills, diuretics, and aspirin. An elevated or borderline level should be further tested with a **postprandial glucose** and possibly with a **glucose tolerance test.** Causes of low glucose (hypoglycemia) include an overdose of insulin or other medications for diabetes, some cancers, intestinal malabsorption, liver disease, and alcoholism. If hypoglycemia is suspected, the blood specimen should be drawn during symptoms.

Blood sugar, fasting glucose, fasting blood sugar, FBS.

□ □ □

□ Glucose tolerance test

WHAT IT IS AND WHY IT'S OBTAINED

The glucose tolerance test (GTT) is used to diagnose diabetes and hypoglycemia. It is usually obtained after an abnormal blood **glucose** or **postprandial blood glucose**. The GTT is not essential for the diagnosis of diabetes if other tests show a very high blood sugar and should *not* be performed if you already know you have diabetes.

HOW IT WORKS

You will be asked to provide a **venous blood sample** which will be analyzed for glucose. You will then be given a high–glucose containing drink, the dose of which is calculated on the basis of your weight. A urine sample may or may not be obtained, depending upon the doctor and the laboratory. At thirty minutes (usually) and then at hourly intervals another **venous blood sample** and possibly urine will be obtained and analyzed for glucose. The total duration of the test is usually three hours, but may be more depending upon the preferences of your doctor.

BEFORE THE TEST

Follow the instructions given to you by the laboratory for a pretest diet. This usually consists of a 600 carbohydrate-calorie diet for three days. You should fast overnight.

AFTER THE TEST

Follow **venous blood sample** aftercare. Resume your normal diet.

SIGNIFICANCE OF RESULTS

The interpretation of the GTT has been controversial and is best left to your doctor. This is because there is a fuzzy line between diabetes and "impaired glucose tolerance." Many things influence blood sugar, including food intake, smoking, steroids, birth control pills, diuretics, aspirin, and other substances.

SYNONYMS AND INCLUDED TESTS

Oral glucose tolerance test.

□ □ □

☐ Glucose-6-phosphate dehydrogenase

WHAT IT IS AND WHY IT'S OBTAINED

Glucose-6-phosphate dehydrogenase (G6PD) is an enzyme which is important in maintaining the ability of **hemoglobin** to transport oxygen. Red blood cell levels of G6PD are used to detect deficiency of this enzyme, either to investigate certain anemias or prior to starting therapy with certain drugs.

HOW IT WORKS

You will be asked to provide a **venous blood sample.** Both screening and quantitative laboratory methods are available.

BEFORE THE TEST

Avoid nonessential medications and others as directed by your doctor.

AFTER THE TEST

Follow **venous blood sample** aftercare.

SIGNIFICANCE OF RESULTS

A positive test means a low level of G6PD was found, the term for which is G6PD deficiency, a common disorder. Twenty percent of female African-Americans are estimated to carry the trait, but symptoms occur in males, since the disease is carried on the X chromosome. While usually causing no symptoms, some conditions, such as infections, can bring about anemia. Other precipating factors are the ingestion of fava beans, acetanilid, doxorubicin, furazolidone, methylene blue, nalidixic acid, niridazole, nitrofurantoin, phenazopyridine, primaquine, and sulfa drugs. High G6PD is found in pernicious anemia* and idiopathic thrombocytopenic purpura*.

□ □ □

□ Glycohemoglobin

WHAT IT IS AND WHY IT'S OBTAINED

Glycohemoglobin (GHb) is **hemoglobin** in red blood cells which has become bound up with sugar **(glucose)**. The amount of this GHb depends upon the concentration of blood glucose. Because red blood cells live for about ninety days, during which time they circulate in the blood and pick up glucose, GHb determinations measure the *average* level of blood glucose over the past ninety days. Thus, unlike blood glucose, which varies from hour to hour, blood levels of GHb are used to monitor the degree of long term (ninety-day) control of diabetes mellitus.

HOW IT WORKS

You will be asked to provide a **venous blood sample** from which serum* will be separated. Several laboratory methods are available for the assay.

BEFORE THE TEST

No special preparation is required.

Follow **venous blood sample** aftercare.

SIGNIFICANCE OF RESULTS

GHb results are given in terms of good, fair, and poor control of diabetes, depending upon the level of GHb. The other test used to assess long term control of diabetes is **fructosamine.**

SYNONYMS AND INCLUDED TESTS

Glycosylated hemoglobin.

□ □ □

□ Gram stain

WHAT IT IS AND WHY IT'S OBTAINED

The Gram stain of potentially infectious material is used to determine quickly the general class of bacteria causing an infection. It is used most often to evaluate lung infections and meningitis, conditions where rapid and accurate treatment are important.

HOW IT WORKS

Although any body fluid may be tested it is usually a **sputum sample** or cerebrospinal fluid* obtained during a **spinal tap.** The specimen is placed on a glass slide, subjected to a series of stains, then examined under a microscope. Gram positive organisms show up as blue; Gram negative organisms show up as red.

BEFORE THE TEST

No special preparation is required.

AFTER THE TEST

No special aftercare is needed.

SIGNIFICANCE OF RESULTS

The main value of this test is that it can give a general indication of the type of bacterial infection within minutes of obtaining a specimen so that an appropriate antibiotic may be selected. Definitive identification of the organism causing an infection is made through **bacterial culture.**

SYNONYMS AND INCLUDED TESTS

Bacterial smear.

□ □ □

□ Growth hormone

WHAT IT IS AND WHY IT'S OBTAINED

Growth hormone (GH) is produced by the pituitary gland and, as its name implies, stimulates growth of tissues, most notably bones. Blood levels are used to evaluate abnormally short stature or abnormally tall stature.

HOW IT WORKS

You will be asked to provide a **venous blood sample** from which serum* will be separated. The level of GH is measured by immunoassay*. Since the level of GH is generally low and may fluctuate a great deal, a number of resting measurements may be taken. After a baseline level is determined, you may be given drugs to stimulate GH, such as insulin, arginine, glucagon, vasopressin, levodopa, or sermorelin, or to suppress GH, such as sugar.

BEFORE THE TEST

You should fast overnight and be at rest for at least thirty minutes.

AFTER THE TEST

Follow **venous blood sample** aftercare.

SIGNIFICANCE OF RESULTS

GH levels are increased in acromegaly, gigantism, and starvation. High levels of GH in those with acromegaly will not be suppressed by oral sugar. Low levels of GH are seen in dwarfism due to insufficiency of the pituitary gland and in obesity. Drugs that cause high levels of GH are birth control pills, amphetamines, levodopa, and nicotinic acid. Drugs that cause low levels are steroids and phenothiazines. **Somatomedin-C** may be obtained to confirm abnormal results.

SYNONYMS AND INCLUDED TESTS

Somatotropin.

□ □ □

□ Ham test

WHAT IT IS AND WHY IT'S OBTAINED

The Ham test is used to diagnose paroxysmal nocturnal hemoglobinuria (PNH), a type of anemia which is due to defective red blood cells. It is most often used to confirm the diagnosis after a positive **sugar water test.**

HOW IT WORKS

You will be asked to provide a **venous blood sample** from which the red blood cells will separated. The red cells will be washed, mixed with acid and normal blood serum*, incubated, and observed for disruption (hemolysis).

BEFORE THE TEST

No special preparation is required.

AFTER THE TEST

Follow **venous blood sample** aftercare.

SIGNIFICANCE OF RESULTS

A positive test is seen in PNH but certain other blood diseases may cause false positive reactions.

SYNONYMS AND INCLUDED TESTS

Acid hemolysis test, paroxysmal nocturnal hemoglobinuria test, PNH test.

□ □ □

□ Haptoglobin

WHAT IT IS AND WHY IT'S OBTAINED

Haptoglobin is a substance which binds strongly to **hemoglobin.** In conditions where there is excessive red blood cell death (hemolysis) hemoglobin is released into the bloodstream where it takes up much or all of the haptoglobin which is there. Thus, blood levels of haptoglobin are obtained to evaluate anemia and to monitor blood transfusion reactions. Determining the haptoglobin type is also sometimes used to establish paternity because the substance exists in several distinct genetic forms.

HOW IT WORKS

You will be asked to provide a **venous blood sample** from which serum* will be separated. Many methods are available for the assay.

BEFORE THE TEST

No special preparation is required.

AFTER THE TEST

Follow **venous blood sample** aftercare.

SIGNIFICANCE OF RESULTS

Low or absent levels occur as a result of rapid red blood cell destruction. Low levels can also occur in mononucleosis, liver disease, and as a congenital defect. High haptoglobin is seen with some infections and inflammations and with advanced cancer.

□ □ □

□ Hearing test

WHAT IT IS AND WHY IT'S OBTAINED

Included under this heading are a number of tests which are designed to detect hearing loss and evaluate its extent.

HOW IT WORKS

There are many variations which are possible. For a typical test you will be placed inside a soundproof enclosure and will be asked to wear headphones. The audiologist will tell you what to do when you hear a tone, such as to say, "Yes," to point to the ear in which you hear the tone, to keep time to the beat of the tone, and so forth. You will hear a series of tones of varying frequency and intensity. The test relies completely upon your cooperation and response. At some point, you may be asked to put on a device which transmits sounds through bone. For this, a vibrator will be placed on the bones located behind your ears. Follow instructions as before. In the speech reception threshold test you will hear words with two syllables at different intensities. In the speech discrimination test you will hear single syllable words at the same loudness. You simply repeat the words as you hear them. Graphs are constructed from your responses.

BEFORE THE TEST

No special preparation is required. Your ears should be free from accumulated wax.

AFTER THE TEST

No special aftercare is needed.

SIGNIFICANCE OF RESULTS

By means of the hearing test your doctor will be able to evaluate the extent of hearing loss, which ear is more severely affected, which frequencies are involved, and whether a hearing aid might help you. In addition, it is often possible to distinguish between various types of hearing loss, such as that due to noise, inner ear disease, or nerve disease. The "speech threshold" and "speech discrimination" tests can give a good profile of how your hearing affects your day-to-day function.

SYNONYMS AND INCLUDED TESTS

Audiogram, pure tone audiometry, speech testing, speech reception threshold, speech discrimination.

□ □ □

□ Heart scan

WHAT IT IS AND WHY IT'S OBTAINED

Included under this heading are a host of tests designed to provide images of the heart in order to evaluate symptoms such as chest pain or shortness of breath, particularly when coronary artery disease (CAD) is suspected. Heart scans are also used to monitor the progress and treatment of heart disease, and to obtain more information when tests such as the **electrocardiogram** (ECG) or **echocardiogram** are abnormal.

HOW IT WORKS

Heart scan procedures are carried out in the nuclear medicine laboratory of a hospital, clinic, or private physician's office. The test is usually performed simultaneously with an ECG and an exercise treadmill. If so, a technician will place electrodes on your arms and legs. You will then receive an injection of a very small amount of a radioactive isotope, called a tracer, designed to reveal the desired information. Technetium or thallium tracers, for example, have an affinity for healthy heart muscle or for heart muscle damaged by a heart attack. Radioactively labeled red blood cells, on the other hand, produce an image of blood within the heart chambers. The vein puncture is usually only mildly uncomfortable. A specialized computer-based instrument called a gamma camera will then take the pictures, either by remaining stationary or moving over your chest. This is painless and you should try to remain as still as possible during the procedure.

BEFORE THE TEST

A three-hour fast is usually recommended. Follow carefully any instructions from your doctor regarding medications.

AFTER THE TEST

No special aftercare is needed. Although safe, this test does involve the injection of a radioactive compound.

SIGNIFICANCE OF RESULTS

The heart scan is used in conjunction with other tests of heart function to provide information about how well your heart is moving blood into your circulation. Interpretation must take into consideration your underlying problem, whether it be CAD, cardiomyopathy, congestive heart failure, or a heart attack.

Cardiac scan, cardiac scintigram, cardiac positron emission tomography, hot spot myocardial imaging, infarct avid imaging, thallium imaging, cold spot myocardial imaging, thallium scintigraphy, persantine-thallium imaging, cardiac blood pool imaging.

◻ ◻ ◻

◻ Heelstick blood sample

WHAT IT IS AND WHY IT'S OBTAINED

The heelstick is a standard method for obtaining blood samples from infants. Although a smaller amount of blood is obtained than with the **venous blood sample,** almost any blood test can be performed using this method. The **fingerstick blood sample** is similar but cannot be used in infants because the bones are too close to the skin.

HOW IT WORKS

The skin over the inner or outer aspect of the heel (not the back of the heel) is cleansed with alcohol. A sharp stylet* is used to puncture the skin quickly and blood allowed to flow. A sample is drawn up into a hollow glass cylinder called a capillary tube.

BEFORE THE TEST

No special preparation is required.

AFTER THE TEST

The site of the heelstick can be cleansed with soap and water or alcohol. A Band-Aid is not recommended since it may loosen and become lodged in the infant's mouth or throat.

SIGNIFICANCE OF RESULTS

Results are reported depending upon the nature of the tests.

SYNONYMS AND INCLUDED TESTS

Skin puncture blood collection, capillary blood collection, heelstick blood collection.

□ □ □

□ Heinz bodies

WHAT IT IS AND WHY IT'S OBTAINED

Heinz bodies are fragments of **hemoglobin** which have become attached to the walls of red blood cells. Testing for them is used to investigate anemia.

HOW IT WORKS

You will be asked to provide a **venous blood sample** which will be smeared on a glass slide, stained, and examined under a microscope. Heinz bodies appear as purple shapes within the red cells.

BEFORE THE TEST

Avoid nonessential medications.

AFTER THE TEST

Follow **venous blood sample** aftercare.

SIGNIFICANCE OF RESULTS

Heinz bodies are found in the type of anemia known as "hemolytic," in which red blood cells break apart. They may be present in **glucose-6-phosphate dehydrogenase** deficiency, in disorders caused by hereditary abnormal hemoglobin, or after splenectomy. Drugs used against malaria, furazolidone, nitrofurans, Dilantin, phenacetin, procarbazine, sulfa drugs, fava beans, and other substances may cause them to form.

□ □ □

□ *Helicobacter pylori* antibody

WHAT IT IS AND WHY IT'S OBTAINED

Helicobacter pylori is a bacterium found in the stomachs of those suffering from ulcers. Blood levels of antibody (a blood protein important to the immune system) to it are used to investigate ulcer symptoms.

HOW IT WORKS

You will be asked to provide a **venous blood sample** from which serum* will be separated. Immunoassay* is used for the laboratory analysis.

BEFORE THE TEST

No special preparation is required.

AFTER THE TEST

Follow **venous blood sample** aftercare.

SIGNIFICANCE OF RESULTS

The presence of *Helicobacter pylori* antibodies in the blood is strong evidence in favor of an infection with this organism. Definitive diagnosis is by a "urease" test (occasionally by **bacterial culture)** using **biopsy** material obtained from **upper gastrointestinal endoscopy.** A breath test is available to monitor the activity of infection once it has been diagnosed.

□ □ □

☐ Hematocrit

WHAT IT IS AND WHY IT'S OBTAINED

The hematocrit is the volume of the red blood cells in blood, expressed as a percentage. It is commonly obtained as part of the **complete blood count** and is used in a wide variety of situations to evaluate bleeding, anemia, polycythemia (in which there are increased amounts of red blood cells), and hydration.

HOW IT WORKS

You will be asked to provide a **venous blood sample.** In infants a **heelstick blood sample** may be used. Most hematocrits are performed by machine, but it can be done manually by simply centrifuging the blood sample. The level of the packed red blood cells at the bottom of the tube is then compared to the level of the serum* at the top of the tube.

BEFORE THE TEST

No special preparation is required.

AFTER THE TEST

Follow **venous blood sample** or **heelstick blood sample** aftercare.

SIGNIFICANCE OF RESULTS

A low hematocrit is found in anemia, recent hemorrhage, and excess fluid intake. Additional tests helpful in the evaluation of anemia include **ferritin, red blood cell indices, reticulocyte count,** and possibly a **bone marrow.** A high hematocrit is seen in polycythemia and dehydration.

SYNONYMS AND INCLUDED TESTS

Crit.

☐ ☐ ☐

☐ Hemoglobin

WHAT IT IS AND WHY IT'S OBTAINED

Hemoglobin is the iron-containing compound in red blood cells which transports oxygen. Blood levels are routinely obtained as part of the **complete blood count** and are used to evaluate anemia, blood loss, and other disorders.

HOW IT WORKS

You will be asked to provide a **venous blood sample.** Hemoglobin is measured by spectrophotometry*.

BEFORE THE TEST

No special preparation is required.

AFTER THE TEST

Follow **venous blood sample** aftercare.

SIGNIFICANCE OF RESULTS

Low hemoglobin is seen in anemia, hemorrhage, and excess fluid intake. High hemoglobin is seen in polycythemia and dehydration. Additional tests helpful in the evaluation of anemia include **ferritin, red blood cell indices, reticulocyte count,** and possibly a **bone marrow.**

☐ ☐ ☐

☐ Hemoglobin electrophoresis

WHAT IT IS AND WHY IT'S OBTAINED

There are many genetic variations of **hemoglobin,** some of which cause blood disorders such as various types of anemia. Hemoglobin electrophoresis is used to identify abnormal hemoglobin types.

HOW IT WORKS

You will be asked to provide a **venous blood sample**. The specimen is analyzed by electrophoresis*.

BEFORE THE TEST

No special preparation is required.

AFTER THE TEST

Follow **venous blood sample** aftercare.

SIGNIFICANCE OF RESULTS

Normally there are three types of hemoglobin in blood: A, A_2, and F. Other hemoglobins exist, such as hemoglobin S, which causes sickle cell anemia*, hemoglobin H, which causes thalassemia, and hemoglobin M, which causes methemoglobinemia. Many other variations are possible. The abnormal hemoglobins produce symptoms (usually a type of anemia) which range from mild to severe. Investigating the rarer types of hemoglobin requires sophisticated laboratory techniques found only in specialized hospital and university laboratories. The **unstable hemoglobin** test may be used to detect some abnormal hemoglobins missed by hemoglobin electrophoresis.

□ □ □

□ Hepatitis A antibody

WHAT IT IS AND WHY IT'S OBTAINED

Hepatitis A virus (HAV) produces the mildest form of viral hepatitis. Blood levels of antibody (a blood protein important to the immune system) to the virus are included in most typical **hepatitis screening tests.**

You will be asked to provide a **venous blood sample** from which serum* will be separated. Immunoassay* is used to detect the **immunoglobulin M** antibodies.

BEFORE THE TEST

No special preparation is required.

AFTER THE TEST

Follow **venous blood sample** aftercare.

SIGNIFICANCE OF RESULTS

The presence of this antibody indicates recent infection with HAV.

SYNONYMS AND INCLUDED TESTS

Anti-HAV.

□ □ □

□ Hepatitis B tests

WHAT IT IS AND WHY IT'S OBTAINED

Hepatitis B virus (HBV) produces a type of hepatitis which is transmitted by blood or body fluids. A number of blood tests are usually bundled together to evaluate the outlook once the diagnosis of hepatitis B has been established. The panel usually consists of hepatitis B surface antigen, hepatitis B_e antigen, hepatitis B core antibody, hepatitis B surface antigen, and hepatitis B_e antibody.

HOW IT WORKS

You will be asked to provide a **venous blood sample** from which serum* will be separated. Immunoassay* is used for the laboratory analysis.

BEFORE THE TEST

No special preparation is required.

AFTER THE TEST

Follow **venous blood sample** aftercare.

SIGNIFICANCE OF RESULTS

The interpretation of these tests should take into consideration results of **liver function tests.** In addition, it is most helpful if multiple samples have been taken over time so that values may be compared with one another. The following is a general interpretation of the different HBV tests.

The presence of *hepatitis B_e antigen* indicates the most contagious stage of the illness. When the infection resolves, the test becomes negative. In the chronic carrier state of HBV infection, however, hepatitis B_e antigen may remain positive for years.

In general, the **immunoglobulin M** part of *hepatitis B core antibody* signifies early infection and the **immunoglobulin G** part, late infection. The total hepatitis B core antibody usually persists for life. The presence of *hepatitis B surface antibody* is taken to mean recovery from hepatitis B infection but it may remain positive for years or for a lifetime even though you are perfectly healthy.

Hepatitis B_e antibody is a good sign that recovery is taking place. If the hepatitis B surface antibody is also present and if the hepatitis B surface antigen is absent, then convalescence is well under way.

□ □ □

☐ Hepatitis C antibody

WHAT IT IS AND WHY IT'S OBTAINED

Hepatitis C virus (HCV) produces a type of hepatitis which was formerly called non-A non-B. Blood levels of the antibody to HCV are used to diagnose this disease.

HOW IT WORKS

You will be asked to provide a **venous blood sample** from which serum* will be separated. Immunoassay* is used for the laboratory analysis.

BEFORE THE TEST

No special preparation is required.

AFTER THE TEST

Follow **venous blood sample** aftercare.

SIGNIFICANCE OF RESULTS

HCV hepatitis is the most common cause of hepatitis following blood transfusions and often becomes chronic. The disease can be serious; liver failure and liver cancer sometimes occur. Unfortunately, this test may only become positive months after infection. It should be interpreted along with other **liver function tests.**

☐ ☐ ☐

☐ Hepatitis D antibody

WHAT IT IS AND WHY IT'S OBTAINED

Hepatitis D virus (HDV) is an incomplete virus which can only infect those who already have a hepatitis B virus infection. Blood levels of antibody to the virus are used to evaluate those with hepatitis B who are showing signs of liver failure.

HOW IT WORKS

You will be asked to provide a **venous blood sample** from which serum* will be separated. Immunoassay* is used for the laboratory analysis.

BEFORE THE TEST

No special preparation is required.

AFTER THE TEST

Follow **venous blood sample** aftercare.

SIGNIFICANCE OF RESULTS

The presence of this antibody in the presence of **hepatitis B surface antigen** signifies an added infection with the HDV and more significant disease. It should be interpreted along with other **liver function tests.**

SYNONYMS AND INCLUDED TESTS

Delta agent serology.

□ □ □

□ Hepatitis screening tests

WHAT IT IS AND WHY IT'S OBTAINED

Viral hepatitis may be caused by a number of different viruses: hepatitis A (HAV), B (HBV), C (HCV), or E (HEV). Hepatitis D virus (HDV) only infects those who already have an infection with HBV. Each virus is transmitted differently and has a different course and outlook. Blood tests are available for all of them except HEV. Hepatitis screening tests usually consist of **hepatitis A antibody,** several **hepatitis B tests,** and, sometimes, **hepatitis C anti-**

body. Symptoms of hepatitis include weakness, jaundice, and darkening of the urine. HAV produces the mildest disease, but the other four viruses may be serious.

HOW IT WORKS

You will be asked to provide a **venous blood sample** from which serum* will be separated. Immunoassay* is used for the laboratory analysis.

BEFORE THE TEST

No special preparation is required.

AFTER THE TEST

Follow **venous blood sample** aftercare.

SIGNIFICANCE OF RESULTS

A positive test of one of the components of a hepatitis screen is followed by repeat tests at intervals and by confirmatory tests. All tests for hepatitis should be interpreted along with **liver function tests.**

◻ ◻ ◻

◻ Herpes antigen

WHAT IT IS AND WHY IT'S OBTAINED

Herpes simplex virus usually produces mild infections on the skin and mucous membranes, but occasionally life-threatening infections occur in those with defective immune systems. When rapid diagnosis is needed in one of these circumstances, the detection of herpes antigen is used. An antigen is a substance which provokes the formation of an antibody by the immune system.

HOW IT WORKS

Many sources for the specimen may be used, such as scraping, swabbing, or brushing the suspected area of infection. Tissue from a biopsy may also be tested. Immunoassay* is used for the laboratory analysis.

BEFORE THE TEST

No special preparation is required.

AFTER THE TEST

Follow **venous blood sample** aftercare.

SIGNIFICANCE OF RESULTS

A positive test indicates active herpes infection. Although rapid, this test is not so sensitive as **viral culture.** It is best to use both methods when indicated.

□ □ □

□ Herpes blood tests

WHAT IT IS AND WHY IT'S OBTAINED

Herpes simplex virus, of which there are two types, produces infections that are extremely common. Type I usually occurs as a recurrent blistering sore above the waist, particularly the lips ("cold sores" or "fever blisters"), whereas type II usually occurs below the waist as genital herpes. Blood levels of antibodies to these types are used to evaluate herpes infections.

HOW IT WORKS

You will be asked to provide a **venous blood sample** from which serum* will be separated. Several methods of immunoassay* are available.

BEFORE THE TEST

No special preparation is required.

AFTER THE TEST

Follow **venous blood sample** aftercare.

SIGNIFICANCE OF RESULTS

Interpretation of antibody tests to herpes is difficult because most people are positive. In addition, the antibodies to type I and type II herpes are not specific, and a flare of type I herpes on the lips can elevate the type II antibody as well as the type I antibody. Repeat determinations can sometimes clarify the situation, but in general herpes blood tests are not useful at all in individuals, and only determine the general infection rate in large populations. More helpful by far is **viral culture** for herpes.

SYNONYMS AND INCLUDED TESTS

Herpes antibody, herpes serology.

☐ ☐ ☐

☐ Histamine

WHAT IT IS AND WHY IT'S OBTAINED

Histamine is a substance with many functions. It increases stomach acid and produces hives and wheezing in allergic reactions. Blood levels are obtained to evaluate systemic mastocytosis, a disease in which there are large numbers of mast cells (specialized cells which manufacture histamine).

HOW IT WORKS

You will be asked to provide a **venous blood sample** from which serum* will be separated. Chromatography* and other methods are available for the assay. Urine may also be tested.

BEFORE THE TEST

A special diet is required. Check with the laboratory performing the test.

AFTER THE TEST

Follow **venous blood sample** aftercare.

SIGNIFICANCE OF RESULTS

Measurement of histamine is not a sensitive indicator of mastocytosis. Other more sophisticated tests involving waste products of histamine such as methylimizazoleacetic acid may be more useful. Besides mastocytosis, high levels of histamine are found in leukemia, polycythemia, and certain other cancers. Low levels are found in HIV infection.

□ □ □

□ HIV tests

WHAT IT IS AND WHY IT'S OBTAINED

Human immunodeficiency virus (HIV) testing has become a controversial and important public health and legal issue since the first cases of AIDS were discovered in the early 1980s. At the present time there are different laws throughout the United States concerning these tests and many states require counseling before the test can be performed. There has been much debate as to the merits of widespread or mandatory screening and the disclosure of test results; it is safe to say that no consensus has yet been reached. At present HIV testing is used to evaluate infection with HIV and to screen blood and organ donors.

HOW IT WORKS

You will be asked to provide a **venous blood sample** from which serum* will be separated. The usual analysis proceeds in two methods of immunoassay*, the first to screen, and the second, Western blot*, to confirm. Another method (OraSure) involves simply taking a sample of saliva which is absorbed onto a special collection pad.

BEFORE THE TEST

No special preparation is required.

AFTER THE TEST

Follow **venous blood sample** aftercare.

SIGNIFICANCE OF RESULTS

Using both screening and confirmatory methods, HIV testing is over 99 percent accurate. If you are in a low-risk group, a negative test virtually assures that you are not infected. There is a latent period of HIV infection, however, and antibodies to HIV may not appear in the blood for over two years. If you are in a high-risk group such as a homosexual or bisexual male, intravenous drug user, sexual contact of an intravenous drug user, prostitute, or hemophiliac who has been exposed to certain blood products, a negative antibody test for HIV may be confirmed by an HIV antigen (p24) test. Another test helpful in the diagnosis of HIV infection is a CD4 cell count by **lymphocyte typing.**

SYNONYMS AND INCLUDED TESTS

Human immunodeficiency virus test, AIDS screen, HIV antibody.

□ □ □

☐ Hollander test

WHAT IT IS AND WHY IT'S OBTAINED

The Hollander test is used to evaluate the success of the surgical operation known as vagotomy, in which the vagus nerve is cut in order to slow stomach acid production in ulcer disease. The Hollander test is a variant of **gastric intubation,** in which the response of stomach acid to insulin is measured. Normally, an injection of insulin causes a drop in blood sugar and the drop in blood sugar causes the vagus nerve to stimulate the stomach to produce acid. If the nerve is cut, this process is interrupted.

HOW IT WORKS

The test is usually performed in a special room. You will be asked to sit in a chair and will have an intravenous fluid drip started. A soft flexible tube will be lubricated and inserted into one of your nostrils and guided down your throat and into your esophagus. It helps greatly to cooperate in this procedure, to swallow when instructed, and to remain calm; you will not choke. The insertion of the tube is not painful but may stimulate a gag reflex. The tube will be gently pushed down into your stomach. You may then be asked to lie on your side or back while the tube is attached to a suction device which will withdraw stomach fluids for approximately one and a half hours. Then you will be given an injection of insulin intravenously. Your blood **glucose** will be obtained at intervals over the next two hours as your gastric fluid continues to be sampled.

BEFORE THE TEST

You should fast overnight and avoid smoking and alcohol. For a day or two before the procedure you should avoid antacids and ulcer medications if directed to do so.

AFTER THE TEST

You may experience a transient nosebleed and some soreness of your nose and throat. You will be fed soon after the procedure to avoid the effects of hypoglycemia* from the insulin. Although safe in most people, this test can be hazardous in the elderly or in those with heart disease.

SIGNIFICANCE OF RESULTS

A positive test means that stomach acid increased in response to insulin and that your vagus nerve is intact, at least in part. This test, however, is subject to some error, and negative tests have been known to become positive with time.

SYNONYMS AND INCLUDED TESTS

Insulin-induced peak acid output.

□ □ □

□ Holter monitor

WHAT IT IS AND WHY IT'S OBTAINED

The Holter monitor is a type of **electrocardiogram** (ECG) which is used to study heartbeat irregularities (arrhythmias) over a period of time.

HOW IT WORKS

You will be asked to undress from the waist up. Electrodes as for an ECG will be pasted to your chest and the wires attached to a small device which is strapped around your waist. You will wear the apparatus for twenty-four hours and will be provided with a diary in which to record your activities, such as exercise, work, eating, and sex. You will return to the laboratory or doctor's office the next day and the device will be removed and the recording analyzed. The recordings may be made on magnetic tape or stored digitally in computer memory.

BEFORE THE TEST

No special preparation is required.

AFTER THE TEST

No special aftercare is needed.

SIGNIFICANCE OF RESULTS

Heartbeat irregularities are often sporadic and may not occur just at the time of your visit to the doctor for the ECG. The Holter monitor in essence is a day-long ECG. The report will include any irregularities which occured during the day, and these will be analyzed. Further studies may include a **stress test** or, on occasion, **invasive electrophysiologic studies.**

SYNONYMS AND INCLUDED TESTS

Ambulatory electrocardiography.

□ □ □

□ Homocysteine

WHAT IT IS AND WHY IT'S OBTAINED

Homocysteine is a substance involved in amino acid and protein production. Blood levels are used to evaluate the risk of coronary artery disease (CAD).

HOW IT WORKS

You will be asked to provide a **venous blood sample** from which serum* will be separated. Chromatography* and other methods may be used for the laboratory measurement.

BEFORE THE TEST

You should fast overnight.

AFTER THE TEST

Follow **venous blood sample** aftercare.

SIGNIFICANCE OF RESULTS

High homocysteine is found in those with sedentary life-styles, **folic acid** deficiency, high blood pressure, and high **cholesterol.** It is also increased in cigarette smokers. Thus, it is associated with an increased risk of CAD. Because it is also elevated in the rare genetic disease called homocysti-nuria, in which CAD is pronounced, homocysteine itself may be responsible for some of the damage to blood vessels. This, however, has not been proven.

□ □ □

□ Homovanillic acid

WHAT IT IS AND WHY IT'S OBTAINED

Homovanillic acid (HVA) is a waste product of dopamine, one of the **catecholamines.** Urine levels are used to diagnose and monitor the course of certain tumors which usually occur in children and adolescents.

HOW IT WORKS

You will be asked to provide a **24-hour urine sample** which should be kept refrigerated. Several methods are available for the assay.

BEFORE THE TEST

Avoid aspirin, disulfiram, reserpine, pyridoxine, and levo-dopa or do as directed by your doctor.

AFTER THE TEST

No special aftercare is needed.

SIGNIFICANCE OF RESULTS

Elevated urine HVA is found in the presence of neuroblastomas, ganglioneuromas, pheochromocytomas, and the Riley-Day syndrome (dysautonomia). A normal HVA, however, does not rule out the presence of these conditions.

□ □ □

□ 24-hour urine sample

WHAT IT IS AND WHY IT'S OBTAINED

The 24-hour urine sample is used when the concentration of a substance in blood or in a random urine specimen is too small to test or when substances are found in the blood intermittently during the day and a more representative level is desired.

HOW IT WORKS

You will be provided with a plastic urine container. Void at a specified time in the morning, for example 8 A.M., and discard the specimen. Then collect all urine for the following twenty-four hours including the final specimen at 8 A.M. the following day. For some tests you will be asked to refrigerate the specimen bottle during collection. For other tests, preservatives may be included in the container which make this unnecessary. Follow instructions regarding fluid, medication, diet, and physical activity carefully. It is very important to collect *all* urine.

BEFORE THE TEST

Follow instructions for the individual test.

Follow instructions for the individual test.

SIGNIFICANCE OF RESULTS

See individual test listing.

□ □ □

□ Human chorionic gonadotropin

WHAT IT IS AND WHY IT'S OBTAINED

Human chorionic gonadotropin (HCG) is a hormone produced during pregnancy. It is the same hormone which is tested for in a **pregnancy test.** Blood levels can be used to detect pregnancy and to diagnose and monitor certain tumors.

HOW IT WORKS

You will be asked to provide a **venous blood sample** from which serum* will be separated. Many immunoassay* methods of analysis are available.

BEFORE THE TEST

No special preparation is required.

AFTER THE TEST

Follow **venous blood sample** aftercare.

SIGNIFICANCE OF RESULTS

A negative test means that little or no HCG was detected in the blood. High values are found in pregnancy and with some tumors. Although many cancers, such as those of the lung, stomach, colon, or breast, are capable of producing HCG, there are several others, such as choriocarcinoma, embryonal cell carcinoma, and gestational trophoblastic tumor, in which its production is highly characteristic. Blood HCG is considerably elevated if you are having twins.

◻ ◻ ◻

◻ Human T-cell leukemia virus antibody

WHAT IT IS AND WHY IT'S OBTAINED

There are two types of human T-cell leukemia virus (HLV). Type I causes a type of leukemia and type II causes a muscle disease. Blood levels of antibody (a blood protein important to the immune system) to these viruses are used mainly to screen blood donors.

HOW IT WORKS

You will be asked to provide a **venous blood sample** from which serum* will be separated. Immunoassay* proceeds in two parts, the first to screen, and the second, the Western blot*, to confirm.

BEFORE THE TEST

No special preparation is required.

AFTER THE TEST

Follow **venous blood sample** aftercare.

SIGNIFICANCE OF RESULTS

A positive test signifies infection with HLV. Diseases caused by this virus are uncommon and there is usually a very long incubation period.

SYNONYMS AND INCLUDED TESTS

HTLV antibody.

◻ ◻ ◻

☐ Hydrogen breath test

WHAT IT IS AND WHY IT'S OBTAINED

This test is based on the principle that carbohydrates such as sugar or starch are digested in the small intestine. If they pass undigested into the large intestine they are fermented and hydrogen gas is produced. Most of this is expelled as intestinal gas but some is absorbed back into your blood and into your lungs, where it is exhaled and can be measured. The hydrogen breath test is used to evaluate intestinal function.

HOW IT WORKS

The test is usually performed in a special laboratory. You will be given an oral dose of lactose or another carbohydrate, after which your breath will be analyzed. There are a number of methods for collecting exhaled gas, including tubes and bags. Some doctors prefer using a plastic tube inserted into your nostrils. Your exhaled air may be collected quickly or over a matter of hours at intervals.

BEFORE THE TEST

You should fast overnight. Do not take antibiotics for a week unless directed otherwise.

AFTER THE TEST

No special aftercare is needed.

SIGNIFICANCE OF RESULTS

Increased breath hydrogen signifies that carbohydrates are not being digested properly in the small bowel or that they are being fermented prematurely in the small bowel by bacteria which should not be there. The **lactose tolerance test** is a variant of this test.

Breath hydrogen analysis, breath analysis.

❏ ❏ ❏

❏ 17-hydroxycorticosteroids

WHAT IT IS AND WHY IT'S OBTAINED

17-hydroxycorticosteroids (17-HCS) are waste products of **cortisol,** the main hormone produced by the adrenal gland. Urine levels are obtained to evaluate symptoms which suggest over- or underactivity of the adrenal gland, such as weight loss or gain, weakness, and high or low blood pressure.

HOW IT WORKS

You will be asked to provide a **24-hour urine sample** which you should keep refrigerated during collection. The Porter Silber reaction (phenylhydrazine in an acidic solution producing a yellow color) is used for the laboratory assay.

BEFORE THE TEST

Withhold nonessential medications for several days or do as directed by your doctor. Avoid stress during the collection period.

AFTER THE TEST

No special aftercare is needed.

SIGNIFICANCE OF RESULTS

Low levels urine 17-HCS are found in adrenal gland insufficiency (Addison's disease), pituitary insufficiency, and the adrenogenital syndrome. Increased values are found in pituitary gland tumors, adrenal gland tumors, congenital adrenal hyperplasia, some cancers (such as lung and thyroid cancer), and in the condition called pseudo-Cushing's disease. Many medications interfere with this test, both in falsely lowering and increasing values. Drugs which may elevate 17-HCS include tranquilizers, spironolactone, ascorbic acid, chloral hydrate, glutethimide, penicillin, quinidine, quinine, iodine compounds, and methenamine. Drugs which may decrease 17-HCS include hydralazine, hydrochlorothiazide, nalidixic acid, and reserpine. A more accurate test of adrenal function can be obtained by directly measuring urine **cortisol.**

□ □ □

□ 5-hydroxyindoleacetic acid

WHAT IT IS AND WHY IT'S OBTAINED

5-hydroxyindoleacetic acid (5-HIA) is the major waste product of **serotonin.** Urine levels are obtained to diagnose certain tumors, called carcinoids, which produce large amounts of serotonin. The "carcinoid syndrome" includes flushing, diarrhea, difficulty breathing, liver enlargement, and heart disease.

HOW IT WORKS

You will be asked to provide a **24-hour urine sample** which you should refrigerate during collection. Several methods are used in the laboratory assay.

BEFORE THE TEST

Avoid avocados, bananas, chocolate, eggplant, pineapples, plums, tomatoes, and walnuts for several days. Discontinue all nonessential medications or do as directed by your doctor.

AFTER THE TEST

No special aftercare is needed.

SIGNIFICANCE OF RESULTS

Elevated 5-HIA suggests a carcinoid tumor, but normal values do not rule it out. Levels may be falsely low in kidney disease and falsely high with malabsorption (in which there is failure to absorb nutrients properly). Blood **serotonin** may be obtained if results are ambiguous.

□ □ □

□ 17-hydroxyprogesterone

WHAT IT IS AND WHY IT'S OBTAINED

17-hydroxyprogesterone (17-HP) is produced by the adrenal gland during the formation of **cortisol**. Blood levels are used to evaluate virilization (the appearance of male characteristics) in women, both in infants and adults, and are sometimes included as part of infertility studies. Amniotic fluid levels are used to diagnose congenital adrenal hyperplasia, in which an enzyme deficiency leads to an accumulation of male hormones in the fetus.

HOW IT WORKS

Either a **venous blood sample, heelstick blood sample,** or amniotic fluid obtained by **amniocentesis** may be used. The serum* is separated and laboratory measurement is by immunoassay*.

BEFORE THE TEST

No special preparation is required.

AFTER THE TEST

Follow **venous blood sample, heelstick blood sample,** or **amniocentesis** aftercare.

SIGNIFICANCE OF RESULTS

17-HP is increased in congenital adrenal hyperplasia, a disease which is usually caused by an enzyme (21-

hydroxylase) deficiency and which causes female hermaphroditism—difficulty in determining the sex of a female infant because of enlargement of the clitoris. 17-HP is also increased in a variant of this disease, late onset 21-hydroxylase deficiency, which has several forms.

◻ ◻ ◻

◻ Hydroxyproline

WHAT IT IS AND WHY IT'S OBTAINED

Hydroxyproline is an important component of collagen. Urine levels are obtained to evaluate conditions in which bone is being broken down or metabolized abnormally.

HOW IT WORKS

You will be asked to provide a **24-hour urine sample,** although a two-hour collection is sometimes used. Colorimetry* or chromatography* may be employed for the assay.

BEFORE THE TEST

Do not eat meat (including poultry and fish) or gelatin (including Jell-O, candies, jelly, or ice cream) for twenty-four hours before the collection begins.

AFTER THE TEST

No special aftercare is needed.

SIGNIFICANCE OF RESULTS

Urine hydroxyproline is increased in osteoporosis, Paget's disease, hyperthyroidism, hyperparathyroidism, prolonged bed rest, pregnancy, cancer which has spread to bone, and broken bones as they heal. It is also high in children and adolescents, especially during growth spurts.

◻ ◻ ◻

☐ Hysterosalpingogram

WHAT IT IS AND WHY IT'S OBTAINED

The hysterosalpingogram is an **X-ray contrast study** which is usually obtained as part of an infertility evaluation. It is used to detect abnormalities in the fallopian tubes (which lead from the ovaries to the uterus), although the uterus is also visualized.

HOW IT WORKS

The test is usually performed in the X-ray department of a hospital or in a private radiologist's office. You will probably be given a mild sedative, especially if you are apprehensive. You will be asked to undress from the waist down, to wear a hospital gown, and to lie on the examining table as for a gynecological examination. A speculum will be inserted into your vagina and a small tube passed into your cervix through which a contrast agent will be allowed to flow into your uterus. This may produce some cramping. The table will be tilted or you will be asked to change position as the flow of the liquid is observed with fluoroscopy* and as **X rays** are taken.

BEFORE THE TEST

No special preparation is required.

AFTER THE TEST

Discomfort from this test is temporary. If you have been given a sedative make sure you have someone drive you home. Rarely the contrast agent (if oil-based) may form pockets of inflammation within the fallopian tubes which may require surgical intervention.

SIGNIFICANCE OF RESULTS

Abnormal findings may include partial or complete blockage of the fallopian tubes from strictures, tumors, or adhesions. Further information may be obtained by means of **laparoscopy.**

SYNONYMS AND INCLUDED TESTS

Uterogram.

◻ ◻ ◻

◻ Immunofixation electrophoresis

WHAT IT IS AND WHY IT'S OBTAINED

Immunofixation electrophoresis (IE) is performed when a **protein electrophoresis** has revealed an increase in one of the protein fractions. It is mainly used to diagnose multiple myeloma, a cancer of plasma cells, a type of cell which is usually found in the bone marrow.

HOW IT WORKS

Either blood or urine may be tested. For blood, you will be asked to provide a **venous blood sample.** For urine, a random sample is sufficient. Analysis is by immunoassay* and electrophoresis*.

BEFORE THE TEST

No special preparation is required.

AFTER THE TEST

If blood was used follow **venous blood sample** aftercare.

SIGNIFICANCE OF RESULTS

Interpretation of IE is performed by a pathologist. Findings may suggest a benign abnormality or multiple myeloma, which will require further testing. Immunofixation electrophoresis is more sensitive than immunoelectrophoresis and is in general the better test.

Immunoelectrophoresis.

□ □ □

□ Immunoglobulin A

WHAT IT IS AND WHY IT'S OBTAINED

Immunoglobulin A (IgA) is an antibody containing protein associated with the intestinal tract. Blood levels are used to evaluate the immune system and to monitor treatment of IgA multiple myeloma, a cancer of plasma cells, a type of cell which is usually found in the bone marrow.

HOW IT WORKS

You will be asked to provide a **venous blood sample** from which serum* will be separated. Immunoassay* is used for the laboratory analysis.

BEFORE THE TEST

No special preparation is required.

AFTER THE TEST

Follow **venous blood sample** aftercare.

SIGNIFICANCE OF RESULTS

Increased IgA levels are found in IgA multiple myeloma, some lymphomas (lymphatic cancers), liver disease, chronic infections, and following exercise. Low IgA is seen in ataxia-telangiectasia, some leukemias, hereditary IgA deficiency, non-IgA multiple myeloma, and pregnancy.

□ □ □

☐ Immunoglobulin A antibodies

WHAT IT IS AND WHY IT'S OBTAINED

Antibodies to **immunoglobulin A** (IgA) are formed during some blood transfusion reactions. Blood levels of these antibodies are used to monitor such reactions.

HOW IT WORKS

You will be asked to provide a **venous blood sample** from which serum* will be separated. Immunoassay* is used for the laboratory analysis.

BEFORE THE TEST

No special preparation is required.

AFTER THE TEST

Follow **venous blood sample** aftercare.

SIGNIFICANCE OF RESULTS

About one out of every 500 or 1,000 people is deficient in IgA and has circulating antibodies to this protein. If you are such a person and receive blood with IgA in it (the usual case), an allergic reaction can develop.

☐ ☐ ☐

☐ Immunoglobulin E

WHAT IT IS AND WHY IT'S OBTAINED

Immunoglobulin E (IgE) is an antibody (a blood protein important to the immune system) containing protein which is associated with allergies. Blood levels are used to evaluate allergic diseases.

HOW IT WORKS

You will be asked to provide a **venous blood sample** from which serum* will be separated. Immunoassay* is used for the laboratory analysis.

BEFORE THE TEST

No special preparation is required.

AFTER THE TEST

Follow **venous blood sample** aftercare.

SIGNIFICANCE OF RESULTS

IgE is high in allergic disorders such as asthma, hay fever, and eczema, infestations with parasites, and in IgE multiple myeloma. Low IgE is found in hereditary IgE deficiency, ataxia-telangiectasia, and non-IgE multiple myeloma.

□ □ □

□ Immunoglobulin G

WHAT IT IS AND WHY IT'S OBTAINED

Immunoglobulin G (IgG) is the most important and plentiful antibody containing protein in the body. Blood levels of it are used to evaluate the immune system, to investigate recurrent infections, and to monitor treatment of IgG multiple myeloma, a cancer of plasma cells, a type of cell which is usually found in the bone marrow.

HOW IT WORKS

You will be asked to provide a **venous blood sample** from which serum* will be separated. Immunoassay* is used for the laboratory analysis.

BEFORE THE TEST

No special preparation is required.

AFTER THE TEST

Follow **venous blood sample** aftercare.

SIGNIFICANCE OF RESULTS

Decreases in total IgG are seen in congenital or acquired IgG deficiency, non-IgG multiple myeloma, pregnancy, and whenever excess amounts of protein are lost. Increase in total IgG is found in AIDS, IgG multiple myeloma, chronic liver disease, chronic infections, infestations with parasites, sarcoidosis, and autoimmune disease (in which the immune system reacts against the body's own tissues). It should be noted that *total* IgG consists of many different and distinct antibodies. These different IgG antibodies, in fact, form the basis of many of the blood tests in this book which are used to diagnose infectious diseases. Thus, the HIV screening test depends upon the detection of specific IgG antibodies to HIV.

□ □ □

□ Immunoglobulin G subclasses

WHAT IT IS AND WHY IT'S OBTAINED

There are four types of **immunoglobulin G** (IgG). Blood levels of these types are used to investigate recurrent infections.

HOW IT WORKS

You will be asked to provide a **venous blood sample** from which serum* will be separated. Immunoassay* is used for the laboratory analysis.

BEFORE THE TEST

No special preparation is required.

Follow **venous blood sample** aftercare.

SIGNIFICANCE OF RESULTS

IgG$_1$ deficiency is associated with Epstein-Barr virus infections. IgG$_2$ deficiency is found in chronic sinus and respiratory infections. Low IgG$_3$ is seen with sinus and ear infections, and IgG$_4$ is decreased in allergies, ataxia-telangiectasia, and chronic sinus and respiratory infections.

□ □ □

□ Immunoglobulin M

WHAT IT IS AND WHY IT'S OBTAINED

Immunoglobulin M (IgM) is the antibody (a blood protein important to the immune system) which is formed first in response to most infections. Blood levels of it are used to evaluate the immune system.

HOW IT WORKS

You will be asked to provide a **venous blood sample** from which serum* will be separated. Immunoassay* is used for the laboratory analysis.

BEFORE THE TEST

No special preparation is required.

AFTER THE TEST

Follow **venous blood sample** aftercare.

SIGNIFICANCE OF RESULTS

Low total IgM is found in hereditary IgM deficiency, multiple myeloma, in infancy, and whenever excessive amounts of protein are lost. It is increased in liver disease, infections, inflammations, Waldenstrom's macroglobuline-mia, and in the hyper-IgM immunodeficiency syndrome. Total IgM consists of different antibodies which may be distinguished in the laboratory. Because the IgM antibody is the first to form in response to an infectious agent—the **immunoglobulin G** (IgG) response coming later—obtaining both IgM- and IgG-specific antibodies can be used to differentiate recent from chronic infections.

□ □ □

□ Infectious mononucleosis screen

WHAT IT IS AND WHY IT'S OBTAINED

As its name implies, this test is used to diagnose infectious mononucleosis, a disease which causes fever, fatigue, sore throat, and enlarged lymph nodes.

HOW IT WORKS

You will be asked to provide a **venous blood sample** from which serum* will be separated. Immunoassay* is used for the laboratory analysis.

BEFORE THE TEST

No special preparation is required.

AFTER THE TEST

Follow **venous blood sample** aftercare.

SIGNIFICANCE OF RESULTS

A positive infectious mononucleosis screening test is very good evidence that you have active infectious mononucleosis, but a negative test does not rule it out. The test becomes positive a week or two after infection and remains so for one to six months, but may persist up to a year. If your symptoms are suggestive of mononucleosis the test may be repeated if negative. The **white blood cell differential** is often helpful, and **viral antibodies** to the Epstein-Barr virus (EBV), which causes mononucleosis, may be obtained. Although it is possible to culture EBV by **viral culture,** the process is technically complex.

SYNONYMS AND INCLUDED TESTS

Mono test, Monospot™, heterophile test.

□ □ □

□ Insect identification

WHAT IT IS AND WHY IT'S OBTAINED

Although many insects are capable of biting or stinging, only a few warrant laboratory identification. Among these are lice, ticks, mites, spiders, fleas, and bedbugs.

HOW IT WORKS

Either the insect itself, an egg (nit) in the case of suspected head lice, or a skin scraping (for scabies) may be used. The specimen is examined under a microscope.

BEFORE THE TEST

No special preparation is required.

AFTER THE TEST

No special aftercare is needed.

SIGNIFICANCE OF RESULTS

Laboratory identification of an insect is occasionally helpful in evaluating a given set of symptoms, but the patterns of bites are often sufficient to make a diagnosis. Flea bites, for example, almost always occur from the knee down; those suffering from bedbugs will often awake with bloody sheets; scabies infestation produces intense itching in the middle of the night between the fingers, at the elbows, groin, and breast; and lice can be seen crawling around with the naked eye.

□ □ □

□ Insulin

WHAT IT IS AND WHY IT'S OBTAINED

Insulin is a hormone produced in the pancreas which regulates sugar **(glucose)** metabolism. Although the most common disease associated with insulin is diabetes mellitus, caused by insufficient amounts of it, insulin blood levels are used to detect *overproduction* of insulin, which occurs in certain tumors and which produces symptoms of hypoglycemia.

HOW IT WORKS

You will be asked to provide a **venous blood sample** from which serum* will be separated. Both **glucose** and insulin are measured at the same time, the latter by immunoassay*.

BEFORE THE TEST

You should fast overnight. Discontinue nonessential medications or other medications as directed by your doctor.

AFTER THE TEST

Follow **venous blood sample** aftercare.

SIGNIFICANCE OF RESULTS

High insulin is found in insulinomas (tumors producing insulin), Cushing's syndrome, steroid use, acromegaly, obesity, and in those taking insulin by injection and in those taking birth control pills. The definitive test for an insulinoma is hypoglycemia and increased insulin after an injection of tolbutamide.

□ □ □

☐ Insulin antibody

WHAT IT IS AND WHY IT'S OBTAINED

Impurities in **insulin** used to treat diabetes, particularly that obtained from beef, can cause allergic reactions in diabetics. The allergy may result in a resistance to insulin, which makes it difficult to control blood sugar **(glucose).** The blood insulin antibody (a blood protein important to the immune system) test is used to detect this situation. It is also sometimes obtained to diagnose the condition known as factitious hypoglycemia, in which someone secretly injects insulin to mimic low blood sugar.

HOW IT WORKS

You will be asked to provide a **venous blood sample** from which serum* will be separated. Immunoassay* is used for the laboratory analysis.

BEFORE THE TEST

No special preparation is required.

AFTER THE TEST

Follow **venous blood sample** aftercare.

SIGNIFICANCE OF RESULTS

Small amounts of insulin antibody are common in diabetics taking insulin and are insignificant. Large amounts may signify the need to adjust therapy. **C-peptide** is helpful in determining factitious hypoglycemia.

☐ ☐ ☐

248

☐ Intrinsic factor antibody

WHAT IT IS AND WHY IT'S OBTAINED

Intrinsic factor is a substance produced by the stomach which helps the absorption of vitamin B_{12}. Blood levels of antibodies to it are used to evaluate anemia.

HOW IT WORKS

You will be asked to provide a **venous blood sample** from which serum* will be separated. Immunoassay* is used for the laboratory analysis.

BEFORE THE TEST

No special preparation is required.

AFTER THE TEST

Follow **venous blood sample** aftercare.

SIGNIFICANCE OF RESULTS

The presence of antibodies to intrinsic factor is common in pernicious anemia, which is caused by failure to adequately absorb vitamin B_{12}. Other tests for pernicious anemia include **red blood cell indices** and blood **vitamin B_{12}.**

☐ ☐ ☐

☐ Invasive electrophysiologic studies

WHAT IT IS AND WHY IT'S OBTAINED

This test is used to evaluate heartbeat irregularities (arrhythmias) with more detail than can be obtained by the **electrocardiogram** or **Holter monitor**.

HOW IT WORKS

The procedure is carried out in a special laboratory with the necessary equipment. You may be given a mild sedative if you are apprehensive. You will be asked to undress, to wear a hospital gown, and to lie down on the examining table. **Electrocardiogram** electrodes will be then be pasted to your chest and you may or may not have intravenous fluids in order to administer medications. Sometimes a temporary cardiac pacemaker may be placed in your chest using local anesthesia. Your groin will be shaved, a local anesthetic injected, and the catheter will be introduced into the femoral vein and then into the heart, where electrical measurements will be taken. Except for the slight stinging from the local anesthetic, the procedure is not uncomfortable.

BEFORE THE TEST

Follow your doctor's instructions carefully regarding the taking of medications and the withholding of foods and liquids.

AFTER THE TEST

You will be placed on bed rest for several hours in a recovery area, during which time your vital signs (pulse, blood pressure, respiration, and temperature) will be measured at intervals and the site of catheter insertion checked for bleeding. This test is generally safe. Complications include bleeding and infection, both of which are uncommon.

SIGNIFICANCE OF RESULTS

Interpretation of this test is performed by a cardiologist. It is usually possible to pinpoint the source of the dysfunction and to evaluate the relative merits of drug treatment or a permanent pacemaker.

HIS bundle recordings.

□ □ □

□ Iron and iron binding capacity

WHAT IT IS AND WHY IT'S OBTAINED

Iron is crucial for the transport of oxygen in red blood cells. It circulates in the blood bound to proteins, but only a portion of the total amount of protein which can bind iron (the iron binding "capacity") normally does so. This test measures the total amount of iron in the blood, the iron binding capacity, and how much of this capacity is being used. It is obtained to evaluate anemia and nutritional status.

HOW IT WORKS

You will be asked to provide a **venous blood sample** from which serum* will be separated. Many laboratory methods are used for the assays.

BEFORE THE TEST

You should fast overnight.

AFTER THE TEST

Follow **venous blood sample** aftercare.

SIGNIFICANCE OF RESULTS

Blood *iron* is increased in hemochromatosis, hepatitis, excessive intake of iron, after multiple blood transfusions, and in hemolytic anemia. It is decreased in iron deficiency and in many chronic diseases. *Iron binding capacity* is increased in iron deficiency, with birth control pills, and in pregnancy. It is decreased in protein deficiency and in chronic diseases. A common problem is differentiating the anemia which comes from iron deficiency from the anemia which occurs as a consequence of chronic and debilitating diseases. Other tests are often obtained to distinguish between the two, including, besides iron and iron binding capacity, **ferritin,** which is the best single test for iron deficiency other than a **bone marrow.**

□ □ □

□ Joint fluid analysis

WHAT IT IS AND WHY IT'S OBTAINED

Joint fluid analysis is used to investigate the cause of joint symptoms such as pain, swelling, or stiffness.

HOW IT WORKS

A joint fluid specimen obtained from a **joint tap** is used. The type of analysis depends upon the laboratory, but commonly multiple studies are performed, including cell count, microscopic examination, **bacterial culture** or other culture, **uric acid,** and **rheumatoid factor.** Your doctor will specify the studies to be performed.

BEFORE THE TEST

No special preparation is required.

AFTER THE TEST

Follow **joint tap** aftercare.

SIGNIFICANCE OF RESULTS

The fact that fluid can be removed from a joint is evidence of disease, since there is normally such a small amount of it. The presence of **uric acid** in the fluid, particularly in greater concentration than blood uric acid, is strong evidence for gout. The presence of cartilage cells is evidence for osteoarthritis ("wear and tear" arthritis) or an injury. Positive rheumatoid factor is evidence for rheumatoid arthritis. Specific bacteria may be cultured in cases of infectious arthritis. Other findings can be interpreted along with other blood tests, **X rays,** or **magnetic resonance imaging.**

SYNONYMS AND INCLUDED TESTS

Synovial fluid analysis.

□ □ □

□ Joint tap

WHAT IT IS AND WHY IT'S OBTAINED

A joint tap refers to removing fluid from a joint, most commonly the knee. It is used to evaluate joint swelling of unknown cause, arthritis, and gout. It may also be employed as treatment to reduce pain or to remove pus in the case of arthritis caused by an infection.

HOW IT WORKS

Any joint can be tapped, and different doctors use slightly different approaches. The following is for the knee. You will be asked to lie on your back with your knee slightly bent. After cleansing with an antiseptic solution, a small amount of local anesthetic will be injected into your skin. This will sting or burn slightly. One or the other side of the kneecap is most commonly selected, but sites above or below the kneecap may be used as well. A needle and syringe will then be inserted into the anesthetized area. The needle is advanced slowly with gentle suction. As soon as fluid is encountered it will be withdrawn. If the volume is large the syringe may have to be changed several times. The procedure is only mildly uncomfortable.

BEFORE THE TEST

No special preparation is required.

AFTER THE TEST

Your doctor will instruct you on aftercare based upon your symptoms. This may range from bed rest to immediate full activity. You may feel some discomfort afterward, but it is usually mild. Complications such as joint infection, bleeding into the joint, persistent pain, tendon rupture, or nerve damage are very rare.

SIGNIFICANCE OF RESULTS

The joint fluid is sent for **joint fluid analysis.**

SYNONYMS AND INCLUDED TESTS

Arthrocentesis.

□ □ □

□ 17-ketogenic steroids

WHAT IT IS AND WHY IT'S OBTAINED

17-ketogenic steroids refer to a group of substances produced by the adrenal glands, testicles, and ovaries. Although still sometimes used to evaluate the adrenal gland, better tests are available (see below).

HOW IT WORKS

You will be asked to provide a **24-hour urine sample** which should be kept refrigerated during collection. A color reaction is used for the laboratory assay.

BEFORE THE TEST

Withhold nonessential drugs and medications for several days before the test or do as directed by your doctor.

AFTER THE TEST

No special aftercare is needed.

Many consider this test to be obsolete because newer and more specific tests of adrenal gland function, such as **cortisol** and **17-hydroxyprogesterone,** are available.

□ □ □

□ 17-ketosteroids

WHAT IT IS AND WHY IT'S OBTAINED

17-ketosteroids (17-KS) are a group of compounds which are derived from the adrenal gland, testicles, and ovaries. Urine levels are used to assess abnormalities of the adrenal gland and reproductive organs.

HOW IT WORKS

You will be asked to provide a **24-hour urine sample** which should be refrigerated during collection. A color reaction is used for the assay.

BEFORE THE TEST

Withhold nonessential drugs and medications for several days before the test or do as directed by your doctor.

AFTER THE TEST

No special aftercare is needed.

SIGNIFICANCE OF RESULTS

Low levels of 17-KS are found in adrenal gland insufficiency (Addison's disease), pituitary insufficiency, hypothyroidism, testicular insufficiency, and ovarian insufficiency. Increased values are found in pituitary gland tumors, adrenal gland tumors, congenital adrenal hyperplasia, interstitial cell tumor of the testicle, and stress. Many medications interfere with this test, both in lowering and elevating values. Because of newer and more accurate tests, such as

testosterone, dehydroepiandosterone, and **androstenedione,** many consider this test, when used to measure *total* 17-KS, to be obsolete. The various hormones which make up 17-KS, however, can be isolated, and this is sometimes helpful in studying difficult hormonal problems.

□ □ □

□ Kidney biopsy

WHAT IT IS AND WHY IT'S OBTAINED

A kidney biopsy is the surgical removal of a portion of kidney tissue for laboratory analysis. It is used to distinguish between kidney diseases and to determine the health of transplanted kidneys. The indications for this procedure are controversial, and many kidney specialists rely upon other **kidney function tests,** kidney **ultrasound** and **computed tomography,** which, although not providing the same information, are safer.

HOW IT WORKS

The procedure is carried out in a special room under sterile conditions. Your vital signs (pulse, blood pressure, respiration, and temperature) will be taken and usually an intravenous drip of fluids will be started. You may be given a sedative if you are anxious. You will be asked to lie facedown and a towel or pillow will be positioned under your abdomen. The location of one kidney (either may be selected) is determined with **ultrasound** and the site cleansed with an antiseptic. Your skin will then be injected with a local anesthetic and an incision made with a scalpel. More anesthetic may be injected and the incision carried deeper. A needle—either the biopsy needle itself or a "finder" needle—will then be advanced into the incision. During this time you will alternately be asked to hold your breath and then to resume normal breathing. The needle is only advanced when you hold your breath because the kidney moves up and down as you breathe. When the membrane surrounding the kidney is located the biopsy itself will be taken as you hold your breath. You will feel some discomfort but it is momentary. Two or three specimens may be obtained.

BEFORE THE TEST

Follow instructions carefully regarding medications. Avoid aspirin for at least a week and ibuprofen, ketoprofen, or naproxen for one day.

AFTER THE TEST

In most cases you will be asked to stay in the hospital overnight for observation. Avoid strenuous activity. Kidney biopsy can be risky. Complications, such as serious hemorrhage and infection, occur at the rate of about 2 percent. Fatalities have been reported to be about one in a thousand.

SIGNIFICANCE OF RESULTS

The specimen of kidney tissue provided by this test is examined by a pathologist and the results will be integrated with other findings. A normal biopsy, it should be remembered, may have missed the disease, because certain kidney diseases only affect portions of the gland. Even abnormal biopsies may not be diagnostic, being reported, for example, as "consistent with" a certain disorder. Many kidney diseases produce similar changes under the microscope.

SYNONYMS AND INCLUDED TESTS

Closed renal biopsy.

□ □ □

□ Kidney function tests

WHAT IT IS AND WHY IT'S OBTAINED

As its name implies, this is a battery of tests which are used to evaluate kidney function in those who need frequent monitoring of their kidney status. The tests usually include

blood urea nitrogen, creatinine, glucose, and **electrolytes (sodium, chloride, potassium,** and **carbon dioxide).**

HOW IT WORKS

You will be asked to provide a **venous blood sample** from which serum* will be separated. A number of methods are used for the analysis.

BEFORE THE TEST

You should fast overnight.

AFTER THE TEST

Follow **venous blood sample** aftercare.

SIGNIFICANCE OF RESULTS

For interpretation, see the individual tests.

SYNONYMS AND INCLUDED TESTS

Kidney profile.

□ □ □

□ Kidney scan

WHAT IT IS AND WHY IT'S OBTAINED

This is a type of **radionuclide scan** used to visualize and assess the function of the kidneys or detect obstruction of the flow of urine. It is often obtained to evaluate the reasons for abnormal **kidney function tests.**

HOW IT WORKS

The test is carried out in the nuclear medicine department of a hospital, clinic, or private physician's office, sometimes as part of a radiology facility. You will receive an injection of a very small amount of a radioactive isotope ("tracer") designed for this test. The vein puncture is usually only mildly uncomfortable. The images are taken with a gamma camera, a computerized device which may stand still or may move over your back to produce pictures. The actual scanning is painless and takes about fifteen minutes. You should try to remain as still as possible for the duration.

BEFORE THE TEST

No special preparation is required. Follow instructions regarding fluid intake; in general it is encouraged.

AFTER THE TEST

No special aftercare is needed. Although safe, this test does involve injection of a radioactive compound.

SIGNIFICANCE OF RESULTS

A negative test means that the images of the kidneys were within normal limits. Abnormal findings may include an obstructed kidney or decreased circulation to one or both kidneys due to kidney disease or to previous injuries, infection, or inflammation. Results should be interpreted along with other tests such as kidney **ultrasound,** kidney **X-ray contrast studies,** and a kidney **angiogram.**

□ □ □

□ Kidney stone analysis

WHAT IT IS AND WHY IT'S OBTAINED

Knowing the chemical composition of a kidney stone helps to determine its cause and may prevent its recurrence. Kidney stones may cause excruciating back and side pain or may be painless, producing only blood in the urine.

HOW IT WORKS

Since kidney stones range greatly in size it may be necessary to strain your urine in order to retrieve them. Place them into a plastic or other container and transport them to the laboratory or doctor's office. In the laboratory they are usually subjected to chemical analysis, but infrared spectroscopy or X-ray diffraction may also be used.

BEFORE THE TEST

No special preparation is required.

AFTER THE TEST

No special aftercare is needed.

SIGNIFICANCE OF RESULTS

Most kidney stones are composed of a mixture of substances, the most common of which is calcium oxalate. These are sometimes found in those who excrete excessively large amounts of **calcium** in their urine, but often no underlying cause is found. Testing urine for **oxalate** is also helpful. Other stones may be caused by primary hyperparathyroidism, primary cystinuria, gout, dehydration, and kidney infections.

SYNONYMS AND INCLUDED TESTS

Urinary calculus composition.

□ □ □

□ Kleihauer-Betke test

WHAT IT IS AND WHY IT'S OBTAINED

The Kleihauer-Betke test is used to detect a special type of **hemoglobin** (hemoglobin F) in the blood. Hemoglobin F is also called fetal hemoglobin, because it is prevalent in the developing fetus. The test is used most commonly to determine how much fetal-maternal hemorrhage has taken place after birth, that is, how much blood from a baby is present in the mother. This is important in the disease called hemolytic disease of the newborn, in which an Rh-negative mother gives birth to an Rh-positive infant. In these cases this test is used to calculate the dose of Rh immune globulin to be given to the mother. The test can also be used to aid in the diagnosis of certain types of anemia, for example thallasemia.

HOW IT WORKS

You will be asked to provide a **venous blood sample** which will be treated with a citric acid phosphate buffer. Adult hemoglobin is soluble in this substance, whereas fetal hemoglobin is not. Any precipitate is measured and represents fetal hemoglobin.

BEFORE THE TEST

No special preparation is required.

AFTER THE TEST

Follow **venous blood sample** aftercare.

SIGNIFICANCE OF RESULTS

Fetal hemoglobin normally represents a minute fraction of adult hemoglobin, whereas in newborn infants it is the major portion. Thus, even a small elevation may signify fetal-maternal hemorrhage. Certain otherwise normal adults, however, have persistent fetal hemoglobin, and this must be taken into consideration.

SYNONYMS AND INCLUDED TESTS

Acid elution for fetal hemoglobin.

□ □ □

□ KOH preparation

WHAT IT IS AND WHY IT'S OBTAINED

The KOH (potassium hydroxide) preparation is a rapid test for the diagnosis of fungus infections. It is used most often to evaluate skin, nail, and hair diseases but may be performed on body fluids.

HOW IT WORKS

A superficial scraping of your skin or a nail or hair clipping will be placed on a glass slide with a few drops of potassium hydroxide solution. This will be heated and examined under a microscope for the presence of organisms.

BEFORE THE TEST

No special preparation is required.

AFTER THE TEST

No special aftercare is needed.

SIGNIFICANCE OF RESULTS

A positive test means that infection with a fungus is present, but a negative test does not rule it out. A **fungal culture** is more definitive and provides specific identification of the fungus.

SYNONYMS AND INCLUDED TESTS

Wet mount for fungus.

□ □ □

□ Lactic acid

WHAT IT IS AND WHY IT'S OBTAINED

Lactic acid is a waste product of carbohydrate metabolism which accumulates when oxygen is deficient. Blood levels are obtained most often in critical situations, such as coma.

HOW IT WORKS

You will be asked to provide a **venous blood sample** from which serum* will be separated. Several methods may be used for the analysis.

BEFORE THE TEST

You should be resting for about an hour.

AFTER THE TEST

Follow **venous blood sample** aftercare.

SIGNIFICANCE OF RESULTS

Although high blood lactic acid may be associated with nothing more than strenuous exercise, it usually signifies a more serious problem which can result from shock, severe hemorrhage, infections, heart attacks, dehydration, poisoning, and any condition characterized by lack of oxygen. It can also result from kidney disease, liver disease, diabetes, leukemia, lymphoma, and certain enzyme deficiencies. The resulting condition is called metabolic (or lactic) acidosis, and is often marked by deep, rapid breathing as the body tries to compensate for the accumulation of acid by eliminating **carbon dioxide.**

◻ ◻ ◻

◻ Lactic dehydrogenase

WHAT IT IS AND WHY IT'S OBTAINED

Lactic dehydrogenase (LD) is an enzyme which is found in all cells of the body. Blood levels are obtained to diagnose heart attacks, blood clots in the lung (pulmonary embolism), liver disease, kidney disease, blood disease, and cancer. LD is most widely used, however, in evaluating chest pain, especially in diagnosing heart attacks. LD exists in five forms, called isoenzymes. LD_1 and LD_2 are mainly found in heart muscle and red blood cells, LD_3 in the lungs, and LD_4 and LD_5 in liver and muscle other than heart muscle.

HOW IT WORKS

You will be asked to provide a **venous blood sample** from which serum* will be separated. The different isoenzymes are separated by electrophoresis*.

BEFORE THE TEST

No special preparation is required.

AFTER THE TEST

Follow **venous blood sample** aftercare.

SIGNIFICANCE OF RESULTS

Both the total LD level and the levels of the different LD forms are important. Normally the LD_2 is higher than the LD_1, but in cases of heart attacks this ratio is reversed, called the LD "flip." This is significant even in the presence of a normal *total* LD value, although in some heart attacks the flip does not occur, the only change being an increase in total LD. LD is not used by itself to diagnose heart attacks, however, and the **electrocardiogram** and **creatine kinase** are usually evaluated at the same time. In the typical heart attack the LD rises later than the creatine kinase. High levels of total LD with a normal isoenzyme pattern can also be seen in cancer, other heart and lung diseases, thyroid disease, kidney disease, and other inflammatory diseases. LD_5 levels are increased in liver disease and after muscle injury.

SYNONYMS AND INCLUDED TESTS

LDH.

□ □ □

☐ Lactose tolerance test

WHAT IT IS AND WHY IT'S OBTAINED

Lactose is a sugar present in milk and other dairy products. Normally, the enzyme lactase converts lactose into ordinary sugar **(glucose).** People who are lactase deficient have trouble with this conversion and develop diarrhea, abdominal distension (bloating), and cramps after drinking dairy products. The lactose tolerance test (LTT) evaluates this condition.

HOW IT WORKS

You will first be asked to provide a **venous blood sample** from which serum* will be separated and analyzed for glucose. You will then be given a dose of liquid lactose to drink. More **venous blood samples** are then drawn at intervals, up to about four hours. The intervals vary according to doctor and laboratory. All samples are tested for glucose. You should remain seated or in bed until all blood samples have been taken. The **hydrogen breath test** is a variation of this test.

BEFORE THE TEST

You should fast overnight. Avoid nonessential medications or do as directed by your doctor.

AFTER THE TEST

If you are lactose intolerant you may develop abdominal symptoms during or after the test. These are transitory but can be uncomfortable.

SIGNIFICANCE OF RESULTS

A negative test means that your blood glucose rose normally after taking the lactose. Lactose intolerance is suggested by a decreased blood glucose level, signifying poor conversion of lactose to glucose. If the breath test is performed, an increase in exhaled hydrogen is considered a positive test. Drugs and medications which alter blood glucose may interfere with this test. You may avoid an LTT if you can keep a careful record of your diet and symptoms. By staying away from dairy products for several days, then ingesting milk, you can reproduce for yourself the symptoms of lactose intolerance if they exist.

□ □ □

□ Laparoscopy

WHAT IT IS AND WHY IT'S OBTAINED

Laparoscopy is used to examine the internal organs. The liver, peritoneum, gallbladder, diaphragm, spleen, and intestines can be directly visualized. In women the ovaries, fallopian tubes, and uterus can be seen. The introduction of laparoscopy provided a great advance in medical diagnosis and is indicated in a variety of situations to evaluate abdominal symptoms, fluid buildup (ascites), liver disease, cancer, and gynecological disease. Many surgical procedures are also possible during laparoscopy, including tubal ligation and gallbladder operations.

HOW IT WORKS

Laparoscopy is generally performed in a surgical room under local or general anesthesia. Gastroenterologists are usually inclined to local anesthesia, whereas surgeons and gynecologists often prefer general anesthesia. If you are to be awake you will be given a sedative by mouth or injection and wheeled into the procedure room on a gurney. Your vital signs (pulse, blood pressure, respiration, and temperature) will be taken, the blood pressure cuff will remain on your arm, and an intravenous drip of fluids will be started. If the procedure is being performed for gynecologic reasons, a pelvic examination will be performed. The skin around your navel will be cleansed with an antiseptic and injected with a local anesthetic. A small incision will then be made near your navel and a needle introduced. This will pump a gas, usually carbon dioxide, into your abdomen and you will experience a feeling of fullness but no real pain. This needle is withdrawn and the sleeve of the laparoscope is guided through the same incision. The laparoscope itself is then advanced through the sleeve and into your abdomen. If you are awake you may be asked to move, breathe, or to perform certain maneuvers during the examination. Biopsies, cultures, or cauterization may be performed.

BEFORE THE TEST

You should fast overnight and follow instructions carefully regarding medications. Avoid aspirin for at least a week and ibuprofen, ketoprofen, or naproxen for one day.

AFTER THE TEST

You will be taken to a recovery area where your vital signs will be taken until they stabilize. Unless a liver biopsy was taken, an overnight stay in the hospital is usually not required. Although generally a safe procedure, perforation of the bowel or other internal organs can occur, as well as laceration of blood vessels. As in any invasive procedure, infection is always a possibility. Abdominal and shoulder pain are common and should go away in a day or two. Report any abnormal pain, bleeding, or fever to your doctor. Follow instructions regarding physical activity.

SIGNIFICANCE OF RESULTS

Many abnormalities may be discovered at laparoscopy, including growths, cysts, adhesions, abscesses, and fistulas. The results of cultures or biopsies may take a week or more to be returned.

SYNONYMS AND INCLUDED TESTS

Peritoneoscopy, peritoneal endoscopy.

□ □ □

☐ LE cell test

WHAT IT IS AND WHY IT'S OBTAINED

The LE cell test was the first laboratory test designed to diagnose lupus erythematosus (LE), the most well-known autoimmune disease. When this test is positive it demonstrates graphically the general principles of autoimmune disease, in which the body produces antibodies and reacts against itself.

HOW IT WORKS

You will be asked to provide a **venous blood sample.** The sample will be shaken with glass beads to rupture some of the white blood cells and expose their DNA. The specimen is then incubated and examined under a microscope. A positive test is indicated by the digestion of DNA by the remaining white blood cells.

BEFORE THE TEST

No special preparation is required.

AFTER THE TEST

Follow **venous blood sample** aftercare.

SIGNIFICANCE OF RESULTS

A positive LE test can be found not only in LE but also in other autoimmune diseases. Furthermore, a number of drugs can cause a positive LE test, such as penicillin, sulfa drugs, and birth control pills. The LE cell test is now considered obsolete. A better test is the **antinuclear antibody.**

SYNONYMS AND INCLUDED TESTS

LE prep, lupus test.

☐ ☐ ☐

☐ Leucine aminopeptidase

WHAT IT IS AND WHY IT'S OBTAINED

Leucine aminopeptidase is an enzyme found in the liver. Blood levels are used to evaluate an elevated **alkaline phosphatase.**

HOW IT WORKS

You will be asked to provide a **venous blood sample** from which serum* will be separated. Several methods are available for the laboratory assay.

BEFORE THE TEST

You should fast overnight.

AFTER THE TEST

Follow **venous blood sample** aftercare.

SIGNIFICANCE OF RESULTS

Leucine aminopeptidase is elevated in diseases of the liver but normal in diseases of bone, thus helping to distinguish between the two major causes of an elevated **alkaline phosphatase.** The **gamma glutamyl transferase,** however, provides similar information, and this test is seldom used.

SYNONYMS AND INCLUDED TESTS

Arylamidase.

☐ ☐ ☐

☐ Leukemia and lymphoma panel

WHAT IT IS AND WHY IT'S OBTAINED

As its name implies, this battery of tests is used to classify leukemia and lymphoma (cancer of the lymphatics).

HOW IT WORKS

The tests may be performed on a **venous blood sample** or **bone marrow.** The white cells are tested for differences ("cell surface markers") by flow cytometry*. There are over two dozen of these markers and they are usually included in a panel in order to classify the malignancy in question.

BEFORE THE TEST

No special preparation is required.

AFTER THE TEST

Follow **venous blood sample** or **bone marrow** aftercare.

SIGNIFICANCE OF RESULTS

Leukemias and lymphomas can be classified into acute or chronic, myelocytic or lymphocytic, and T or B types, with multiple subclassifications. Treatment and outlook vary with each type. This panel of tests can also help in cases where leukemia or lymphoma suddenly takes a turn for the worse (crisis) by determining if a change in the type of cells is causing the problem.

☐ ☐ ☐

☐ Leukocyte alkaline phosphatase

WHAT IT IS AND WHY IT'S OBTAINED

Alkaline phosphatase is an enzyme which is widely distributed in the body. White blood cell (leukocyte) levels of it

(LAP) are used to differentiate leukemia from disorders which mimic leukemia, both of which may produce a high **white blood cell count.**

HOW IT WORKS

You will be asked to provide a **venous blood sample** which will be smeared on glass slides. The smears are treated in a multiple stage chemical procedure.

BEFORE THE TEST

No special preparation is required.

AFTER THE TEST

Follow **venous blood sample** aftercare.

SIGNIFICANCE OF RESULTS

Low levels of LAP are found in chronic myelocytic leukemia whereas high levels are found in disorders which may mimic leukemia, such as polycythemia (in which there are large numbers of red blood cells) and some infections.

□ □ □

□ Lip biopsy for Sjögren's syndrome

WHAT IT IS AND WHY IT'S OBTAINED

Sjögren's syndrome is an autoimmune disease (in which the immune system reacts against the body's own tissues) which produces dry mouth and dry eyes. Lip biopsy is sometimes needed to prove the diagnosis.

HOW IT WORKS

You will be seated in a dental chair and your lower lip will be anesthetized with a local anesthetic. This will sting or burn slightly. An incision will be made into the inside of your lower lip and several salivary glands (at least five) will be removed. Stitches will be used to close the wound. The glands are then sent to the laboratory where they will be examined for signs of inflammation.

BEFORE THE TEST

Avoid aspirin for at least a week and ibuprofen, ketoprofen, or naproxen for one day.

AFTER THE TEST

There will be minor pain which will resolve in a few days. Take acetaminophen for pain if needed. If bleeding develops apply direct pressure for five minutes, watching the clock. Follow instructions for return to the office for stitch removal. This is a safe procedure but persistent numbness of the lower lip can develop from the cutting of nerves. Even if this does happen, however, it usually improves with time.

SIGNIFICANCE OF RESULTS

A positive test means that inflammation of the salivary glands was found. Other causes of inflammation, however, may lead to false positive results. Dry eyes and dry lips are very common symptoms and most people who suffer from them do not have Sjögren's syndrome. Function of the glands which produce saliva may also be evaluated by **radionuclide scan** or **X-ray contrast study**. The **Schirmer test** is used to detect eye involvement in Sjögren's syndrome.

SYNONYMS AND INCLUDED TESTS

Labial salivary gland biopsy.

□ □ □

□ Lipase

WHAT IT IS AND WHY IT'S OBTAINED

Lipase is an enzyme produced in the pancreas which aids fat digestion. Blood levels are used to diagnose pancreatitis (inflammation of the pancreas), which can cause abdominal pain.

HOW IT WORKS

You will be asked to provide a **venous blood sample** from which serum* will be separated. Several laboratory methods of analysis are available.

BEFORE THE TEST

You should fast overnight.

AFTER THE TEST

Follow **venous blood sample** aftercare.

SIGNIFICANCE OF RESULTS

Lipase is elevated in pancreatitis but may also be increased in kidney failure, liver disease, and alcoholism. Certain drugs, such as diuretics and narcotics, also elevate blood lipase. Multiple lipase and **amylase** determinations may be necessary over a period of time to diagnose pancreatitis. The lipase tends to be elevated longer than the amylase after an acute attack.

□ □ □

□ Lipid profile

WHAT IT IS AND WHY IT'S OBTAINED

Lipids are body fats. Since lipids cannot dissolve in blood (oil and water don't mix), they must travel with proteins, the resulting substances being called lipoproteins. These lipoproteins differ in density and can be separated into certain classes. **Cholesterol,** the best known and most important lipid, is found mostly in the low-density lipoprotein (LDL) fraction, but a certain amount is also found in the high-density lipoprotein (HDL) fraction. The lipid profile is a battery of tests used to evaluate the risk of coronary artery

273

disease (CAD) and usually consists of HDL cholesterol, LDL cholesterol, total cholesterol, and **triglycerides.** The very–low density lipoprotein (VLDL) fraction is also sometimes included. The lipid profile predicts CAD better than a simple blood cholesterol.

HOW IT WORKS

You will be asked to provide a **venous blood sample** from which serum* will be separated. Several methods may be used for the assay.

BEFORE THE TEST

You should fast overnight. Don't drink alcohol for twenty-four hours and avoid nonessential medications or do as directed by your doctor.

AFTER THE TEST

Follow **venous blood sample** aftercare.

SIGNIFICANCE OF RESULTS

Lipoproteins transport cholesterol, and can carry it *to* a blood vessel where it may be deposited, or can carry it *away* from a blood vessel for elimination. In fact, HDL cholesterol (also known as "good cholesterol") helps to clear cholesterol from blood and tissue, decreasing and reversing arteriosclerosis. Thus, high relative levels of HDL cholesterol are more important than low total cholesterol levels in determining the risk of CAD. Although the results of a lipid profile are reported as numbers, it is easier to understand the numbers by relying on the computer's calculation, which takes into account your age and sex. This is often reported as "average risk" of CAD, "half average risk," "two times average risk," or "three times average risk," and so on. There are several medications which will interfere with this test, including, most obviously, drugs which lower cholesterol. Steroids, estrogens, and certain diuretics (water pills) may also change lipid levels.

Coronary heart disease risk index.

□ □ □

□ Lipoprotein (a)

WHAT IT IS AND WHY IT'S OBTAINED

Lipoprotein (a) is a substance composed of fat (lipid) and **protein** which is similar to low-density lipoprotein (LDL), the type of lipoprotein which is associated with "bad" cholesterol. Blood levels of lipoprotein (a) are used to evaluate the risk of coronary artery disease (CAD).

HOW IT WORKS

You will be asked to provide a **venous blood sample** from which serum* will be separated. Immunoassay* is used for the laboratory analysis.

BEFORE THE TEST

You should fast overnight.

AFTER THE TEST

Follow **venous blood sample** aftercare.

SIGNIFICANCE OF RESULTS

Increased lipoprotein (a) is associated with a higher risk of CAD *if* your **cholesterol** is high. If your cholesterol is normal, a high lipoprotein (a) is not so significant.

□ □ □

❑ Lipoprotein electrophoresis

WHAT IT IS AND WHY IT'S OBTAINED

Lipids (fats) are insoluble in blood (oil and water don't mix) and must travel as lipid-protein complexes called lipoproteins. These lipoproteins differ in density and can be separated into certain classes. Lipoprotein electrophoresis separates these lipoproteins and can be used to classify certain inherited diseases which cause increased blood lipoproteins (familial hyperlipoproteinemias).

HOW IT WORKS

You will be asked to provide a **venous blood sample** from which serum* will be separated. The different lipoprotein fractions are separated by electrophoresis*.

BEFORE THE TEST

You should fast overnight. It is also helpful to be on a stable diet for two to three weeks.

AFTER THE TEST

Follow **venous blood sample** aftercare.

SIGNIFICANCE OF RESULTS

Lipoprotein electrophoresis has mostly been replaced by the **lipid profile,** except for diagnosing type III hyperlipoproteinemia.

SYNONYMS AND INCLUDED TESTS

Lipoprotein phenotyping.

❑ ❑ ❑

☐ Liver and spleen scan

WHAT IT IS AND WHY IT'S OBTAINED

This is a type of **radionuclide scan** designed to visualize the liver and the spleen. It is used to evaluate abdominal diseases and injuries along with abdominal X rays, **computed tomography, magnetic resonance imaging,** and **ultrasound.**

HOW IT WORKS

The test takes about thirty minutes and is carried out in the nuclear medicine department of a hospital, clinic, or private physician's office, sometimes as part of a radiology facility. You will receive an injection of a very small amount of a radioactive isotope ("tracer") designed for this test. The vein puncture is usually only mildly uncomfortable. The images are taken with a gamma camera, a computerized device which may stand still or may move over your abdomen to produce pictures. The actual scanning is painless. Follow instructions regarding breathing carefully, since an important part of the study is determining how well your liver moves as you breathe.

BEFORE THE TEST

No special preparation is required.

AFTER THE TEST

No special aftercare is needed. Although safe, this test does involve the injection of a radioactive compound.

SIGNIFICANCE OF RESULTS

A negative test means that the images of the liver and the spleen were within normal limits and that the amount of radioactive tracer picked up by each organ was roughly the same. Abnormalities may include liver or spleen enlargement or shrinkage, tumors, hemorrhage, or generalized liver disease such as cirrhosis.

SYNONYMS AND INCLUDED TESTS

Liver scan, spleen scan.

□ □ □

□ Liver biopsy

WHAT IT IS AND WHY IT'S OBTAINED

Liver biopsy is the removal of liver tissue by needle in order to help diagnose liver disease. It is used in selected cases after **liver function tests** have been shown to be abnormal and after visualizing techniques, such as a **liver and spleen scan, computed tomography, magnetic resonance imaging,** or liver **ultrasound** indicate that it may be helpful. The indications for liver biopsy are varied. Although it is invasive, liver biopsy is able to provide valuable information which is not available by other means.

HOW IT WORKS

There are several methods and needles available, but the technique falls basically into two categories, a quick method and a slow method. In both, but especially the slow method, it is important to follow instructions carefully. The procedure is done in a special room but may be performed in your bed if you are hospitalized. You will be asked to lie on your back with your right arm behind your head. Your abdomen will be examined and the site of the proposed biopsy marked. The skin of your right lower chest will then be cleansed with an antiseptic and a local anesthetic will be injected at a location between two of the lower ribs. This will sting or burn slightly. A small incision is sometimes made in the numb area. Just before the biopsy is taken you will be told to take a deep breath, and then exhale. In the quick technique, the biopsy needle is thrust into your liver and the specimen taken in that instant. You may experience a transient pain in your right shoulder. In the slower method, you will have to hold your breath for five to ten seconds while the needle is advanced and the several steps necessary to cut the tissue are performed. These procedures may be repeated two or three times to obtain an adequate specimen.

BEFORE THE TEST

Avoid aspirin for at least a week and ibuprofen, ketoprofen, or naproxen for one day. You should fast overnight. In some hospitals you will be given a glass or two of milk before the test in order to empty your gallbladder. Take or discontinue other medications as your doctor directs.

AFTER THE TEST

If you are in good health you may be allowed to go home; otherwise an overnight stay in the hospital is required. In general, you will spend a few hours lying on your right side and your vital signs (pulse, blood pressure, respiration, and temperature) will be checked frequently. After a time you will be allowed to sit up, but bed rest is advisable for about a day. If you do go home, have a friend or family member available to take you back to the hospital if needed. Mild pain in your right shoulder is common and need cause you no concern. It usually goes away in a day or two. Hemorrhage is the most common serious complication. It is usually minor and confined to some bleeding from the biopsy site, but it may be internal. Report any severe abdominal or chest pain, shortness of breath, or fever.

SIGNIFICANCE OF RESULTS

Possible findings include cirrhosis, hepatitis, liver cancer, lymphoma (lymphatic cancer), and infections. The major disadvantage to a needle liver biopsy is that it is "blind," and although multiple samples may be taken, it is possible for all of them to miss the disease. This can be partially overcome by doing a liver biopsy during **laparoscopy.**

Needle biopsy of the liver.

□ □ □

□ Liver function tests

WHAT IT IS AND WHY IT'S OBTAINED

Because assessment of liver disease requires multiple tests, they are often bundled together. Different laboratories include different studies in their liver function tests (LFTs), but a common list would include **lactic dehydrogenase, aspartate aminotransferase, alanine aminotransferase, gamma glutamyl transferase, bilirubin,** and **alkaline phosphatase.** Repeat LFTs are often obtained to monitor the progress of liver disease.

HOW IT WORKS

You will be asked to provide a **venous blood sample** from which serum* will be separated. Various methods are used for the laboratory analyses.

BEFORE THE TEST

You should fast overnight.

AFTER THE TEST

Follow **venous blood sample** aftercare.

SIGNIFICANCE OF RESULTS

For interpretation, see the individual tests. It should be noted that these tests do not include a **liver biopsy,** nor any visualizing technique such as a **liver and spleen scan, computed tomography, magnetic resonance imaging, ultrasound,** or **laparoscopy,** all of which can provide valuable information about the liver.

Liver screen, liver battery, liver panel, liver profile.

◻ ◻ ◻

◻ Lung scan

WHAT IT IS AND WHY IT'S OBTAINED

The lung scan is a type of **radionuclide scan** which is used when a pulmonary embolism (blood clot in the lung) is suspected.

HOW IT WORKS

The test takes about thirty minutes and is carried out in the nuclear medicine department of a hospital, clinic, or private physician's office, sometimes as part of a radiology facility. There are two portions to the test, the *ventilation* part, which measures how well air reaches the lungs, and the *perfusion* part, which measures how well blood reaches the lungs. For the ventilation portion, you will be asked to breathe through a mouthpiece while a radioactive substance, called a "tracer," is added to the air you are breathing. The substance may be a technetium isotope aerosol, or a xenon or krypton gas isotope. Depending upon the substance, you may be asked to hold your breath for a few seconds. The images are taken with a gamma camera, a computerized device which takes pictures in six or eight views from different angles. This should take about fifteen minutes. For the perfusion part you will receive an intravenous injection of a very small amount of a radioactive isotope, also a "tracer," designed for this test. The multiple view scanning procedure is then repeated.

BEFORE THE TEST

No special preparation is required.

AFTER THE TEST

No special aftercare is needed. Although safe, this test does involve the injection of a radioactive compound.

SIGNIFICANCE OF RESULTS

A negative test means that both the ventilation and perfusion images were uniform throughout the lungs. If *perfusion* to one part of the lung is decreased, a blood clot is indicated, whereas if *ventilation* is decreased, a disease of the lungs themselves, such as pneumonia, may be the problem.

SYNONYMS AND INCLUDED TESTS

Ventilation/perfusion scan.

□ □ □

□ Luteinizing hormone

WHAT IT IS AND WHY IT'S OBTAINED

Luteinizing hormone (LH) is a hormone produced by the pituitary gland which stimulates the ovaries in women and the testicles in men. In women, blood levels are used to evaluate infertility and menstrual disturbances. In men, they are used to investigate problems such as low **testosterone.**

HOW IT WORKS

You will be asked to provide a **venous blood sample** from which serum* will be separated. Because LH is secreted intermittently some laboratories perform multiple tests with analysis of the pooled blood sample. A **24-hour urine sample** may also be analyzed. Immunoassay* is used for the laboratory analysis.

BEFORE THE TEST

No special preparation is required. It is important for women to carefully note the time of their menstrual periods and inform the laboratory, since levels of LH vary during the menstrual cycle.

AFTER THE TEST

Follow **venous blood sample** aftercare.

SIGNIFICANCE OF RESULTS

In general, LH is low if the pituitary gland itself is not functioning well or if the hypothalamus in the brain is not stimulating it enough. LH tends to be high (because of insufficient feedback suppression) if either the ovaries or the testicles are not producing sufficient sex hormones. LH should be interpreted along with **follicle stimulating hormone** (FSH) and usually with **estrogen** and **testosterone.** Most often LH and FSH parallel each other, but if one is high and the other is low a pituitary tumor may be present. If level of LH is more than three times higher than that of FSH, the Stein-Leventhal syndrome (polycystic ovaries) is indicated.

◻︎ ◻︎ ◻︎

◻︎ Lyme disease antibody

WHAT IT IS AND WHY IT'S OBTAINED

Lyme disease is caused by a germ called *Borrelia burgdorferi.* Blood levels of antibody (a blood protein important to the immune system) to this organism are obtained in suspected cases of Lyme disease, a disease which is transmitted by ticks, and which causes arthritis, fatigue, and a large round circular rash.

HOW IT WORKS

The test may be performed on serum* obtained by **venous blood sample,** joint fluid obtained by **joint tap,** or cerebrospinal fluid* (CSF) obtained by **spinal tap.** The fluid is tested by one of several methods of immunoassay* and the Western blot* is often used to confirm the results.

BEFORE THE TEST

No special preparation is required.

AFTER THE TEST

Follow **venous blood sample** aftercare.

SIGNIFICANCE OF RESULTS

Results of the *blood* test can be variable and sometimes unreliable. If antibody is found in CSF or joint fluid, however, Lyme disease can be diagnosed with much more certainty. In general a positive result is only of value if you have symptoms of Lyme disease. Furthermore, it is estimated that Lyme antibody is detected in only 40 percent of those with Lyme disease in the first few weeks of infection, when treatment is most likely to be of value. However, as a general rule, if three consecutive Lyme antibody tests taken three weeks apart have proven negative, Lyme disease can be excluded. The real problem with the Lyme antibody test is that "weakly positive" results are very common because many people carry benign organisms which cross react with the the *Borrelia* germ. DNA tests using the **polymerase chain reaction** are showing promise in the detection of Lyme disease but are not yet in widespread use.

SYNONYMS AND INCLUDED TESTS

Lyme arthritis serology.

□ □ □

☐ Lymph node biopsy

WHAT IT IS AND WHY IT'S OBTAINED

Lymph node **biopsy** is the surgical removal of one or more lymph nodes ("glands"), either partly or completely, to evaluate their enlargement. It is also of value, however, in determining the spread of cancer in lymph nodes which appear to be normal.

HOW IT WORKS

The location of the procedure depends upon the lymph node or nodes being tested. Common sites include the neck, armpits, and groin, although concentrations of lymph nodes are found in other areas, such as above the collarbone and around the elbow joints. It is usually performed under local anesthesia in a properly equipped surgical room. For a *needle* biopsy the skin over the node in question will be cleansed with an antiseptic and injected with a local anesthetic. This will sting or burn slightly. The doctor will then grasp the node with one hand while inserting a special biopsy needle into it with the other hand. A small core of tissue will be removed. For an *excisional* biopsy the area will be similarly prepared and anesthetized but an incision will be made in your skin and the gland(s) removed in their entirety. Stitches will be used to close the wound.

BEFORE THE TEST

Avoid aspirin for at least a week and ibuprofen, ketoprofen, or naproxen for one day.

AFTER THE TEST

Observe the site for abnormal pain, redness, pus, or bleeding. Lymph node biopsy is generally a safe procedure. Return to the doctor for stitch removal if an excisional biopsy was performed.

SIGNIFICANCE OF RESULTS

The main question to be answered by the pathologist is whether the lymph nodes are involved with cancer, either that which has spread from somewhere else, such as the breast, or that which is primary to the lymphatic system itself, such as Hodgkin's disease and other lymphomas. A **lymphangiogram** may provide valuable information in the latter case. Lymph node biopsy specimens in the abdomen may be obtained by **laparoscopy**.

SYNONYMS AND INCLUDED TESTS

Lymph gland biopsy.

□ □ □

□ Lymphangiogram

WHAT IT IS AND WHY IT'S OBTAINED

The lymphangiogram is an **X-ray contrast study** designed to visualize the lymph vessels and the lymph nodes ("glands"). It is used to evaluate the spread of tumors and to find the cause of enlarged lymph nodes.

HOW IT WORKS

The test is performed in a procedure room with **X ray** and surgical equipment. You will be asked to lie on your back. The skin of your feet will be cleansed with an antiseptic and a blue dye will be injected between your toes. This will cause the superficial lymph vessels in your foot to become visible. A small amount of local anesthetic will sting or burn slightly as it is injected into your skin and an incision will then be made over one of the lymphatic vessels. A needle will be inserted into a lymph vessel and an X-ray contrast agent will be dripped into it slowly. At first there may be some discomfort in your legs as the dye is dripped in, but this should pass. When the infusion is complete the needles will be removed and the wound will be stitched closed. The procedure may take several hours to complete. X rays of your pelvis and abdomen will be taken immediately, and a day later.

BEFORE THE TEST

No special preparation is required.

AFTER THE TEST

Follow instructions regarding activity. Your skin, urine, and vision will be blue for several days. Return as directed to the doctor for removal of stitches. Allergic reactions to the X-ray contrast dye are possible and may range from mild to severe.

SIGNIFICANCE OF RESULTS

Abnormal findings may include lymph channels which are blocked by tumors, injury, or inflammation. In evaluating lymphoma (cancer of the lymphatics), the lymphangiogram can give a general picture of the extent of disease. More specific information can be obtained with **computed tomography, ultrasound,** and lymph node **biopsy.**

SYNONYMS AND INCLUDED TESTS

Lymphangiography.

□ □ □

□ Lymphocyte transformation test

WHAT IT IS AND WHY IT'S OBTAINED

The lymphocyte transformation test is used to evaluate the immune system.

HOW IT WORKS

You will be asked to provide a **venous blood sample.** In the laboratory the lymphocytes will be cultured and incubated with substances designed to stimulate T and B lymphocytes. The uptake of radioactive thymidine by the cells indicates they are working.

BEFORE THE TEST

No special preparation is required.

AFTER THE TEST

Follow **venous blood sample** aftercare.

SIGNIFICANCE OF RESULTS

A low lymphocyte transformation rate is seen in AIDS, the DiGeorge syndrome, Wiskott-Aldrich syndrome, combined immunodeficiency, sarcoidosis, lymphomas, burns, chemotherapy, malnutrition, and in the aged. Because this test is nonspecific it has largely been replaced by **lymphocyte typing**.

□ □ □

□ Lymphocyte typing

WHAT IT IS AND WHY IT'S OBTAINED

Lymphocytes are white blood cells which are crucial to the immune system. Lymphocyte typing is used to evaluate the immune system and to classify leukemias and lymphomas (cancer of the lymphatics).

HOW IT WORKS

You will be asked to provide a **venous blood sample** from which serum* will be separated. Flow cytometry* and a variety of other methods are used to determine the lymphocyte subsets.

BEFORE THE TEST

No special preparation is required.

AFTER THE TEST

Follow **venous blood sample** aftercare.

SIGNIFICANCE OF RESULTS

There are at least fifty types of lymphocyte, each with its own function in the immune system. One of these types, CD4, has been found to be deficient in AIDS. Counts of CD4 lymphocytes, therefore, are valuable in determining the course and outlook in AIDS and are often used in treatment decisions. The interpretation should take into consideration the specific disease being evaluated.

SYNONYMS AND INCLUDED TESTS

Immunodeficiency profile, lymphocyte subset enumeration, T- and B-cell count.

□ □ □

□ Magnesium

WHAT IT IS AND WHY IT'S OBTAINED

Magnesium is a mineral which is particularly important to the nerves and muscles. Blood levels are obtained when magnesium deficiency or toxicity is suspected. The symptoms of low magnesium include twitching, tremors, muscle cramps, seizures, or unexplained irregularities of the heartbeat. High magnesium produces muscle weakness, sweating, low blood pressure, and flushing of the skin.

HOW IT WORKS

You will be asked to provide a **venous blood sample** from which serum* will be separated. Spectrophotometry* and other methods of analysis are available. Urine levels may also be obtained. For this purpose you will be asked to provide a **24-hour urine sample.**

BEFORE THE TEST

Avoid antacids or laxatives which contain magnesium.

AFTER THE TEST

Follow **venous blood sample** aftercare.

SIGNIFICANCE OF RESULTS

Low magnesium is found in malnutrition, alcoholism, diabetes, intestinal malabsorption (in which the intestines fail to absorb nutrients properly), an overactive parathyroid gland (hyperparathyroidism), pregnancy, and kidney dialysis. High magnesium is seen in kidney failure, Addison's disease, and increased intake in the form of products which contain magnesium.

□ □ □

□ Magnetic resonance imaging

WHAT IT IS AND WHY IT'S OBTAINED

Magnetic resonance imaging (MRI) can be used to produce images of virtually any area of the body, such as the abdomen, chest, skull, bones, and heart. It is most valuable in providing clear views of the brain and spinal cord. Like **computed tomography** the pictures are multiple cross sections which can produce a three-dimensional effect. The popularity of the MRI stems from its safety, since no X rays are involved. It cannot replace conventional X rays, however, because of certain limitations, foremost of which is that metal reacts unfavorably within the MRI device. Thus, if you have had recent surgery in which some form of metallic device was placed in your body, such as a heart valve or clip to stop the flow of blood, the object may become dislodged. Furthermore, you cannot have an MRI if you have a cardiac pacemaker.

HOW IT WORKS

The principle of MRI relies upon the properties of the hydrogen nucleus, since hydrogen in water is present everywhere in the body. The technique involves aligning all the hydrogen atoms in your body in the same direction by putting you into an intense magnetic field. Radio waves are then transmitted into your body, causing the hydrogen nuclei to spin. When the radio waves are stopped, the hydrogen nuclei emit their own radio waves which are sensed and processed by a computer. The MRI study is conducted by placing you into an enclosed structure, of which there are various types. Previously these were very small and unsuitable to those weighing more than about 300 pounds, but larger models and more open models have been developed. Unless you have severe claustrophobia, being inside the machine is not uncomfortable. The apparatus whines and clanks loudly as it works but the test is painless. You should remain as still as possible during each scan to avoid blurred images. There are a number of modifications of the MRI. These include the "magnetic resonance angiogram," in which a contrast agent which outlines blood vessels is injected intravenously. Another modification is "magnetic resonance spectroscopy," in which chemicals are injected and imaged as they are metabolized. "Diffusion-perfusion imaging" requires a stronger magnetic field and provides rapid diagnosis of strokes. The "neurogram" shows nerves as three-dimensional structures. "Fast MRI" shows a picture of the blood as it flows through the circulation.

BEFORE THE TEST

You will be asked detailed questions regarding previous surgery and medical conditions, all with the idea that the presence of any kind of metal either on or in your body can produce disastrous results. This includes jewelry, metallic foreign bodies, surgically implanted metallic devices, pacemakers, or prosthetic heart valves. Shrapnel wounds, bullets, and orthopedic prostheses usually do not present a problem unless they are in the area to be scanned, in which case the image may be poor. You will also be scanned for metal prior to the study. Tell your doctor if you are particularly claustrophobic, in which case you will be given a mild sedative. The reason for this is that image quality suffers if you move during the scanning process.

AFTER THE TEST

No special aftercare is needed. If you received a contrast agent you may experience an allergic reaction which may range from mild to severe, but reactions are extremely rare. If you develop a rash, itching, or shortness of breath you should contact your doctor.

SIGNIFICANCE OF RESULTS

Interpreting an MRI is done both by the radiologist and your doctor, although once you have an idea of the anatomy involved and are oriented properly, abnormalities can be seen clearly by anyone. It is most useful in giving an accurate picture and location of growths which may be present. When performed with a contrast agent or with the "fast" technique on the heart, abnormalities in the walls, valves, and blood vessels may be revealed. MRI of the brain may show areas of decreased blood flow from a stroke or the site of bleeding in the case of a cerebral hemorrhage.

SYNONYMS AND INCLUDED TESTS

Magnetic resonance scan.

□ □ □

□ Malaria smear

WHAT IT IS AND WHY IT'S OBTAINED

This test is used to diagnose malaria.

HOW IT WORKS

You will be asked to provide a **venous blood sample** or **fingerstick blood sample** which will be smeared on a microscope slide. It will be stained and examined under a microscope for organisms within the red blood cells.

BEFORE THE TEST

Blood should be obtained just before a fever spike is anticipated. This is often possible because of the episodic nature of fever in malaria.

AFTER THE TEST

Follow **venous blood sample** or **fingerstick blood sample** aftercare.

SIGNIFICANCE OF RESULTS

A positive result confirms the diagnosis of malaria and usually can differentiate between the four types of parasite *Plasmodium* which cause it: *vivax, falciparum, ovale,* and *malariae.*

□ □ □

□ Mammogram

WHAT IT IS AND WHY IT'S OBTAINED

The mammogram is an **X ray** for detecting breast cancer. Current recommendations for routine screening mammography in women are: one study between the ages of thirty-five and thirty-nine, one every one to two years between the ages of forty and forty-nine, and one every year thereafter.

HOW IT WORKS

You will be seated in a chair with one of your breasts resting upon the X-ray table. A plate will then compress your breast and the X ray will be taken. The machine will be rotated and the same process repeated from the side. The other breast will be tested the same way. The degree of discomfort from breast compression will vary depending upon the size of your breasts but is temporary.

BEFORE THE TEST

Cleanse the skin of your breasts and armpits with soap and water and dry thoroughly. Avoid talcum powder and deodorants because they may cause shadows to appear on the X-ray film.

AFTER THE TEST

No special aftercare is needed.

SIGNIFICANCE OF RESULTS

A negative mammogram means that no suspicious lesions were found. Mammography, like any other test, is not foolproof, and a **breast biopsy** is needed to confirm whether a suspicious area is benign or malignant. High-definition **ultrasound** can be used to gain more information prior to biopsy.

SYNONYMS AND INCLUDED TESTS

Breast X ray.

□ □ □

□ Manganese

WHAT IT IS AND WHY IT'S OBTAINED

Manganese is a metal which is essential to many enzymes in the body. Blood levels are used to diagnose manganese toxicity, which may cause nausea, vomiting, headache, and psychiatric disturbances.

HOW IT WORKS

You will be asked to provide a **venous blood sample** with special metal-free equipment. Laboratory measurement is by spectrophotometry*. Urine may also be tested, usually with a **24-hour urine sample.**

BEFORE THE TEST

No special preparation is required.

AFTER THE TEST

Follow **venous blood sample** aftercare.

SIGNIFICANCE OF RESULTS

High manganese occurs in industrial exposure and after liver transplantation (due to decreased excretion). Some water supplies are contaminated with it. The nerve damage may be permanent.

□ □ □

□ Metanephrines

WHAT IT IS AND WHY IT'S OBTAINED

Metanephrines are waste products of epinephrine (adrenalin) and norepinephrine, hormones which are produced by the adrenal gland as part of the "flight or fight" response to stress. Large amounts of these substances may be produced by certain tumors which characteristically cause "crises" — headache, palpitations, or perspiration—because of bouts of high blood pressure. Urine metanephrine levels are used to diagnose those tumors.

HOW IT WORKS

You will be asked to provide a **24-hour urine sample** which should be kept refrigerated during collection. Rather than beginning your collection at 8 A.M., however, it is better to start with a "crisis," and collect urine for the next twenty-four hours. Chromatography* is used for the laboratory analysis.

BEFORE THE TEST

Avoid excessive physical activity and stress during the collection period. Check with your doctor for any medications which may influence the test.

AFTER THE TEST

Resume normal activity and medications.

SIGNIFICANCE OF RESULTS

High urine metanephrines strongly suggest pheochromocytoma. **Catecholamines** or **vanillylmandelic acid** may be used to confirm the results.

◻ ◻ ◻

◻ Methemoglobin

WHAT IT IS AND WHY IT'S OBTAINED

Methemoglobin is a chemical form of **hemoglobin** that cannot carry oxygen. Blood levels are used to diagnose methemoglobinemia, which causes blue skin, headache, and difficulty breathing. Death can result.

HOW IT WORKS

You will be asked to provide a **venous blood sample** from which serum* will be separated. Spectrophotometry* is used for the analysis.

BEFORE THE TEST

No special preparation is required.

AFTER THE TEST

Follow **venous blood sample** aftercare.

SIGNIFICANCE OF RESULTS

There are two reasons for high levels of methemoglobin. The first is inherited, either as an enzyme deficiency or as an abnormal form of hemoglobin. The second—and more common—is as a result of drugs or chemicals, such as smoke, car exhausts, aniline dyes, nitrites, nitrates, sulfa drugs, and ferrous sulfate.

□ □ □

□ Methylene blue stain

WHAT IT IS AND WHY IT'S OBTAINED

This test is used to evaluate diarrhea.

HOW IT WORKS

You will be asked to provide a **stool specimen,** a portion of which will be smeared on a glass slide and stained. It will then be examined under a microscope for the presence of white blood cells.

BEFORE THE TEST

No special preparation is required.

AFTER THE TEST

No special aftercare is needed.

SIGNIFICANCE OF RESULTS

A positive test is associated with diarrhea due to bacteria, such as *Shigella, Salmonella, Helicobacter,* and *Yersinia.* The methylene blue stain in diarrhea due to viruses, toxins, or parasites is usually negative. **Bacterial culture** may demonstrate the specific organism. Ulcerative colitis produces a positive test, but symptoms and other signs are usually different from bacterial diarrhea.

SYNONYMS AND INCLUDED TESTS

Stool for white cells.

□ □ □

□ **Metyrapone test**

WHAT IT IS AND WHY IT'S OBTAINED

Metyrapone is a substance which blocks **cortisol** production by the adrenal gland. If it is given to a normal individual, cortisol production goes down, but one of the precursors to cortisol, 11-deoxycortisol, goes up. Since this sequence depends upon a functioning pituitary gland and "feedback" between it and the adrenal gland, metyrapone can be used to test how well the pituitary gland and the adrenal gland are interacting with each other. It is mainly used to evaluate Cushing's syndrome, which is caused by an overactive adrenal and which can cause obesity, "moon face," diabetes, and acne, among other symptoms.

HOW IT WORKS

You will be given an oral dose of metyrapone to be taken at night. The next morning you will be asked to provide **venous blood sample.** This will be analyzed in the laboratory by immunoassay* for 11-deoxycortisol and cortisol. **Adrenocorticotropic hormone** may also be measured.

BEFORE THE TEST

Other tests, for example the **cosyntropin test,** are done first to make certain that your adrenal glands are functioning. If they are not, metyrapone might be dangerous because of the further decrease in cortisol production.

298

AFTER THE TEST

Follow **venous blood sample** aftercare. Metyrapone may cause nausea, abdominal pain, headache, fatigue, and low blood pressure. Allergic reactions such as hives may also occur.

SIGNIFICANCE OF RESULTS

Since this test is always performed as part of a battery of tests designed to test the endocrine system, interpretion must take the other results into consideration. In general, if this test was done to discover the cause of Cushing's syndrome, an increase in 11-deoxycortisol suggests the presence of a tumor of the pituitary, whereas no increase in 11-deoxycortisol suggests the presence of a tumor of the adrenal gland.

□ □ □

□ Mixed lymphocyte culture

WHAT IT IS AND WHY IT'S OBTAINED

The mixed lymphocyte culture is used to match donors and recipients for organ transplantation.

HOW IT WORKS

If you are to be an organ recipient you will be asked to provide a **venous blood sample.** The proposed donor will also provide a blood sample, and lymphocytes (a type of white blood cell) from both of your samples will be mixed together. If the donor is a good match your lymphocytes will not become stimulated. The way this is measured is by inactivating the donor's lymphocytes and adding a radioactive compound to the mixture. If your cells become activated they will pick up the radioactivity.

BEFORE THE TEST

No special preparation is required.

AFTER THE TEST

Follow **venous blood sample** aftercare.

SIGNIFICANCE OF RESULTS

A low degree of stimulation of your cells indicates a good match and increased organ survival.

□ □ □

□ Molybdenum

WHAT IT IS AND WHY IT'S OBTAINED

Although the trace element molybdenum is important to several enzymes in the body, diseases caused by its deficiency or excess are very rare. Blood levels are occasionally obtained to evaluate nutritional status and to diagnose molybdenum toxicity, which may produce liver disease, kidney disease, and arthritis.

HOW IT WORKS

You will be asked to provide a **venous blood sample** with special metal-free equipment. The serum* will be separated and atomic absorption will be used for the assay.

BEFORE THE TEST

No special preparation is required.

AFTER THE TEST

Follow **venous blood sample** aftercare.

SIGNIFICANCE OF RESULTS

The interpretation of high or low molybdenum blood levels is still being studied, since this test is relatively new and infrequently used. Overexposure may occur in certain industries or in certain geographical locations with a high content of the element in the soil.

□ □ □

□ Myelogram

WHAT IT IS AND WHY IT'S OBTAINED

A myelogram is an **X-ray contrast study** designed to visualize the spinal cord. It is used to evaluate symptoms such as numbness, pain, or muscle weakness which may be caused by nerve compression.

HOW IT WORKS

This test is conducted in a procedure room with surgical and X-ray equipment. You will be asked to lie on your side, to flex your back as much as possible, to place your chin on your chest, and to draw your knees to your chest. A site over your lower back will be cleansed with an antiseptic and you will feel a burning sensation as the area is anesthetized using a local anesthetic. A needle will then be inserted between two vertebrae, usually with the aid of fluoroscopy*. Some spinal fluid may be removed for analysis as in a **spinal tap.** You will then be asked to move carefully to a face-down position and straps will be used to hold you in place. You will also be asked to tilt your head backward as far as you can. The X-ray contrast agent will then be injected and you may feel a pressure in your back or neck. These symptoms may recur when the study is started. The head of the table is then slowly tilted downward to allow the dye to move toward your head as X rays are taken. Fluoroscopy will be used to prevent the dye from entering the space around your brain.

BEFORE THE TEST

You should take nothing by mouth for several hours; follow instructions given by the laboratory or your doctor. Discon-

tinue medications as directed, especially drugs in the phenothiazine class (such as Thorazine and Compazine).

AFTER THE TEST

You will be placed on strict bed rest with your head elevated
for at least twelve hours during which time your vital signs
(pulse, blood pressure, respiration, and temperature) will be
monitored. Drink plenty of fluids to avoid dehydration.
Backache, headache, vomiting, neck stiffness, and fever
may occur. Meningitis and seizures are also possible.

SIGNIFICANCE OF RESULTS

A myelogram may detect tumors, herniated disks, bone
spurs, and injuries. **Computed tomography** and **magnetic
resonance imaging** are non invasive techniques which may
be very helpful in localizing abnormalities of the spinal
cord.

□ □ □

□ Myoglobin

WHAT IT IS AND WHY IT'S OBTAINED

Myoglobin is a **protein** found in muscle which is released
when muscle is injured. Blood levels are mainly used to help
diagnose recent heart attacks.

HOW IT WORKS

You will be asked to provide a **venous blood sample** from
which serum* will be separated. Immunoassay* is used for
the laboratory analysis.

BEFORE THE TEST

No special preparation is required.

AFTER THE TEST

Follow **venous blood sample** aftercare.

Blood myoglobin is one of the earliest laboratory signs of a heart attack. It begins to rise about an hour after the attack and reaches its highest level within twelve hours. It is very sensitive, but not specific, because elevations may be seen after injections, strenuous exercise, or other muscle injury. High myoglobin also occurs with kidney failure, shock, and after heart surgery. The diagnosis of heart attacks must be made in conjunction with other tests, such as the **electrocardiogram, lactic dehydrogenase,** and **creatine kinase.**

□ □ □

□ Nailfold capillary microscopy

WHAT IT IS AND WHY IT'S OBTAINED

This test is used to evaluate autoimmune diseases (in which the immune system reacts against the body's own tissues).

HOW IT WORKS

A drop of oil will be placed on the skin around one or more of your fingernails. A variety of devices can be used to enlarge the view, such as microscopes or magnifying glasses. The skin is observed for abnormalities of the capillaries.

BEFORE THE TEST

No special preparation is required.

AFTER THE TEST

No special aftercare is needed.

SIGNIFICANCE OF RESULTS

Certain abnormal findings in the skin capillaries, such as widening, reduction in number, disrupted architecture, or hemorrhage, are associated with the development of scleroderma, in which the skin becomes hard and inelastic. Normal findings indicate a more benign course.

□ □ □

□ Nasal endoscopy

WHAT IT IS AND WHY IT'S OBTAINED

Nasal endoscopy is used to examine the nose and throat and to evaluate nasal discharge, postnasal drip, nosebleeds, sinus infections, difficulty breathing, and snoring. Many ear, nose, and throat specialists consider this to be a routine part of their examination.

HOW IT WORKS

You will be seated in an examining chair and an anesthetic mixture may be sprayed into your nostrils and back of your throat. You may also be asked to gargle with an anesthetic. A small flexible tube with a magnifying eyepiece will be inserted into one nostril and advanced slowly backward, then downward into your throat. This is not painful and rarely causes gagging unless you are extremely sensitive. When the examination through one nostril is completed the tube is withdrawn and inserted into the other nostril, with the same procedure being repeated. This test is for examination only; the tube is too small to permit biopsy or cauterization.

BEFORE THE TEST

Avoid aspirin for at least a week and ibuprofen, ketoprofen, or naproxen for one day.

AFTER THE TEST

Do not eat or drink until your gag reflex returns. Your nose and throat may be sore for one or two days. Although rare, complications include nosebleeds, swelling and closure

of the voicebox or bronchial tubes, fainting, and arrhythmia*.

SIGNIFICANCE OF RESULTS

Visible abnormalities may include a deviated nasal septum,
polyps, cysts, tumors, ulcers, and abscesses. Further testing
by means of **X ray, computed tomography, magnetic resonance imaging,** or biopsy may be indicated.

□ □ □

□ Nerve conduction studies

WHAT IT IS AND WHY IT'S OBTAINED

Nerve conduction studies are used to diagnose nerve diseases and to distinguish between nerve and muscle disease.
When not functioning well, both muscles and nerves can
cause similar symptoms, such as muscle weakness or pain.

HOW IT WORKS

The testing procedure varies slightly from laboratory to
laboratory, but the general principle is the same: to stimulate a nerve at one point with an electrical current and then
to detect the current at another point. Both the velocity and
the character of the conduction will be noted. The test is
usually performed in a special laboratory in a hospital,
clinic, or private doctor's office. You will be asked either to
sit in a chair or lie down on an examining table. The skin
over the nerve to be tested will be cleansed and an electrode
pressed against it, although some laboratories use small
needles, which are slightly uncomfortable. The experience
you will have depends upon the specific nerve being tested,
but is only mildly uncomfortable; you will sense a mild
electric shock when the stimulus is being applied. It is usual
to test each nerve at more than one site. If your problem is
localized, only the nerves in that area need testing, but if
your symptoms are more generalized, multiple sites may be
evaluated.

BEFORE THE TEST

No special preparation is required. There is some controversy regarding the use of nerve conduction studies if you have a cardiac pacemaker, especially if testing is to be performed on the chest. Discuss this with your doctor.

AFTER THE TEST

No special aftercare is needed.

SIGNIFICANCE OF RESULTS

Normal nerve conduction studies usually rule out nerve disease. If the studies are abnormal, the pattern will often suggest whether the problem is in the nerve fiber itself (axon) or in its covering (myelin sheath).

SYNONYMS AND INCLUDED TESTS

Nerve conduction velocity.

□ □ □

□ Neuron-specific enolase

WHAT IT IS AND WHY IT'S OBTAINED

Neuron-specific enolase is an enzyme found in nerve tissue. Blood levels are used to diagnose or monitor treatment of tumors derived from nerve tissue.

HOW IT WORKS

You will be asked to provide a **venous blood sample** from which serum* will be separated. Immunoassay* is used for the laboratory analysis.

BEFORE THE TEST

No special preparation is required.

AFTER THE TEST

Follow **venous blood sample** aftercare.

SIGNIFICANCE OF RESULTS

High levels are seen in certain tumors such as neuroblastoma and small cell carcinoma of the lung. Its level generally corresponds to the severity of the illness. It is not specific, however, since elevations also occur in kidney failure and other tumors.

☐ ☐ ☐

☐ Nitroblue tetrazolium test

WHAT IT IS AND WHY IT'S OBTAINED

The nitroblue tetrazolium test is used to study the function of white blood cells, specifically to evaluate recurrent infections in childhood.

HOW IT WORKS

A **venous blood sample** is obtained and incubated with nitroblue tetrazolium dye. Adequately functioning white blood cells (neutrophils) will change the color of the dye.

BEFORE THE TEST

No special preparation is required.

AFTER THE TEST

Follow **venous blood sample** aftercare.

SIGNIFICANCE OF RESULTS

A positive test signifies chronic granulomatous disease of childhood, an inherited disease, but the test is prone to many false positives and false negatives, especially in the presence of some infections and cancer. Chronic granulomatous disease of childhood can be diagnosed using **DNA probe testing.**

SYNONYMS AND INCLUDED TESTS

NBT test.

□ □ □

□ 5′ nucleotidase

WHAT IT IS AND WHY IT'S OBTAINED

5′ nucleotidase is an enzyme found in the liver. Blood levels are used to evaluate an elevated **alkaline phosphatase.**

HOW IT WORKS

You will be asked to provide a **venous blood sample** from which serum* will be separated. Several methods are available for the laboratory assay.

BEFORE THE TEST

You should fast overnight.

AFTER THE TEST

Follow **venous blood sample** aftercare.

SIGNIFICANCE OF RESULTS

5′ nucleotidase is elevated in diseases of the liver but normal in diseases of bone, thus helping to distinguish between the two major causes of an elevated **alkaline phosphatase.** Blood **gamma glutamyl transferase,** however, provides similar information, and the 5′ nucleotidase test is seldom used.

□ □ □

☐ Ophthalmoscopy

WHAT IT IS AND WHY IT'S OBTAINED

Ophthalmoscopy is used to examine the retina of the eye. A small, handheld instrument is usually employed as part of a routine physical examination, whereas eye specialists (ophthalmologists) often employ a more sophisticated device, called an indirect ophthalmoscope.

HOW IT WORKS

You will be seated in a chair in a darkened room and will probably have had eyedrops instilled to dilate your pupils as much as possible. The examiner will shine a light from the ophthalmoscope into each eye in turn while you are looking straight ahead. You will hear a clicking sound as the lenses within the instrument are adjusted and the light brought very close to your eye. You will be asked to look in different directions in order for the examiner to look at each section of your retina. Indirect ophthalmoscopy is somewhat different in that the light is part of a device that the examiner wears on his head while holding a lens close to your eye. The light in this case is much brighter and may cause some temporary discomfort.

BEFORE THE TEST

No special preparation is required.

AFTER THE TEST

If eyedrops have been instilled your vision will be blurry for a few hours. Some doctors instill another drop which will reverse the dilation, usually within an hour. These drops may sting when instilled.

SIGNIFICANCE OF RESULTS

A number of eye disorders can be diagnosed with this test, including blood vessel disease caused by high blood pressure or diabetes, an inflamed optic nerve, a damaged optic nerve as is found in glaucoma, swelling of the optic disk from increased pressure within the skull, and retinal holes, tears, or detachment. Even AIDS may sometimes be suspected based upon this examination. Blood vessel diseases may be further studied with **fluorescein angiography.**

□ □ □

□ Osmolality

WHAT IT IS AND WHY IT'S OBTAINED

The osmolality of a solution is a measure of how concentrated it is. Blood osmolality is used to evaluate acid-base balance and the state of hydration. It is useful in cases of unexplained coma. Urine osmolality is used to measure kidney function.

HOW IT WORKS

For blood osmolality you will be asked to provide a **venous blood sample** from which serum* will be separated. For urine a random or timed urine specimen is obtained. In either event, freezing point depression is most often used for the assay.

BEFORE THE TEST

No special preparation is required.

AFTER THE TEST

Follow **venous blood sample** aftercare for the blood test.

SIGNIFICANCE OF RESULTS

High *blood* osmolality is found in excessive salt intake, dehydration, increased blood sugar, kidney failure, very low birth weight infants, and alcohol poisoning. Low *blood* osmolality is seen in excessive fluid intake and the syndrome of inappropriate secretion of antidiuretic hormone, which sometimes occurs in lung cancer. Low *urine* osmolality means that the kidneys are having difficulty in concentrating urine. High *urine* osmolality is seen in dehydration.

□ □ □

□ Osmotic fragility

WHAT IT IS AND WHY IT'S OBTAINED

Osmosis is the movement of water across a membrane. In the osmotic fragility test osmosis is used to measure the strength of the red blood cell membrane to evaluate anemia.

HOW IT WORKS

You will be asked to provide a **venous blood sample** which will be incubated with varying dilutions of saline. The degree of red blood cell breakup (hemolysis*) is noted at each dilution.

BEFORE THE TEST

No special preparation is required.

AFTER THE TEST

Follow **venous blood sample** aftercare.

SIGNIFICANCE OF RESULTS

Increased osmotic fragility is seen in hereditary spherocytosis (in which the red blood cells are spheres rather than disks) and some other anemias in which red blood cells are disrupted (hemolytic anemias). Decreased osmotic fragility is found in iron deficiency anemia, thalassemia, and sickle cell anemia.

□ □ □

☐ Otoscopy

WHAT IT IS AND WHY IT'S OBTAINED

Otoscopy is used to examine the ear canal and eardrum. It should be a part of every complete physical examination.

HOW IT WORKS

Your ear will be pulled upward and backward while the tip of the otoscope is gently inserted into your ear canal. The otoscope is a device with a light source, a conical tube, magnifying lens, and, sometimes, an air bulb and hose. The examiner will look through the instrument and possibly blow a small amount of air through it to see how well your eardrum moves.

BEFORE THE TEST

No special preparation is required.

AFTER THE TEST

No special aftercare is needed.

SIGNIFICANCE OF RESULTS

Abnormal findings may include inflammation (otitis), foreign bodies, a perforated or scarred eardrum, tumors, fluid collections, or excessive wax buildup.

☐ ☐ ☐

☐ Oxalate

WHAT IT IS AND WHY IT'S OBTAINED

Oxalate is a waste product which, with calcium, forms the most common type of kidney stone. The amount of oxalate in the urine is used to evaluate kidney stone formation.

312

HOW IT WORKS

You will be asked to provide a **24-hour urine sample** specimen. Chromatography* and other methods are available for laboratory measurement.

BEFORE THE TEST

No special preparation is required.

AFTER THE TEST

No special aftercare is needed.

SIGNIFICANCE OF RESULTS

High urine oxalate is sometimes found with increased dietary intake of beans, beets, chocolate, cocoa, green pepper, rhubarb, okra, spinach, berries, tea, and nuts. It is also elevated in malabsorption (in which the intestines fail to absorb nutrients properly), in poisoning with antifreeze solutions (ethylene glycol), and in the rare hereditary disease called primary hyperoxaluria.

□ □ □

□ Pancreatic peptide

WHAT IT IS AND WHY IT'S OBTAINED

Pancreatic peptide (PP) is a hormone produced by the pancreas. Blood levels are used to diagnose certain tumors of the pancreas which release increased amounts of it.

HOW IT WORKS

You will be asked to provide a **venous blood sample** from which serum* will be separated. Immunoassay* is used for the laboratory analysis. Two studies are done, one fasting and the other after you have eaten. You may also be given the drug atropine in a suppression test.

BEFORE THE TEST

You should fast overnight. Follow the instructions of your doctor or the laboratory regarding food intake for the second test.

AFTER THE TEST

Follow **venous blood sample** aftercare.

SIGNIFICANCE OF RESULTS

High PP is found in certain tumors of the pancreas as well as in kidney failure, hypoglycemia, diabetes, and after eating. Because PP is not specific, other studies are often indicated in evaluating suspected tumors of the pancreas, including **glucagon, gastrin,** and **vasoactive intestinal peptide.**

□ □ □

□ Pap smear

WHAT IT IS AND WHY IT'S OBTAINED

The Pap smear is the most common medical test using **cytology.** It is mainly used to screen for cancer and precancerous conditions of the cervix, but it is also used to diagnose vaginal infections. Pap smears should be obtained every year if you are a woman of childbearing age. If you are taking birth control pills or other hormones your gynecologist may suggest one every six months.

HOW IT WORKS

A Pap smear is often performed as part of a routine pelvic examination. You will be given a drape and be asked to disrobe from the **waist** down. Leave your shoes on since it is more comfortable. **You** will be asked to lie on a table on your back and to place your feet in stirrups. Bring your buttocks as far down toward the edge of the table as you can since it makes the procedure easier. A metal or plastic speculum will then introduced into your vagina. The speculum should not be lubricated but may be moistened with warm water or saline solution to make insertion easier. Using a wooden spatula or cotton swab the cervix or vagina will be scraped and the material transferred to a glass microscope slide and sprayed or dipped into a fixative. It is then transported to the laboratory for microscopic examination.

BEFORE THE TEST

Do not douche or use vaginal suppositories for twenty-four hours before the test. It is best to perform Pap smears between menstrual periods.

AFTER THE TEST

No special aftercare is needed.

SIGNIFICANCE OF RESULTS

Pap smears are examined and interpreted by pathologists or trained and licensed technicians. Formerly, the results of Pap smears were given as classes 1 through 5, with 1 being normal, and 5 being cancer, but recently the "Bethesda System" has become more common. The most benign category, formerly category 1, is called "within normal limits," and the most malignant category, formerly 5, has been broken down and further described by specifying the type of cancer. The intermediate classifications refer to grades of dysplasia (irregularity in the appearance of the cells), inflammation, or infection. Infections with herpes, papillomavirus, yeasts, *Trichomonas,* and others may be specified. Recommendations for follow-up of Pap smear results vary among doctors, but a typical program is the following:

Result	Recommendation
Within normal limits	Repeat Pap smear in one year
Inflammation or infection	Confirm the result, treat the underlying condition, and repeat Pap smear
Low-grade dysplasia	Repeat Pap smear in three months
High-grade dysplasia	**Colposcopy** and **cervical punch biopsy**
Cancer	Confirm with biopsy and treat

SYNONYMS AND INCLUDED TESTS

Cervical smear, cervical/vaginal cytology.

□ □ □

◻ Paracentesis

WHAT IT IS AND WHY IT'S OBTAINED

Paracentesis is the withdrawal of excess fluid—called ascites—from the abdominal cavity. It is most commonly used to find the cause of the fluid accumulation and to diagnose infections of the fluid.

HOW IT WORKS

The procedure will be performed in a procedure room or at your bedside if you are in a hospital. You will usually be lying on your back with your head slightly raised, but if only a small amount of fluid is present you may be asked to get on your hands and knees in order for the fluid to collect at its lowest point. The skin just beneath your navel will be cleansed with an antiseptic and injected with a local anesthetic. This will sting or burn slightly. Then a needle on a syringe will be introduced into your abdomen. When fluid is encountered it will be withdrawn and placed in suitable containers for transport to the laboratory. Multiple tests can be performed on the fluid, including **cytology, bacterial culture,** and chemical studies.

BEFORE THE TEST

No special preparation is required.

AFTER THE TEST

You will be placed on bed rest and your vital signs (pulse, blood pressure, respiration, and temperature) will be taken until they are stable. This is generally a safe procedure but there have been instances of perforation of the liver, spleen, intestines, or a blood vessel. Infection of the ascites fluid may occur.

SIGNIFICANCE OF RESULTS

The presence of fluid in the abdomen—ascites—is always abnormal. Although ascites is almost always caused by severe liver disease, there are other diseases which can produce it, including heart failure, kidney failure, and cancer. Analysis of fluid obtained by paracentesis can help distinguish among these problems. A positive **bacterial culture** is particularly helpful in detecting the disease called spontaneous bacterial peritonitis.

SYNONYMS AND INCLUDED TESTS

Ascites fluid tap.

☐ ☐ ☐

☐ Parasite antibodies

WHAT IT IS AND WHY IT'S OBTAINED

A parasite is a living creature, usually an animal such as a tapeworm, which lives inside the body. Blood levels of antibody to a parasite measure the response of the immune system to such infestations. A variety of creatures can be tested for in this manner.

HOW IT WORKS

You will be asked to provide a **venous blood sample** from which serum* will be separated. Several methods of immunoassay* may be used for the laboratory analysis.

BEFORE THE TEST

No special preparation is required.

AFTER THE TEST

Follow **venous blood sample** aftercare.

SIGNIFICANCE OF RESULTS

The presence of antibody to a specific parasite, and in particular a rise in the concentration (titer) of that antibody suggests the presence of the parasite. As with all antibody tests, however, a positive test does not prove infestation, since the same antibody will often react to several organisms. A negative test, similarly, does not disprove a diagnosis, because unless the parasite has actually invaded living tissue no response of the immune system is possible. Intestinal parasites can be diagnosed with **stool for ova and parasites.**

□ □ □

□ Parathyroid hormone

WHAT IT IS AND WHY IT'S OBTAINED

Parathyroid hormone (PTH) is produced by the parathyroid glands in the neck and acts upon the bones, kidneys, and intestines to increase blood **calcium**. Blood levels of PTH are used to evaluate the parathyroid, particularly when there is a high blood calcium.

HOW IT WORKS

You will be asked to provide a **venous blood sample** from which serum* will be separated. Several methods are available for the analysis. Several forms of PTH circulate in the blood and to be most accurate a "two-site" analysis is performed.

BEFORE THE TEST

You should fast overnight.

AFTER THE TEST

Follow **venous blood sample** aftercare.

SIGNIFICANCE OF RESULTS

A blood **calcium** is necessary to evaluate PTH results. In *primary* hyperparathyroidism (caused by benign or malignant enlargement of the parathyroids), PTH is high and calcium is normal or high. In *secondary* hyperparathyroidism (caused by kidney disease, vitamin D deficiency, or failure to absorb calcium properly), PTH is high and calcium is low. If calcium is high and PTH is normal, the problem is not parathyroid gland dysfunction. In hypoparathyroidism (usually caused by surgical removal of the parathyroid glands), both PTH and calcium are low.

SYNONYMS AND INCLUDED TESTS

Parathormone.

□ □ □

□ Parathyroid scan

WHAT IT IS AND WHY IT'S OBTAINED

This is a type of **radionuclide scan** designed to visualize the parathyroid glands located in the neck. It is usually obtained to evaluate overactive parathyroids, which may cause hyperparathyroidism. Parathyroid diseases often involve abnormal **calcium** metabolism.

HOW IT WORKS

The test is carried out in the nuclear medicine laboratory of a hospital, clinic, or private physician's office, sometimes as part of a radiology facility. You will be given an intravenous injection of two radioactive tracer compounds, the first based on thallium and the second based on technetium. The vein puncture is usually only mildly uncomfortable. The two compounds are needed for a "subtraction technique" to differentiate parathyroid from thyroid* tissue. After a short time your neck will be scanned with a computer-driven device called a gamma camera that detects the compound's radioactive emissions. The actual scanning is painless and takes about fifteen minutes. You should try to remain as still as possible. This part of the test is painless.

BEFORE THE TEST

No special preparation is required.

AFTER THE TEST

No special aftercare is needed. Although safe, this test does involve the injection of a radioactive compound.

SIGNIFICANCE OF RESULTS

An abnormal result will generally fall into one of two categories: *diffuse* increased function of the parathyroids or *localized* increased function in one gland. These findings are particularly useful in planning surgery for removal and testing of the diseased portions. Thyroid diseases, however, can interfere with obtaining good images.

□ □ □

☐ Parietal cell antibody

WHAT IT IS AND WHY IT'S OBTAINED

Parietal cells are located in the stomach and produce hydrochloric acid. Blood levels of antibodies to them are used to evaluate anemia and diseases of the stomach.

HOW IT WORKS

You will be asked to provide a **venous blood sample** from which serum* will be separated. Immunoassay* is used for the laboratory analysis.

BEFORE THE TEST

No special preparation is required.

AFTER THE TEST

Follow **venous blood sample** aftercare.

SIGNIFICANCE OF RESULTS

Parietal cell antibodies are found in pernicious anemia, chronic gastritis, stomach ulcers, stomach cancer, and auto-immune diseases (in which the immune system reacts against the body's own tissues).

SYNONYMS AND INCLUDED TESTS

Antiparietal cell antibody.

☐ ☐ ☐

☐ Paroxysmal cold hemoglobinuria test

WHAT IT IS AND WHY IT'S OBTAINED

This test is used to diagnose a rare type of anemia called paroxysmal cold hemoglobinuria (PCH).

HOW IT WORKS

You will be asked to provide a **venous blood sample** from which serum* will be separated. The serum* is chilled, remixed with your red blood cells, and observed for breakdown (hemolysis*) of those cells.

BEFORE THE TEST

No special preparation is required.

AFTER THE TEST

Follow **venous blood sample** aftercare.

SIGNIFICANCE OF RESULTS

A positive result indicates PCH, which may be seen with syphilis or viral illnesses.

SYNONYMS AND INCLUDED TESTS

Cold hemolysin test.

□ □ □

□ Partial thromboplastin time

WHAT IT IS AND WHY IT'S OBTAINED

The partial thromboplastin time (PTT) is a screening test for bleeding disorders. It is used most often before surgery and in monitoring treatment with blood thinners (anticoagulants, particularly heparin). It is most useful when obtained with a **prothrombin time** and **platelet count**.

HOW IT WORKS

You will be asked to provide a **venous blood sample** from which plasma* will be separated. The plasma is incubated with an activator, after which thromboplastin and calcium are added and a timer is started. The timing stops with the formation of a clot. A handheld device using a **fingerstick blood sample** is available.

BEFORE THE TEST

No special preparation is required.

AFTER THE TEST

Follow **venous blood sample** aftercare.

SIGNIFICANCE OF RESULTS

A long PTT is seen generally in bleeding disorders from "intrinsic factor" deficiencies of the blood clotting system—factors VIII, IX, XI, and XII (see **coagulation factor screen**)—which include the most common type of hemophilia, and with heparin treatment. Other defects in the clotting system, however, if severe enough, will also prolong the PTT.

SYNONYMS AND INCLUDED TESTS

Activated partial thromboplastin time, APTT.

□ □ □

□ Patch test

WHAT IT IS AND WHY IT'S OBTAINED

Patch tests are used to diagnose contact dermatitis, a disease in which the skin becomes inflamed as a result of direct contact with some external substance. The best example of contact dermatitis is poison ivy, but many other possibilities exist, such as nickel metal in jewelry, rubber in gloves, preservatives in lotions, and fragrances in cosmetics. Patch testing is usually performed by dermatologists or allergists.

HOW IT WORKS

Several techniques and commercial kits are available. The general principle is to apply suspected chemicals on pieces of paper, gauze, or cellulose in strips on your back. You will remove these yourself (or your doctor may prefer to have you come into the office) in two days. At forty-eight and seventy-two hours you should return to the office for an examination of the sites. Reactions, if any, are graded by severity.

BEFORE THE TEST

No special preparation is required.

AFTER THE TEST

There may be itching for several days if any of the tests were positive. Although this is transient, your doctor will usually give you a topical steroid preparation to reduce symptoms.

SIGNIFICANCE OF RESULTS

The interpretation of patch test results, as with all allergy tests, can be difficult. No test can exactly mimic the conditions required for contact dermatitis to develop. If you have a dermatitis (redness, scaling, itching, or blisters), for example, on both ear lobes and you wear earrings, the odds are overwhelming that you are allergic to nickel. Yet the patch test to nickel may or may not be positive because your back skin is different from your ear skin. The same holds true for allergies to rubber, hair dye, lanolin, benzocaine, and the host of other substances which can produce contact dermatitis.

SYNONYMS AND INCLUDED TESTS

Contact dermatitis skin test.

□ □ □

☐ Pemphigus/pemphigoid antibody

WHAT IT IS AND WHY IT'S OBTAINED

Pemphigus and pemphigoid are severe blistering diseases of the skin. Blood levels of antibody (a blood protein important to the immune system) to various skin components are used to support each diagnosis and to monitor treatment.

HOW IT WORKS

You will be asked to provide a **venous blood sample** from which serum* will be separated. Immunoassay* is used for the laboratory analysis.

BEFORE THE TEST

No special preparation is required.

AFTER THE TEST

Follow **venous blood sample** aftercare.

SIGNIFICANCE OF RESULTS

The antibody in pemphigus is directed against the area between the cells of the epidermis, whereas the antibody in pemphigoid is directed against the membrane beneath the epidermis. Presence of either antibody is strong evidence for the respective disease but a **skin biopsy** is necessary to confirm the diagnosis.

☐ ☐ ☐

☐ Penile blood flow

WHAT IT IS AND WHY IT'S OBTAINED

This test is used to evaluate impotence and is usually obtained if results of **sleep erection monitoring** are abnormal.

HOW IT WORKS

A tiny blood pressure cuff will be wrapped around the base of your penis and the blood flow measured with **ultrasound.** This is uncomfortable, but the discomfort lasts only a short time. If results are normal, the test is repeated after exercise.

BEFORE THE TEST

No special preparation is required.

AFTER THE TEST

No special aftercare is needed.

SIGNIFICANCE OF RESULTS

A normal result is evidence that the cause of your erectile difficulty is not from diseases of the blood vessels. The evaluation of impotence, however, can be difficult and many physical and emotional factors must be taken into consideration. The **penile injection test** may be helpful.

SYNONYMS AND INCLUDED TESTS

Penile Doppler studies.

□ □ □

□ Penile injection test

WHAT IT IS AND WHY IT'S OBTAINED

The penile injection test is used to evaluate impotence (erectile dysfunction).

HOW IT WORKS

This test is performed in a urologist's office. You will be asked to undress from the waist down. One side of your penis will be cleansed with an antiseptic and a small needle will be used to inject a medication into the spongy tissue of your penis. This is moderately uncomfortable. You will be asked to stand and the time it takes for you to get an erection will be observed and recorded, along with its firmness. The substance injected is either a type of prostaglandin (Caverject) or papaverine.

BEFORE THE TEST

No special preparation is required.

AFTER THE TEST

You should remain in the doctor's office until your erection subsides. If it lasts more than several hours, another medication, such as epinephrine, may have to be injected, along with drainage of excess blood. Penile pain occurs often but is transient.

SIGNIFICANCE OF RESULTS

A normal result is the production of a firm erection within a certain amount of time. Absence of an erection suggests an organic cause for your impotence, most likely a blood vessel abnormality, but the results are not definitive.

SYNONYMS AND INCLUDED TESTS

Injection of the corpus cavernosum with pharmacologic agents, papaverine test.

□ □ □

□ Pericardiocentesis

WHAT IT IS AND WHY IT'S OBTAINED

The pericardium is a tough membrane covering the outside of the heart. Under certain circumstances, such as infections or cancer, fluid collects between the heart itself and this membrane and can restrict the pumping action of the heart. This test removes this fluid, called a pericardial effusion, both for testing and treatment. It is highly invasive and some cardiologists recommend that it be employed only in emergencies.

HOW IT WORKS

If you are having this procedure performed you are most likely in a hospital or emergency room. Pericardiocentesis is usually done in a special treatment room or in the cardiac catheterization laboratory by a doctor trained in the technique, usually a cardiologist. Often **right heart catheterization** is performed at the same time and your blood pressure and **electrocardiogram** will be monitored continuosly. An intravenous fluid drip will be running. You will be asked to lie on your back with your head elevated slightly. The skin of your upper abdomen just below your breastbone will be cleansed and injected with a local anesthetic. A larger needle on a syringe will then be inserted and directed toward your left shoulder, sometimes with the aid of an **echocardiogram.** The needle will be advanced until the pericardium is punctured. This should cause no pain. Fluid will then be withdrawn until there is none left. If you have been feeling faint or short of breath because of the fluid you should experience immediate relief. The fluid is sent to the laboratory for **cytology, bacterial culture,** and other studies as indicated.

BEFORE THE TEST

Follow any instructions carefully.

AFTER THE TEST

You will most likely be placed in the intensive care unit in order to monitor your condition carefully. Complications may be serious and include puncture of the heart, laceration of the coronary arteries, collapsed lung, and heartbeat irregularities. Fatalities have occurred.

SIGNIFICANCE OF RESULTS

Analysis of the fluid obtained during this procedure will hopefully determine its cause. Culture may reveal the presence of bacteria, such as that which causes tuberculosis. Cytology may show malignant cells which indicate cancer.

SYNONYMS AND INCLUDED TESTS

Pericardial effusion tap, aspiration of pericardial fluid.

□ □ □

□ **Phenylketonuria screen**

WHAT IT IS AND WHY IT'S OBTAINED

Phenylketonuria (PKU) is a hereditary enzyme deficiency which leads to mental retardation. Prompt diagnosis of PKU and an altered diet can prevent problems from developing. Although newborn screening for this disease is mandatory in most states, the timing of the test is important, since three or four full days of feeding is required to detect a high percentage of cases. Nowadays, however, because of cost controls, many mothers and infants are being discharged before this time, and some cases are slipping through. Since the majority of cases of PKU will still be picked up by earlier testing, the current recommendation is that all infants be screened before discharge from the hospital or soon thereafter.

HOW IT WORKS

A **heelstick blood sample** is obtained and placed on a special piece of paper. The Guthrie test employs a bacterium, *Bacillus subtitlis*, which needs phenylalanine to grow.

BEFORE THE TEST

No special preparation is required.

AFTER THE TEST

Follow **heelstick blood sample** aftercare.

SIGNIFICANCE OF RESULTS

A positive PKU screen is confirmed with blood **phenylalanine** and **tyrosine.** If PKU is present, the former will be high and the latter low. False positive PKU screens sometimes occur in infants who have been given antibiotics, particularly ampicillin.

SYNONYMS AND INCLUDED TESTS

Guthrie test, phenylalanine screen.

□ □ □

□ Phosphate

WHAT IT IS AND WHY IT'S OBTAINED

Phosphate (a salt form of phosphorus) is a major component of bone, where it exists with **calcium.** Blood levels are used to evaluate kidney disease, acid-base balance, and diseases of bone. Urine levels are obtained to investigate calcium-phosphate balance and kidney stones.

HOW IT WORKS

You will be asked to provide a **venous blood sample** or a **24-hour urine sample,** the latter of which should be kept refrigerated during collection. Several methods are used for the analysis.

BEFORE THE TEST

You should fast overnight if the blood test is being taken.

AFTER THE TEST

Follow **venous blood sample** aftercare for the blood test.

SIGNIFICANCE OF RESULTS

Phosphate blood levels must be interpreted along with blood calcium. High *blood* phosphate is found in children, kidney failure, dehydration, hypoparathyroidism, bone disease, excessive vitamin D intake, sarcoidosis, and liver disease. Phosphate is also increased after exercise or after a phosphate-containing enema. Low *blood* phosphate occurs in malnutrition, malabsorption (in which the intestines fail to absorb nutrients properly), and with chronic use of antacids and steroids. Phosphate blood levels also decrease after meals.

High *urine* phosphate is seen in hyperparathyroidism, vitamin D deficiency, and with use of diuretics (water pills). Low *urine* phosphate occurs in hypoparathyroidism, excess vitamin D ingestion, and in some bone diseases. Urine phosphate may be high or low in kidney disease, depending upon the specific problem.

SYNONYMS AND INCLUDED TESTS

Phosphorus.

□ □ □

□ Pinworm identification

WHAT IT IS AND WHY IT'S OBTAINED

This test is used to diagnose infection with *Enterobius vermicularis* (pinworms), which cause itching of the anus, especially at night.

HOW IT WORKS

Since multiple family members are usually affected, a responsible member is designated as the tester, since the best specimens are obtained at home late at night or early in the morning. Commercial kits with instructions are available. The basic method is to attach one end of a piece of clear tape to a glass slide. The tape is rolled back, sticky side out, and pressed against the skin around the anus four times, once in each quadrant. The free end of the tape is then fastened to the other side of the glass slide and transported to the laboratory where it is examined under a microscope.

BEFORE THE TEST

No special preparation is required.

AFTER THE TEST

No special aftercare is needed.

SIGNIFICANCE OF RESULTS

A positive test proves infestation with pinworms, but a negative test does not rule it out. **Stool for ova and parasites** is needed to identify any other intestinal parasites.

SYNONYMS AND INCLUDED TESTS

Scotch tape test.

□ □ □

□ Placental lactogen

WHAT IT IS AND WHY IT'S OBTAINED

Blood levels of placental lactogen in pregnant women have been used to assess the health of the fetus. This test, however, is controversial.

HOW IT WORKS

You will be asked to provide a **venous blood sample** from which serum* will be separated. Immunoassay* is used for the laboratory analysis.

BEFORE THE TEST

No special preparation is required.

AFTER THE TEST

Follow **venous blood sample** aftercare.

SIGNIFICANCE OF RESULTS

Although a low placental lactogen has been taken as a bad sign, it is not reliable. Similarly, a normal level of placental lactogen does not mean that your baby's development is satisfactory. **Ultrasound** or **amniocentesis** is preferred.

□ □ □

□ Plasminogen

WHAT IT IS AND WHY IT'S OBTAINED

Plasminogen is the precursor of plasmin, an enzyme which breaks down blood clots. Blood levels of plasminogen are used to evaluate bleeding disorders and abnormal tendencies to clot (thrombosis). Plasminogen may also be used to monitor treatment with clot-dissolving (thrombolytic) medications.

HOW IT WORKS

You will be asked to provide a **venous blood sample** from which plasma* will be separated. A plasminogen activator is added to the plasma* and the resulting plasmin can be measured by color change.

BEFORE THE TEST

No special preparation is required.

AFTER THE TEST

Follow **venous blood sample** aftercare.

SIGNIFICANCE OF RESULTS

Low plasminogen may occur as a result of a genetic defect, liver disease, surgery, or disseminated intravascular coagulation, a serious disease in which the substances responsible for blood clotting—mainly **fibrinogen**—are depleted, leading to excessive bleeding from multiple sites.

◻ ◻ ◻

◻ Platelet adhesion

WHAT IT IS AND WHY IT'S OBTAINED

Blood platelets are particles in the blood which are crucial to the development of blood clotting. The blood platelet adhesion test is used to evaluate bleeding disorders by measuring how "sticky" the platelets are. Some hematologists do not consider this a valid test because it is difficult to standardize.

HOW IT WORKS

You will be asked to provide a **venous blood sample** which will be divided into two parts. A **platelet count** is performed on each sample, one of the samples first having been filtered through a column of tiny glass beads. If platelets are sticky many should adhere to the glass beads and result in a lower filtered platelet count.

BEFORE THE TEST

Avoid aspirin for at least a week, ibuprofen, ketoprofen, or naproxen for one day, and other nonessential medications, especially antihistamines, as directed by your doctor. You should fast overnight and avoid caffeine on the day of the test.

AFTER THE TEST

Follow **venous blood sample** aftercare.

Poor platelet adhesion is found in von Willebrand's disease, thrombasthenia, storage pool disease, and the Bernard-Soulier syndrome.

□ □ □

□ Platelet aggregation

WHAT IT IS AND WHY IT'S OBTAINED

Blood platelet aggregation is used to evaluate bleeding disorders and measures how well platelets stick together.

HOW IT WORKS

You will be asked to provide a **venous blood sample** from which plasma* will be separated. A chemical which causes platelets to come together, such as collagen, epinephrine, or ristocetin, is added and the reaction observed as the platelets clump and fall to the bottom of the tube.

BEFORE THE TEST

Avoid aspirin for at least a week, ibuprofen, ketoprofen, or naproxen for one day, and other nonessential medications, especially antihistamines, as directed by your doctor. You should fast overnight and avoid caffeine on the day of the test.

AFTER THE TEST

Follow **venous blood sample** aftercare.

SIGNIFICANCE OF RESULTS

Poor platelet aggregation is found in von Willebrand's disease, thrombasthenia, storage pool disease, and the Bernard-Soulier syndrome. Many drugs, particularly aspirin, inhibit platelet aggregation. It is this effect which makes aspirin of value in helping to prevent heart attacks.

□ □ □

□ Platelet count

WHAT IT IS AND WHY IT'S OBTAINED

Counting blood platelets is performed to investigate bleeding disorders, as a screen before surgery, and to monitor chemotherapy. As a screening test it is most valuable when obtained with a **prothrombin time** and a **partial thromboplastin time.**

HOW IT WORKS

You will be asked to provide a **venous blood sample.** The count may be done manually or by machine.

BEFORE THE TEST

No special preparation is required.

AFTER THE TEST

Follow **venous blood sample** aftercare.

SIGNIFICANCE OF RESULTS

Low platelet counts may be associated with abnormal bleeding. If the count is moderately decreased only easy bruisability may be noted, but if severe, spontaneous hemorrhage occurs. Low platelets (called thrombocytopenia) may occur for many reasons, including aplastic anemia, leukemia, cancer, an enlarged spleen, an immune system abnormality, infections, or in some genetic diseases. Many drugs and medications may decrease platelets, including aspirin, antihistamines, penicillin, and diuretics (water pills). Increased platelet counts are less common but are seen in iron deficiency, hemorrhage, recent surgery (particularly after removal of the spleen), autoimmune diseases (in which the immune system reacts against the body's own tissues), polycythemia (in which the number of red blood cells is increased), and some leukemias, cancers, and infections. Birth control pills may increase the platelet count slightly.

□ □ □

□ Platelet sizing

WHAT IT IS AND WHY IT'S OBTAINED

Measuring blood platelet size is sometimes used to study bleeding disorders but is not a common test.

HOW IT WORKS

You will be asked to provide a **venous blood sample** which is analyzed by flow cytometry* to compute volume and average width.

BEFORE THE TEST

No special preparation is required.

AFTER THE TEST

Follow **venous blood sample** aftercare.

SIGNIFICANCE OF RESULTS

In general, large platelets, which tend to be young platelets, work better than small platelets, which tend to be older. Increased platelet volume and size are seen in idiopathic thrombocytopenic purpura and some other conditions. Small platelets are found in the Wiscott-Aldrich syndrome, when the spleen is enlarged, and in low platelets caused by infection.

□ □ □

☐ Pleural biopsy

WHAT IT IS AND WHY IT'S OBTAINED

The pleura is the membrane which coats the lungs and inner chest cavity. A pleural biopsy is the surgical removal of a portion of this membrane and is used to diagnose malignancies of the pleura, to assist in the diagnosis of tuberculosis, and to obtain more information after a **thoracentesis.**

HOW IT WORKS

Pleural biopsy may be performed at the bedside in a hospital or as an outpatient in a clinic or private doctor's office, usually by pulmonary disease specialists or chest surgeons. You will be placed in a comfortable sitting position and will be asked to lean over in order to widen the spaces between your ribs. The skin will be cleansed with an antiseptic and a local anesthetic will burn or sting slightly as it is injected into the site to be biopsied. Next, a small incision with a scalpel will be made and a special needle will be introduced through the opening. Fluid may be removed, after which the actual biopsy, which is painless, will be performed. A specimen of pleura may also be obtained in the operating room during surgery under general anesthesia. This is called an "open" pleural biopsy.

BEFORE THE TEST

No special preparation is required.

AFTER THE TEST

Like thoracentesis, the main complication is puncture and collapse of the lung, called pneumothorax. For this reason a chest **X ray** will be obtained immediately after the biopsy. If the procedure was performed as an outpatient you will be observed for a period of time and your vital signs (pulse, blood pressure, respiration, and temperature) will be taken until they are stable. Report any chest pain or shortness of breath.

A negative test means that the specimen appeared normal. A positive test may indicate malignancy or tuberculosis. The report, however, is often nonspecific, and the pathologist may ask for another specimen. Because the procedure is "blind," the specimen selected may have missed the disease.

SYNONYMS AND INCLUDED TESTS

Closed pleural biopsy, needle pleural biopsy.

□ □ □

□ Polycystic kidney disease DNA detection

WHAT IT IS AND WHY IT'S OBTAINED

This test is used for genetic counseling and prenatal diagnosis in families with a history of polycystic kidney disease, a common and serious inherited disorder.

HOW IT WORKS

Several sources may be tested, such as blood from a **venous blood sample** or amniotic fluid* from an **amniocentesis.** The Southern blot* technique is used for the analysis.

BEFORE THE TEST

No special preparation is required.

AFTER THE TEST

Follow **venous blood sample** or **amniocentesis** aftercare.

SIGNIFICANCE OF RESULTS

Your own test results or those of your baby must be interpreted along with those of other family members since several genes and patterns of inheritance are involved. The report from the laboratory will express the probability of your or your baby's developing polycystic kidney disease.

□ □ □

□ Polymerase chain reaction

WHAT IT IS AND WHY IT'S OBTAINED

The polymerase chain reaction (PCR) is a laboratory technique which is revolutionizing and will continue to revolutionize medical testing. PCR is used in prenatal testing for sickle cell anemia, hemophilia, cystic fibrosis, muscular dystrophy, and other inherited disorders. PCR tests have been devised for hepatitis, AIDS, Lyme disease, tuberculosis, chlamydia, and other diseases caused by germs.

HOW IT WORKS

Any source of DNA can be used, including blood, tissue, hair, semen, amniotic fluid from an **amniocentesis,** pus, and fluid from a **spinal tap.** The general method is to separate the DNA double strands by heating, allow a "primer" to flank the DNA to be amplified, cause the gene DNA to duplicate, and then to repeat the process. The DNA can be amplified a million times or more and is detected by electrophoresis*.

BEFORE THE TEST

No special preparation is required.

AFTER THE TEST

This depends upon the method used to take the sample.

SIGNIFICANCE OF RESULTS

Interpretation of PCR results must take into consideration the extraordinary sensitivity of the test and the requirements for strict quality control. It is possible, for example, to detect one infected cell, or to diagnose a genetic defect with one drop of blood. Along with this sensitivity comes the danger of possible contamination. It should be noted that PCR cannot replace traditional **bacterial culture** because **bacterial sensitivity** tests can only be performed on living organisms.

□ □ □

□ Porphyrins

WHAT IT IS AND WHY IT'S OBTAINED

Porphyrins are a group of chemical compounds which form the building blocks of **hemoglobin.** Normally the porphyrins are metabolized and excreted, but in certain conditions, called porphyrias, the compounds accumulate in tissues and cause disease. Porphyrias can cause many symptoms, including sun sensitivity, abdominal pain, skin rashes, liver damage, and dementia.

HOW IT WORKS

Either urine, blood, or feces may be tested. Often a urine screen will be performed and if positive or questionable, a more detailed assay will be obtained. Except for protoporphyria, urine porphyrins are in general the most useful test. For this you will be asked to provide a **24-hour urine sample.** Keep the specimen refrigerated and protected from light during collection and transportation to the laboratory. Various laboratory methods are used to separate and measure the different porphyrin compounds.

BEFORE THE TEST

Avoid alcohol and nonessential medications before and during collection.

AFTER THE TEST

For blood tests follow **venous blood sample** aftercare.

SIGNIFICANCE OF RESULTS

In congenital erythropoietic porphyria, urine uroporphyrin and coproporphyrin are increased. In acute intermittent porphyria and variegate porphyria, porphobilinogen and delta aminolevulinic acid are increased during attacks. In hereditary coproporphyria, coproporphyrin and porphobilinogen are elevated. In porphyria cutanea tarda there is increased urine uroporphyrinogen, uroporphyrin, and coproporphyrin. Protoporphyria is confirmed by testing blood for protoporphyrin. Red blood cell levels of uroporphyrinogen-I-synthetase are used to confirm the diagnosis of acute intermittent porphyria.

□ □ □

□ Postprandial glucose

WHAT IT IS AND WHY IT'S OBTAINED

The postprandial glucose (PPG) is the best test for the diagnosis of diabetes mellitus (sugar diabetes). It is often obtained if the fasting blood **glucose** (sugar) level is high or if there are symptoms which are suspicious for diabetes, such as increased thirst, increased appetite, increased urination, blurred vision, weakness, frequent infections, neurological symptoms, or positive family history.

HOW IT WORKS

You will be given a liquid containing a concentrated sugar solution, which you should drink within five minutes. Two hours later you will be asked to provide a **venous blood sample** which will be analyzed for glucose. Alternatively, the blood sample may be taken two hours after a normal meal (the original meaning of "postprandial"), but taking a specific amount of sugar is better.

BEFORE THE TEST

No special preparation is required.

AFTER THE TEST

Follow **venous blood sample** aftercare.

SIGNIFICANCE OF RESULTS

The PPG may be normal or may indicate diabetes, particularly if the same results are obtained on more than one occasion. There is a borderline zone, however, which is called "impaired glucose tolerance." Borderline results may be further studied with a **glucose tolerance test.**

SYNONYMS AND INCLUDED TESTS

Two-hour postprandial blood glucose.

□ □ □

□ Potassium

WHAT IT IS AND WHY IT'S OBTAINED

Potassium is one of the major **electrolytes** of the body and is the major positive ion inside cells. It is crucial in maintaining proper acid-base balance and electrical activity within muscle. Potassium levels are a part of most routine blood tests and are particularly important in the elderly and in those with kidney disease.

HOW IT WORKS

You will be asked to provide a **venous blood sample** from which serum* will be separated. Several methods are available for the analysis. Urine may also be tested.

BEFORE THE TEST

No special preparation is required.

AFTER THE TEST

Follow **venous blood sample** aftercare.

High potassium is found in kidney disease, severe injuries, burns, heart attacks, severe diabetes, Addison's disease, excessive potassium intake, and with certain drugs, such as ibuprofen, ketoprofen, or naproxen. Low potassium is common and occurs in vomiting, diarrhea, and with steroids or certain diuretics (water pills).

□ □ □

□ Pregnancy test

WHAT IT IS AND WHY IT'S OBTAINED

Pregnancy testing, whether by laboratory or home kit, relies on **human chorionic gonadotropin** (HCG) in blood or urine. Besides being useful in detecting suspected pregnancy, pregnancy testing is also used before certain procedures, such as **X ray** or surgery on the reproductive organs as well as prior to administering some medications.

HOW IT WORKS

Either a **venous blood sample** or urine may be used, but urine is more common, since levels of HCG in urine are close to those in blood. The first morning specimen is the best because it is most concentrated. A variety of methods for detecting HCG are available, but most involve mixing urine, an antibody (a blood protein important to the immune system) to HCG, and an enzyme which changes color if the antibody binds to the HCG.

BEFORE THE TEST

No special preparation is required.

AFTER THE TEST

No special aftercare is needed.

SIGNIFICANCE OF RESULTS

Although pregnancy testing is both sensitive and specific, there are still false negatives and false positives. Home testing kits, of which there are a number, vary widely in their accuracy but are very popular. The instructions in these kits are detailed and helpful and there is often a toll-free number to call for questions. Laboratory methods of testing are more reliable, the most sensitive ones (using blood) being able to detect pregnancy as early as six days after conception. False positives may occur if you are taking drugs in the phenothiazine class (such as Thorazine), or when there is too much **protein** or blood in your urine. False negatives may occur early in pregnancy or if there is an implantation of the embryo outside of the uterus (ectopic pregnancy).

□ □ □

□ Progesterone

WHAT IT IS AND WHY IT'S OBTAINED

Progesterone is a hormone produced in the ovary by the "corpus luteum," a structure which is formed after an egg is discharged. If the egg is fertilized the corpus luteum persists for months, but if the egg is not fertilized the corpus luteum shrinks and progesterone production falls. During pregnancy, progesterone is produced by the placenta and is important in maintaining the pregnancy. Blood levels of progesterone are used in infertility evaluations to confirm the presence of ovulation and during pregnancy to study how well the placenta is working. It is also used to monitor the effectiveness of medication-induced ovulation.

HOW IT WORKS

You will be asked to provide a **venous blood sample** from which serum* will be separated. Immunoassay* is used for the laboratory analysis. Repeat tests are often necessary.

BEFORE THE TEST

No special preparation is required.

AFTER THE TEST

Follow **venous blood sample** aftercare.

SIGNIFICANCE OF RESULTS

Interpretation of a single progesterone level must take into account the phase of your menstrual cycle or the duration of your pregnancy, as the case may be. Taking hormones or birth control pills may also influence your progesterone level. If you are pregnant, low progesterone may indicate an impending miscarriage. If you are not pregnant, low progesterone may mean failure to ovulate properly. High progesterone is seen in pregnancy, ovulation, certain tumors, and congenital adrenal hyperplasia.

□ □ □

□ Prolactin

WHAT IT IS AND WHY IT'S OBTAINED

Prolactin is a hormone which is produced by the pituitary gland and which stimulates the breasts to secrete milk. In women, blood levels are used to investigate abnormal lactation and menstrual difficulties. In men, it is used to evaluate breast enlargement (gynecomastia) and impotence.

HOW IT WORKS

You will be asked to provide a **venous blood sample** from which serum* will be separated. Immunoassay* is used for the laboratory analysis.

BEFORE THE TEST

You should fast overnight.

AFTER THE TEST

Follow **venous blood sample** aftercare.

SIGNIFICANCE OF RESULTS

Prolactin is usually obtained as part of a battery of tests and should be interpreted along with **follicle stimulating hormone, luteinizing hormone, testosterone, thyroid stimulating hormone,** and **cortisol.** It is high during pregnancy, with lactation, in the presence of certain pituitary tumors (prolactinomas), in hypothyroidism, and with many medications, such as estrogens and antidepressants. It is also increased in those taking DHEA as a dietary supplement and in the benign condition known as "big big prolactin." It is low in pituitary insufficiency.

SYNONYMS AND INCLUDED TESTS

Lactogenic hormone, lactogen.

□ □ □

□ Prostate biopsy

WHAT IT IS AND WHY IT'S OBTAINED

Prostate **biopsy** is the surgical removal of a portion of the prostate gland for laboratory analysis. It is used to diagnose cancer which may be suspected because of an abnormal physical (digital) examination, **ultrasound,** or an elevated **prostate specific antigen.**

HOW IT WORKS

The prostate is most commonly biopsied through the rectum with ultrasound guidance, although an approach through the perineum (the area between your anus and scrotum) is possible. Discuss the options with your doctor. It is performed by a urologist as an outpatient under local anesthesia. For the *rectal* approach you will be asked to lie on your side or back. The doctor will insert the ultrasound probe into your rectum until he sees your prostate on a screen and will guide a needle into the gland. Several specimens are usually taken and you will feel some transient discomfort as this occurs. For the *perineal* approach you will be asked to lie on your back with your legs spread. The perineum will be cleansed with an antiseptic and you will experience stinging or burning as the anesthetic is injected into your skin. The doctor will make a very small incision into your skin, will place his finger into your rectum to immobilize your prostate, and will guide a needle into the gland. Again, you will feel some transient pain as this is done several times to take several specimens.

BEFORE THE TEST

Avoid aspirin for at least a week and ibuprofen, ketoprofen, or naproxen for one day. For the *rectal* approach you will be given enemas to cleanse your bowel and an antibiotic to prevent infection.

AFTER THE TEST

Follow instructions carefully. If the perineal or rectal approach was used report any abnormality in your urine, such as frequency, burning, blood, or inability to void.

SIGNIFICANCE OF RESULTS

A negative test means that no abnormality was found. This usually, but not always, rules out cancer, and if suspicion is high, your doctor might want to repeat the test. Other abnormalities detectable by prostate biopsy include benign enlargement (benign prostatic hypertrophy) or prostatitis (inflammation). If cancer is found, **acid phosphatase, prostate specific antigen, computed tomography,** and a **bone scan** may be used to see if it has spread.

□ □ □

❑ Prostate specific antigen

WHAT IT IS AND WHY IT'S OBTAINED

Prostate specific antigen (PSA) is an enzyme produced by the prostate gland. Blood levels are used to diagnose and monitor the treatment of prostate cancer.

HOW IT WORKS

You will be asked to provide a **venous blood sample** from which serum* will be separated. Immunoassay* is used for the laboratory analysis.

BEFORE THE TEST

No special preparation is required.

AFTER THE TEST

Follow **venous blood sample** aftercare.

SIGNIFICANCE OF RESULTS

A negative test means that the level of PSA was normal but does not completely rule out the possibility of prostate cancer. Moderately high PSA is associated with both benign prostate enlargement and prostate cancer, but very high levels are generally associated with cancer. Small elevations of PSA may be due either to benign or malignant prostate disease or prostate infection and have even been reported after digital rectal examination in otherwise normal men. If blood PSA is elevated when no infection is present, it is best to have a prostate **ultrasound** and **prostate biopsy** to rule out prostate cancer.

❑ ❑ ❑

☐ Protein

WHAT IT IS AND WHY IT'S OBTAINED

Protein is the main building block of most tissues in the body. Blood levels of protein are used to evaluate nutrition and to investigate causes for swelling, particularly swelling about the ankles.

HOW IT WORKS

You will be asked to provide a **venous blood sample** from which serum* will be separated. The biuret test (sodium hydroxide and copper sulfate produce a pink-violet color) is used for the laboratory analysis.

BEFORE THE TEST

No special preparation is required.

AFTER THE TEST

Follow **venous blood sample** aftercare.

SIGNIFICANCE OF RESULTS

High protein may be found in dehydration, multiple myeloma (a cancer of plasma cells, a type of cell which is usually found in the bone marrow), macroglobulinemia, sarcoidosis, leprosy (and some other tropical diseases), and some cases of chronic inflammation. Low protein occurs with excessive fluid intake, pregnancy, prolonged bed rest, heart failure, kidney diseases, severe skin disease, burns, malabsorption (in which the intestines fail to absorb nutrients properly), cancer, and malnutrition. Protein levels in liver disease may be high, low, or normal. **Albumin** is often measured along with total protein and the calculated **albumin/globulin ratio** is sometimes useful. More detailed information about protein status can be obtained with **protein electrophoresis** and **immunofixation electrophoresis**.

☐ ☐ ☐

☐ Protein C

WHAT IT IS AND WHY IT'S OBTAINED

Protein C is a naturally occurring blood thinner (anticoagulant) which acts to prevent blood clots from becoming too large. Blood levels are used to investigate the tendency to form blood clots (thromboses), especially in children and young adults. Protein S is a related substance which may also be tested.

HOW IT WORKS

You will be asked to provide a **venous blood sample** from which plasma* will be separated. There are several methods of assay.

BEFORE THE TEST

No special preparation is required.

AFTER THE TEST

Follow **venous blood sample** aftercare.

SIGNIFICANCE OF RESULTS

Low protein C is seen in certain genetic conditions in which there is a tendency to form blood clots in the veins (thrombophlebitis) and lungs (pulmonary emboli). Protein C may also be decreased in liver disease.

☐ ☐ ☐

☐ Protein electrophoresis

WHAT IT IS AND WHY IT'S OBTAINED

Protein electrophoresis (PE) measures the amounts and types of blood proteins. It is often used to evaluate an abnormal total blood protein or an abnormal **albumin/-globulin ratio.** PE may also be used to study nutrition, liver disease, kidney disease, and cancer.

HOW IT WORKS

You will be asked to provide a **venous blood sample** from which serum* will be separated. The serum* is studied by electrophoresis*. There are five protein fractions: albumin (the largest), alpha$_1$ globulin, alpha$_2$ globulin, beta globulin, and gamma globulin.

BEFORE THE TEST

No special preparation is required.

AFTER THE TEST

Follow **venous blood sample** aftercare.

SIGNIFICANCE OF RESULTS

A negative test means that the PE fell within the normal range. There are many abnormal PE patterns which may be created by the different components. Interpretation may be difficult and additional PE determinations are often needed, particularly when there is an increase in one of the globulin fractions. This is termed a "monoclonal gammopathy" and may either be benign or signify the disease known as multiple myeloma (a cancer of plasma cells, a type of cell which is usually found in the bone marrow). Abnormal PE patterns are found in liver disease, heart disease, stress, Waldenstrom's macroglobulinemia, cancer, ulcers, ulcerative colitis, malnutrition, gallbladder disease, kidney disease, autoimmune diseases (in which the immune system reacts against the body's own tissues), thyroid disease, and diabetes. The various patterns tend to suggest rather than diagnose different diseases and confirmation is necessary.

Serum protein electrophoresis.

□ □ □

□ Prothrombin time

WHAT IT IS AND WHY IT'S OBTAINED

Prothrombin is crucial to the formation of blood clots. The prothrombin time (PT) is a screening test for bleeding disorders which is used before surgery and in monitoring treatment with the blood thinner (anticoagulant) warfarin (Coumadin). As a screening test it is most useful when obtained with a **partial thromboplastin time** and **platelet count.**

HOW IT WORKS

You will be asked to provide a **venous blood sample** from which plasma* will be separated. The plasma* is incubated with citrate, after which thromboplastin and calcium are added and a timer is started. The timing stops with the formation of a clot. A handheld device using a **fingerstick blood sample** is also available.

BEFORE THE TEST

No special preparation is required.

AFTER THE TEST

Follow **venous blood sample** aftercare.

SIGNIFICANCE OF RESULTS

A long PT is seen generally in bleeding disorders due to "extrinsic factor" deficiencies of the blood clotting system—factors II, V, VII, or X (see **coagulation factor screen**)—and with warfarin treatment. The PT is also long in fibrinogen (factor I) insufficiency, liver failure, disseminated intravascular coagulation (a serious disease in which the substances responsible for blood clotting—mainly **fibrinogen**—are depleted, leading to excessive bleeding from multiple sites), and vitamin K deficiency. Many substances influence the PT, both to increase and decrease it, an effect which is very important if you are taking warfarin and the dose is being adjusted. Drugs which may increase the PT include aspirin, steroids, chloral hydrate, chloramphenicol, clofibrate, glucagon, indomethacin, mefenamic acid, methimazole, neomycin, oxyphenbutazone, phenylbutazone, phenyramidol, phenytoin, propylthiouracil, quinidine, quinine, thyroid hormones, and vitamin A. Drugs which decrease the PT include barbiturates, ethchlorvynol, glutethimide, griseofulvin, and vitamin K.

SYNONYMS AND INCLUDED TESTS

Pro time.

□ □ □

□ Pulmonary function tests

WHAT IT IS AND WHY IT'S OBTAINED

Pulmonary function tests are used to evaluate lung diseases. Although there are many ways to do this, the basic principle is to measure your ability to move air in and out of your lungs.

HOW IT WORKS

Pulmonary function testing is done in a special laboratory with a device called a spirometer. You will be provided with a nose clip and a mouthpiece and be asked to inhale and exhale in various ways while the volume of air and the time it takes for the air to move is recorded on a strip of paper. Since accurate results depend upon your full cooperation it is important to follow directions as well as you can. Typically you will be told to breathe normally, to inhale as deeply as you can, to exhale as completely and rapidly as you can, to hold your breath, to breathe slowly, and to pant. These maneuvers may be repeated a number of times, sitting and lying down. At times the air you will be breathing will be changed to include carbon dioxide, helium, nitrogen, or carbon monoxide. A more sophisticated series of tests may be conducted in a special airtight chamber in which the air content and pressure in your surroundings can be monitored. Depending upon your breathing problem, drugs may be administered before testing, both to make it harder to breathe (bronchial challenge test with methacholine or histamine), or easier to breathe (bronchodilators).

BEFORE THE TEST

Avoid heavy meals for three hours prior to the test.

AFTER THE TEST

Do not attempt to walk or stand if you feel dizzy.

SIGNIFICANCE OF RESULTS

Many numbers and graphs may be derived from pulmonary function testing which may be helpful in your case. Figures for the amount of air you move during normal breathing, the amount of air left in your lungs after you exhale completely, the speed with which you can inhale or exhale with maximum effort, and changes which take place if you breathe carbon dioxide, are a few of the measurements available. The two general categories of lung disease are those due to some obstruction of the pathway of air, such as asthma, emphysema, or chronic bronchitis, and those due to restriction to the normal movement of the chest or diaphragm, such as pulmonary fibrosis. Pulmonary function studies are valuable when obtained as serial measurements in order to monitor the course of your disease.

SYNONYMS AND INCLUDED TESTS

Spirometry.

□ □ □

☐ Pyruvate kinase

WHAT IT IS AND WHY IT'S OBTAINED

Pyruvate kinase is an enzyme which is important to red blood cell metabolism. Red blood cell levels of it are used to evaluate anemia.

HOW IT WORKS

You will be asked to provide a **venous blood sample** from which red blood cells will be separated and washed. Spectrophotometry* is used for the assay.

BEFORE THE TEST

No special preparation is required.

AFTER THE TEST

Follow **venous blood sample** aftercare.

SIGNIFICANCE OF RESULTS

A very low level of red blood cell pyruvate kinase is found in the anemia caused by the inherited disease called pyruvate kinase deficiency. Smaller reductions may be seen in leukemia and aplastic anemia.

☐ ☐ ☐

☐ Radioallergosorbent test

WHAT IT IS AND WHY IT'S OBTAINED

The radioallergosorbent test (RAST) is used to evaluate allergic diseases. It is less sensitive and less reliable than skin testing and should be done only if you have severe allergies and cannot tolerate **allergy skin testing.** The RAST consists of many individual tests. It does not substitute for **patch testing.**

HOW IT WORKS

You will be asked to provide a **venous blood sample** from which serum* will be separated. The serum is incubated with radioactive substances (antigens) which have been absorbed into paper disks.

BEFORE THE TEST

No special preparation is required.

AFTER THE TEST

Follow **venous blood sample** aftercare.

SIGNIFICANCE OR RESULTS

Interpretation of RAST tests must take into consideration your symptoms and the history of your disease. The situation can be very complicated. For example, there are people who have allergic reactions to one species of shrimp but not another, the RAST studies being different in both cases. With dog and cat allergies, a negative test means that you are very unlikely to be allergic to dogs and cats, but a positive test does not necessarily mean that you *are* allergic. **Food allergy tests** are a more scientific way of evaluating food allergies.

SYNONYMS AND INCLUDED TESTS

IgE specific antibody, allergy screen.

□ □ □

□ Radionuclide scan

WHAT IT IS AND WHY IT'S OBTAINED

Radionuclide scanning is designed to visualize internal organs. Unlike **X rays, computed tomography** (CT), or **magnetic resonance imaging,** which only show how an organ *looks,* radionuclide images also reveal information about how an organ *works.* Scans may be obtained of the liver, gallbladder, bones, bone marrow, brain, heart, spleen, lung, thyroid gland, parathyroid glands, and kidneys.

HOW IT WORKS

Radionuclide scanning involves administering radioactive "tracer" compounds either by injection or by mouth. The substance is allowed to disperse in the body and in the organs of interest for a variable time. The organ is then scanned from the outside with a computerized camera that detects the tracer's radioactive emissions. The tracer concentrates at a level which depends on the metabolism of the tissue. The actual scanning is painless and takes from five to thirty minutes. A variation of this test is called single-photon emission tomography (SPECT) and provides cross sectional views similar to those of CT.

BEFORE THE TEST

No special preparation is required.

AFTER THE TEST

No special aftercare is needed. Although generally safe, these tests involve exposure to radiation, the actual amount of which varies according to the organ being studied. Sometimes it is less than with conventional X rays and sometimes more.

SIGNIFICANCE OF RESULTS

The information derived from scanning is useful because of its sensitivity: diseases often show up months or years before they produce symptoms or signs. For specific information, see the individual tests.

SYNONYMS AND INCLUDED TESTS

Nuclear medicine, scintigram.

□ □ □

☐ Red blood cell count

WHAT IT IS AND WHY IT'S OBTAINED

The red blood cell (RBC) count is part of the **complete blood count** and is used to evaluate anemia, polycythemia (in which the red cells are increased, the opposite of anemia), and hemorrhage.

HOW IT WORKS

You will be asked to provide a **venous blood sample.** Counts may be performed manually or by machine.

BEFORE THE TEST

No special preparation is required.

AFTER THE TEST

Follow **venous blood sample** aftercare.

SIGNIFICANCE OF RESULTS

A low RBC count is found in anemia, hemorrhage, or excessive fluid intake. The evaluation of anemia is done in steps which take into account the **reticulocyte count, hemoglobin, hematocrit, red blood cell indices, ferritin,** and possibly a **bone marrow.** A high RBC count is seen in polycythemia and dehydration. These may be distinguished by means of **blood volume.**

☐ ☐ ☐

☐ Red blood cell indices

WHAT IT IS AND WHY IT'S OBTAINED

Red blood cell (RBC) indices estimate the general characteristics of red blood cells and are used to evaluate anemia. There are four indices: the size of the average RBC, the concentration of hemoglobin in the average RBC, the weight of hemoglobin in the average RBC, and the variation in size of the RBCs.

HOW IT WORKS

You will be asked to provide a **venous blood sample.** The first three indices (MCV, MCHC, and MCH) can be calculated from a **red cell blood count,** hemoglobin, and **hematocrit,** but are usually analyzed by computerized machines. The fourth index (RDW) must be measured by machine.

BEFORE THE TEST

No special preparation is required.

AFTER THE TEST

Follow **venous blood sample** aftercare.

SIGNIFICANCE OF RESULTS

Patterns of the various RBC indices may indicate a specific type of anemia. For example, in iron deficiency anemia three of four indices are decreased and one is increased. In the anemia due to vitamin B_{12} deficiency (pernicious anemia), on the other hand, all of them tend to be high. Further testing for anemia may include **ferritin, reticulocyte count,** and possibly a **bone marrow.**

□ □ □

□ Red blood cell mass

WHAT IT IS AND WHY IT'S OBTAINED

Red blood cell mass is used to determine the total volume of red blood cells in the body. It is used to evaluate polycythemia, in which red blood cells are increased, and on occasion to monitor chemotherapy. Although accurate, the red cell mass is not commonly obtained because of cost and technical complexity.

HOW IT WORKS

You will be asked to provide a **venous blood sample.** Your red blood cells will then be incubated with a radioactive substance and reinjected intravenously. Blood samples will be obtained at ten and thirty minutes and analyzed for radioactivity. The volume of red blood cells is estimated by calculating how much dilution has taken place.

BEFORE THE TEST

No special preparation is required.

AFTER THE TEST

Follow **venous blood sample** aftercare. Although safe, this test does involve the injection of a radioactive compound.

SIGNIFICANCE OF RESULTS

Increased red cell mass is seen in polycythemia, in some cases of heart disease, living at high altitudes, some inherited disorders of hemoglobin, and overproduction of **erythropoietin,** which may be hereditary or due to certain tumors. Low red cell mass occurs in anemia, hemorrhage, and chronic diseases of many types.

□ □ □

□ Red blood cell survival

WHAT IT IS AND WHY IT'S OBTAINED

Red blood cell survival is an estimate of the average life span of the red blood cell, which is normally about 120 days. This test may be used to evaluate anemia but is not common because of cost and technical complexity.

HOW IT WORKS

You will be asked to provide a **venous blood sample.** Your red blood cells will be incubated with radioactive chromium and reinjected intravenously. A day later and then at several day intervals, more blood samples are obtained and the blood analyzed for residual radioactivity. A graph is then constructed to estimate the rate at which your red cells are being destroyed.

BEFORE THE TEST

No special preparation is required.

AFTER THE TEST

Follow **venous blood sample** aftercare. Although safe, this test does involve the injection of a radioactive compound.

SIGNIFICANCE OF RESULTS

Decreased red blood cell survival is found in anemia due to red blood cell disruption (hemolytic anemia), red blood cell enzyme deficiencies, inherited disorders of **hemoglobin,** and blood loss.

SYNONYMS AND INCLUDED TESTS

Chromium-51 RBC survival.

□ □ □

□ Refraction

WHAT IT IS AND WHY IT'S OBTAINED

The general term "refraction" refers to the bending of light waves as they pass from one substance to another, as from air through glass. It is the method by which corrective lenses are selected for those with some degree of visual impairment. It should be part of every complete eye examination.

HOW IT WORKS

There are two methods of refraction, objective and subjective. Both are usually performed, the objective being first.

Children will often have their eyes dilated with drops when the objective portion of the examination is to be performed. There are two types of objective measurement. In the first, called retinoscopy, you will be asked to sit in a chair and a device containing multiple corrective lenses will be placed in front of your eyes. The examiner will shine a light into one eye and adjust lenses until the reflection from your retina is stable. Then the other eye will be checked the same way. This gives the examiner a general estimate of the lens power you will require. The second type of objective refraction uses an automated refractor which accomplishes the same thing. In the subjective test you will be asked to read from a chart of letters or numbers of decreasing size, again while lenses are changed, until your vision is corrected to the best possible degree.

BEFORE THE TEST

Bring corrective lenses if you have them.

AFTER THE TEST

If eyedrops to dilate your pupils have been instilled, your vision will be blurry for a few hours. Some doctors instill another drop which will reverse the dilation, usually within an hour. These drops may sting when instilled.

SIGNIFICANCE OF RESULTS

A person whose distance vision is less than normal is said to be nearsighted or to have myopia, whereas a person who cannot see close up is said to be farsighted or to have hyperopia. In either case your visual problem may be compounded by astigmatism, in which the light rays are bent more in one plane than another, giving a type of "barrel-shaped" image. Results of refraction are used to fashion lenses which correct the problem.

□ □ □

☐ Renin

WHAT IT IS AND WHY IT'S OBTAINED

Renin is an enzyme found in the kidney. When released into the bloodstream it starts a series of reactions which result in secretion of **aldosterone** by the adrenal gland. Blood renin levels are used to evaluate high blood pressure.

HOW IT WORKS

You will be asked to provide a **venous blood sample** from which serum* will be separated. The renin level may be measured directly or calculated indirectly by means of what is called plasma* renin activity.

BEFORE THE TEST

Follow the instructions of your doctor and the laboratory carefully with regard to drugs and diet. In general, medications to reduce high blood pressure, steroids, birth control pills, diuretics, and licorice should be discontinued for two weeks since they interfere with results.

AFTER THE TEST

Resume medications and diet as directed. Follow **venous blood sample** aftercare.

SIGNIFICANCE OF RESULTS

Increased renin may be seen in the severe form of high blood pressure called malignant hypertension and the high blood pressure found in kidney disease. Decreased levels may be seen in primary aldosteronism (Conn's syndrome), Cushing's syndrome, licorice ingestion, Liddle's syndrome, steroid intake, and congenital adrenal hyperplasia. Results are evaluated along with blood aldosterone.

Primary aldosteronism is confirmed with a **renin stimulation test.**

□ □ □

□ Renin stimulation test

WHAT IT IS AND WHY IT'S OBTAINED

The **renin** stimulation test is used to confirm a diagnosis of primary aldosteronism (Conn's syndrome), a disease which causes high blood pressure and low **potassium.**

HOW IT WORKS

You will be given an intravenous injection of furosemide, a diuretic*, after which you will be asked to lie flat for about an hour. Then you will be asked to stand for about two hours, after which a **venous blood sample** will be obtained and analyzed for renin and **aldosterone.**

BEFORE THE TEST

Follow the dietary instructions given by the laboratory or your doctor. This is usually a low-sodium, high-potassium diet for three days.

AFTER THE TEST

Since the test results in a decrease in your body fluids, you may feel faint or dizzy. This is transient.

SIGNIFICANCE OF RESULTS

A negative test means that blood renin rose appropriately. In a positive test, which confirms primary aldosteronism, renin activity remains low because of unregulated aldosterone production.

☐ Reticulocyte count

WHAT IT IS AND WHY IT'S OBTAINED

Reticulocytes are immature red blood cells. Blood levels of them are used to evaluate anemia and are particularly important since they provide crucial information which may indicate the need for further tests, in particular whether a **bone marrow** should be performed.

HOW IT WORKS

Either a **venous blood sample** or **heelstick blood sample** may be used, and the count may be done manually or by machine. The result is expressed as a percentage of red blood cells which are reticulocytes. The reticulocyte production index is a calculation which gives a good approximation of red blood cell production.

BEFORE THE TEST

No special preparation is required.

AFTER THE TEST

Follow **venous blood sample** or **heelstick blood sample** aftercare.

SIGNIFICANCE OF RESULTS

A high reticulocyte count means that the bone marrow has increased production of red blood cells for some reason. This may be the result of hemorrhage or some cases of anemia. A low reticulocyte count is found either when the bone marrow is not functioning well, as in aplastic anemia, or when some crucial step in red blood cell formation is missing, as in **vitamin B_{12}** deficiency, which causes pernicious anemia.

☐ ☐ ☐

☐ Rheumatoid factor

WHAT IT IS AND WHY IT'S OBTAINED

Rheumatoid factor (RF) is an antibody (a blood protein important to the immune system) which is formed in certain autoimmune diseases (in which the immune system is directed against the body's own tissues). Blood levels are used to evaluate arthritis, particularly to diagnose rheumatoid arthritis.

HOW IT WORKS

You will be asked to provide a **venous blood sample** from which serum* will be separated. Several methods may be used for the assay.

BEFORE THE TEST

No special preparation is required.

AFTER THE TEST

Follow **venous blood sample** aftercare.

SIGNIFICANCE OF RESULTS

Although RF is present in most people with rheumatoid arthritis, it also can be found in many other diseases, including bacterial endocarditis (infection of the heart valves), malaria, syphilis, tuberculosis, hepatitis, leprosy, leishmaniasis, sarcoidosis, and infectious mononucleosis. Furthermore, many normal people, particularly the elderly, often have a positive RF. The concentration of the antibody is helpful, because high levels are more significant. High levels also tend to indicate more severe disease. Children with rheumatoid arthritis often have a negative RF.

☐ ☐ ☐

☐ Right heart catheterization

WHAT IT IS AND WHY IT'S OBTAINED

Right heart catheterization (RHC) is the insertion of a catheter into the pulmonary artery, the blood vessel which carries blood from the right ventricle to the lungs. It is used to monitor blood pressures in specific areas of the heart and blood vessels and to monitor treatment for a variety of heart and lung disorders. It is mainly used in intensive care settings.

HOW IT WORKS

There are several possible sites of catheter insertion, such as the neck (internal jugular vein), below the collarbone (subclavian vein), or in the groin (femoral vein). The site will first be cleansed with an antiseptic. Then, a small amount of local anesthetic will sting or burn slightly as it is injected into your skin. A series of needles, guide wires, dilators, and the catheter itself will then be introduced through the skin area into the desired vein, vena cava, right atrium of the heart, left atrium of the heart, and finally the pulmonary artery, where it may be "wedged" into a smaller blood vessel.

BEFORE THE TEST

No special preparation is required. This is usually an urgent procedure.

AFTER THE TEST

The site of the catheter insertion will be cared for by medical staff. Follow any instructions you may be given after the catheter has been removed.

SIGNIFICANCE OF RESULTS

Results of RHC are given as blood pressure tracings. Results may indicate defects in the heart valves, "holes" in the heart (septal defects), blood clots in the lungs (pulmonary emboli), and various types of heart failure.

SYNONYMS AND INCLUDED TESTS

Swan-Ganz catheterization, pulmonary artery catheterization.

□ □ □

□ Schilling test

WHAT IT IS AND WHY IT'S OBTAINED

The Schilling test is used to diagnose pernicious anemia (caused by inadequate vitamin B_{12}) and to evaluate intestinal absorption.

HOW IT WORKS

The test has three parts. In the first part you will be given an oral dose of radioactive **vitamin B_{12}** followed an hour later by an injection of ordinary vitamin B_{12}. Then you will be asked to provide a **24-hour urine sample** which will be analyzed for radioactivity. If the urine sample shows low radioactivity (inadequate absorption of vitamin B_{12}) the second part of the test is performed. This is identical to the first part but with the addition of "intrinsic factor" taken by mouth. Intrinsic factor is a substance normally produced in the stomach which allows **vitamin B_{12}** to be absorbed. If the intrinsic factor does not correct the problem, the third part is obtained, which repeats the test after a course of antibiotics.

BEFORE THE TEST

No special preparation is required.

AFTER THE TEST

No special aftercare is needed. Although safe, the test does involve exposure to a small amount of radiation.

SIGNIFICANCE OF RESULTS

Interpretation of the Schilling test depends upon the disease being evaluated. For pernicious anemia, inadequate absorption of vitamin B_{12} corrected by intrinsic factor strongly suggests the disease, but other blood studies—such as **red blood cell indices** and **intrinsic factor antibody**—should be used to confirm the diagnosis. For malabsorption (in which the intestines fail to absorb nutrients properly), the **xylose absorption test** and **small bowel biopsy** may be helpful.

SYNONYMS AND INCLUDED TESTS

Vitamin B_{12} absorption test.

□ □ □

□ Schirmer test

WHAT IT IS AND WHY IT'S OBTAINED

The Schirmer test measures tear production and is used to evaluate dry eyes.

HOW IT WORKS

Several methods are in use, all of which involve hooking a special sterile strip of filter paper beneath your lower eyelid, waiting five minutes, and measuring the length of the paper which has become moistened by your tears. The test may also be performed by instilling anesthetic eyedrops before the paper is put into position.

BEFORE THE TEST

Avoid using eyedrops and artificial tears as directed by your doctor.

AFTER THE TEST

No special aftercare is needed.

The Schirmer test provides only a rough approximation of tear production. Further testing can be performed with **slit-lamp examination.** Dry eyes are relatively common and may result from the aging process. More severe forms may be associated with Sjögren's syndrome, lymphoma (lymphatic cancer), leukemia, and rheumatoid arthritis.

□ □ □

□ Scleroderma antibody

WHAT IT IS AND WHY IT'S OBTAINED

Scleroderma (progressive systemic sclerosis) causes widespread hardening of the skin and internal organs. An antibody (a blood protein important to the immune system) to an enzyme involved in DNA metabolism is called scleroderma antibody. Blood levels of it are used to aid the diagnosis of this disease.

HOW IT WORKS

You will be asked to provide a **venous blood sample** from which serum* will be separated. Immunoassay* is used for the laboratory analysis.

BEFORE THE TEST

No special preparation is required.

AFTER THE TEST

Follow **venous blood sample** aftercare.

SIGNIFICANCE OF RESULTS

A positive result suggests scleroderma, particularly in those likely to have severe symptoms. A negative result indicates that no antibody was found but does not rule out scleroderma, since most of those with the disease do not have the antibody.

SYNONYMS AND INCLUDED TESTS

Scl-1 antibody, Scl-70 antibody.

□ □ □

□ Sedimentation rate

WHAT IT IS AND WHY IT'S OBTAINED

The sedimentation rate is a blood test which is used to screen for inflammation, cancer, and infection.

HOW IT WORKS

You will be asked to provide a **venous blood sample**. The specimen will be placed in a special tube and observed. The rate at which the red blood cells settle to the bottom of the tube is noted and expressed in terms of millimeters per hour. A **heelstick blood sample** may be used in infants.

BEFORE THE TEST

No special preparation is required.

AFTER THE TEST

Follow **venous blood sample** or **heelstick blood sample** aftercare.

SIGNIFICANCE OF RESULTS

A high sedimentation rate is found in a wide variety of infectious, inflammatory, and malignant diseases. A high rate is generally taken to indicate the presence of some abnormality which needs further evaluation. A normal sedimentation rate, conversely, is often held to indicate the absence of significant disease. **C-reactive protein** is used for similar purposes. At times no cause can be found for a high sedimentation rate.

SYNONYMS AND INCLUDED TESTS

Erythrocyte sedimentation rate, ESR, sed rate.

□ □ □

□ Selenium

WHAT IT IS AND WHY IT'S OBTAINED

Selenium is an element which is important to several enzyme systems in the body. Blood and urine levels are obtained to evaluate nutritional status and to diagnose selenium poisoning. Selenium deficiency tends to cause muscle weakness, including the heart (cardiomyopathy), whereas selenium toxicity produces nerve diseases, a garlic odor to the breath, and swelling of the hands and feet.

HOW IT WORKS

You will be asked to provide a **venous blood sample** which will be obtained with special metal-free equipment. Either serum* (for recent intake), red blood cells (for long-term intake), or whole blood (for average intake) may be used. Atomic absorption is used for the assay. A **24-hour urine sample** may also be analyzed.

BEFORE THE TEST

No special preparation is required.

AFTER THE TEST

Follow **venous blood sample** aftercare.

SIGNIFICANCE OF RESULTS

Low selenium is usually found in those who have undergone prolonged intravenous feeding in which selenium has not been added to the nutrient mixture. It is also found in geographic areas with low levels of selenium in the soil. High selenium is associated with industrial exposure and in geographic areas with high selenium levels in the soil.

□ □ □

□ Semen analysis

WHAT IT IS AND WHY IT'S OBTAINED

Semen consists of sperm, nutrients for the sperm, and fluids derived from the prostate and other glands. Semen analysis is mainly used to evaluate infertility in men but may also be obtained to see if a vasectomy has been effective.

HOW IT WORKS

The "best" semen sample is the subject of debate among urologists and infertility specialists, some preferring masturbation in the laboratory in which the test will be performed, others claiming that it is better to collect the specimen in a condom during intercourse. However it is obtained, a number of different measurements on the specimen may be made, depending on the laboratory. In general the ejaculate's volume, color, pH, clotting, liquefaction, and viscosity are noted. The concentration of sperm, their ability to move (motility), and their appearance under a microscope are also evaluated, sometimes by computer-driven machines and flow cytometry*.

BEFORE THE TEST

You will be asked to abstain from sexual activity for a few days before providing the specimen, each urologist and laboratory having a personal preference.

AFTER THE TEST

No special aftercare is needed.

SIGNIFICANCE OF RESULTS

For the purposes of evaluating fertility the sperm count is the most important number, the normal being 20 to 150 million per milliliter. Low or absent sperm counts can be found in atrophy of the testicles, which sometimes occurs after mumps, after inflammation of the testicles (orchitis) or other testicular diseases, and sometimes after hernia surgery. Certain substances may also lower sperm counts, most notably chemotherapy drugs. Sperm motility is another important consideration. There are additional problems with semen which may make it difficult to fertilize an egg and which cannot be determined by this basic test. It is sometimes difficult to determine the exact cause of infertility. Additional sperm tests may be needed to detect antibodies on the surface of sperm or to measure the ability of sperm to penetrate vaginal secretions.

SYNONYMS AND INCLUDED TESTS

Sperm count, infertility screen, sperm examination.

□ □ □

□ Sequential multiple analyzer

WHAT IT IS AND WHY IT'S OBTAINED

Diagnostic medicine was revolutionized with the introduction of computerized machines which were able to process many tiny blood samples quickly and inexpensively. Rather than ordering tests individually, doctors could then simplify the process by ordering a battery of them. At wellness or health fairs these tests are popular. Although different laboratories include different tests in their profiles and call them by different names, the terms "sequential multiple analyzer" (SMA) or "sequential multiple analyzer with computer" (SMAC) are almost universally recognized.

HOW IT WORKS

You will be asked to provide a **venous blood sample** from which serum* will be separated. The sample is run through a computer and the results are provided within minutes. The "SMA 12" usually consists of **glucose, cholesterol, albumin, protein, bilirubin, blood urea nitrogen, uric acid, aspartate aminotransferase, lactic dehydrogenase, alkaline phosphatase, calcium,** and **phosphate.** The "SMA 21" in addition to the above usually consists of **triglycerides, sodium, potassium, chloride, carbon dioxide, creatinine, gamma glutamyl transferase, alanine aminotransferase,** and iron. For a "chemistry profile," a thyroid screening test such as **thyroid stimulating hormone** is often included, as well as **ferritin.**

BEFORE THE TEST

You should fast overnight.

AFTER THE TEST

Follow **venous blood sample** aftercare.

SIGNIFICANCE OF RESULTS

See the individual test listings for interpretation. With so many results being generated it is not at all uncommon for one or more to be abnormal. If the findings do not match your symptoms, or if the values are only slightly high or low, the wisest course is usually simply to repeat the test.

SYNONYMS AND INCLUDED TESTS

SMA, SMAC.

□ □ □

☐ Serologic test for syphilis

WHAT IT IS AND WHY IT'S OBTAINED

The serologic test for syphilis (STS) is not one test but refers to several different blood tests used to screen for syphilis. They may be used in cases of suspected syphilis, in cases of contact with known infected persons, as an aid in monitoring treatment, and as a screening test before hospitalization or surgery.

HOW IT WORKS

You will be asked to provide a **venous blood sample** from which serum* will be separated. Each test uses a different method of immunoassay* in the laboratory.

BEFORE THE TEST

No special preparation is required.

AFTER THE TEST

Follow **venous blood sample** aftercare.

SIGNIFICANCE OF RESULTS

The rapid plasma reagin (RPR) test is the most sensitive STS, but as with all screening tests, many false positives occur and are automatically confirmed with another test, usually the **FTA-ABS.** The concentration of the antibody is important, with high concentrations tending to be more significant. False positive reactions occur in malaria, leprosy, infectious mononucleosis, hepatitis, autoimmune diseases (in which the immune system reacts against the body's own tissues), pregnancy, drug addiction, and three diseases related to syphilis: pinta, bejel, and yaws. The STS becomes positive two to three weeks after infection with the germ which causes syphilis *(Treponema pallidum),* and early cases may be missed. If your STS is negative but you have symptoms such as a sore which is suspicious for syphilis, a **darkfield** examination may be helpful.

SYNONYMS AND INCLUDED TESTS

RPR, VDRL (Venereal Disease Research Laboratory), ART (automated reagin test). The Kahn, Kline, Mazzini, and Wasserman tests are no longer used.

◻ ◻ ◻

◻ Serotonin

WHAT IT IS AND WHY IT'S OBTAINED

Serotonin is a powerful constrictor of blood vessels which is widely distributed in the body. Abnormally high amounts of it may be produced by certain tumors called carcinoids. The "carcinoid syndrome" includes flushing of the skin, diarrhea, difficulty breathing, enlarged liver, and heart disease. The usual test for the carcinoid syndrome, however, analyzes urine levels of one of the waste products of serotonin, **5-hydroxyindoleacetic acid** (5-HIA), which is better than measuring serotonin directly. Blood serotonin is only obtained if urinary 5-HIA is equivocal.

HOW IT WORKS

You will be asked to provide a **venous blood sample** from which serum* will be separated. Several methods may be used for the laboratory assay.

BEFORE THE TEST

Avoid avocados, bananas, chocolate, eggplant, pineapples, plums, tomatoes, and walnuts for several days before the test. Discontinue all nonessential medications or do as directed by your doctor.

AFTER THE TEST

Follow **venous blood sample** aftercare.

SIGNIFICANCE OF RESULTS

High serotonin is found in the carcinoid syndrome, but this test is not accurate.

SYNONYMS AND INCLUDED TESTS

5-hydroxytryptamine, 5-HT.

□ □ □

□ Sickle cell test

WHAT IT IS AND WHY IT'S OBTAINED

This test screens for sickle cell anemia, a hereditary disease found mainly in Africans and African-Americans.

HOW IT WORKS

You will be asked to provide a **venous blood sample.** The sample will be analyzed in the laboratory by one of several methods which rely upon the principle that red blood cells which contain hemoglobin S become distorted into a sickle shape when deprived of oxygen and incubated with a chemical reducing agent. A **heelstick blood sample** may be used in infants.

BEFORE THE TEST

No special preparation is required.

AFTER THE TEST

Follow **venous blood sample** or **heelstick blood sample** aftercare.

SIGNIFICANCE OF RESULTS

A positive test strongly suggests the presence of sickle cell disease or a related hereditary anemia. False negatives, however, are possible.

□ □ □

☐ Sigmoidoscopy

WHAT IT IS AND WHY IT'S OBTAINED

The sigmoid colon is that portion of the large intestine located between the descending colon (in the left side of the abdomen) and the rectum. Sigmoidoscopy is used to examine this area. It probes deeper than **anoscopy** but not so deep as **colonoscopy.** It is used to evaluate symptoms such as intestinal bleeding, abdominal pain, and diarrhea. It is also recommended as an aid in screening for bowel cancer. The usual recommendation is that it should be performed on everyone over fifty years of age every three to five years.

HOW IT WORKS

You will be asked to disrobe from the waist down and to lie on your left side on an examining table. Your doctor will first perform a digital rectal examination and then insert a flexible lubricated tube into your anus. As the sigmoidoscope is introduced farther into the rectum and colon you will feel pressure and cramping. During the procedure air is introduced to distend the intestine and this will cause further cramping and a feeling that you have to expel gas. Don't fight the feeling. Suction to remove secretion or feces is noisy but painless. Biopsies, if taken, are also painless. There are two main models of sigmoidoscope, a longer (60 centimeters) and a shorter (35 centimeters). The longer one is better at detecting disease but is also more uncomfortable.

BEFORE THE TEST

Several bowel preparations are in use for this test, and you should follow the specific instructions carefully. Usually one or two enemas are given shortly before the procedure begins.

AFTER THE TEST

No special aftercare is needed. Sedation is usually not given and so you may drive home without difficulty. Your anus may be sore for a day or so and you may note a small amount of bright red blood on the toilet tissue. Perforation of the intestine is rare. Report any abnormal abdominal or rectal pain or bleeding to your doctor.

SIGNIFICANCE OF RESULTS

A negative sigmoidoscopy means that no abnormal findings were encountered. Possible findings may include tumors, polyps, diverticulosis, abscesses, inflammation (colitis), and fissures. Biopsy reports may take a week or more to come back.

□ □ □

□ Sjögren's antibodies

WHAT IT IS AND WHY IT'S OBTAINED

Sjögren's syndrome causes dry mouth, dry eyes, arthritis, and other symptoms. It is an autoimmune disease in which the immune system reacts against the body's own tissues. Antibodies are found in most people with Sjögren's syndrome and this test is used to see if they are present.

HOW IT WORKS

You will be asked to provide a **venous blood sample** from which serum* will be separated. Immunoassay* is used for the laboratory analysis.

BEFORE THE TEST

No special preparation is required.

AFTER THE TEST

Follow **venous blood sample** aftercare.

SIGNIFICANCE OF RESULTS

A negative test means that no antibodies were found. A positive result strongly suggests Sjögren's syndrome but may also occur in other autoimmune diseases.

SYNONYMS AND INCLUDED TESTS

SS-A (same as Ro antibody) and SS-B (same as La antibody).

□ □ □

□ Skeletal muscle antibody

WHAT IT IS AND WHY IT'S OBTAINED

Skeletal muscles are those we commonly think of as muscles, of the arms, legs, back, abdomen, chest, and so forth. Blood levels of antibodies to these muscles are used to investigate muscle disease.

HOW IT WORKS

You will be asked to provide a **venous blood sample** from which serum* will be separated. Immunoassay* is used for the laboratory analysis.

BEFORE THE TEST

No special preparation is required.

AFTER THE TEST

Follow **venous blood sample** aftercare.

SIGNIFICANCE OF RESULTS

A positive test may be found in many autoimmune diseases (in which the immune system reacts against the body's own tissues), but is not specific for any of them. At present the precise significance of finding antibodies to muscles is not known.

□ □ □

□ Skin biopsy

WHAT IT IS AND WHY IT'S OBTAINED

A skin biopsy is the surgical removal of a portion of skin for laboratory examination. It is used most commonly to test whether a growth is benign or malignant but can also be helpful in skin rashes.

HOW IT WORKS

A skin biopsy is almost always performed as an outpatient in a doctor's office. The skin over the site to be biopsied will be cleansed with an antiseptic and a small amount of local anesthetic will sting or burn as it is injected into your skin. The pain depends upon the site of the biopsy: on the back it is relatively mild, whereas on the tip of a finger or nose it can be uncomfortable. In either event the discomfort is transient. "Freezing" the site of injection with a refrigerant does little to reduce the sting, but the use of Emla cream, a topical prescription anesthetic, can be helpful. It is expensive, however, and somewhat cumbersome, since it must be applied an hour before the procedure and covered with an occlusive plastic film. The actual biopsy should be painless, irrespective of its type: in the "shave biopsy," a tangential cut is used to slice off an elevated growth; in the "punch biopsy," a portion of skin is removed with a small circular device which looks like a cookie cutter; in the "excisional" or "incisional biopsy," elliptical samples are taken out with a scalpel and sutures or pieces of tape used to close the wound. After the tissue is removed it is placed in a preservative and sent to the laboratory where it is processed, embedded in paraffin, sliced thinly, stained, and examined under a microscope by a pathologist. Special stains may be used to differentiate among the more uncommon skin diseases.

BEFORE THE TEST

Avoid aspirin for at least a week and ibuprofen, ketoprofen, or naproxen for one day.

AFTER THE TEST

If bleeding develops apply direct pressure for five minutes (watch the clock). Stitches can usually be removed in about a week. Report any abnormal tenderness, pus, or drainage, although a small amount of irritation in the form of redness and mild sensitivity is normal.

SIGNIFICANCE OF RESULTS

If the biopsy was taken to rule out malignancy, the report will usually be straightforward. If it was taken to provide information about a rash, the results will hopefully clarify the situation. The report, however, can be "negative" in the sense that the condition is benign, but one may be no closer to giving the eruption a name. Still, a result which shows a benign inflammation, even if the cause remains obscure, is not entirely bad, since more serious conditions have been ruled out.

□ □ □

□ Sleep erection monitoring

WHAT IT IS AND WHY IT'S OBTAINED

This test is used to evaluate impotence (erectile dysfunction).

HOW IT WORKS

There are several methods for measuring sleep erections. One way is to ask your wife or lover to stay awake all night with a watch and memo pad to observe the status of your erections, both as to time, duration, and intensity. Another technique is to use "postage" stamps, a set of four standardized stamps which you fasten around your penis with adhesive before you go to sleep. In the morning the stamps are examined for breaks along the perforations. A number of commercial devices are available which are more sophisticated, such as monitoring the circumference of the penis by means of an elastic loop, or measuring the rigidity of the penis by means of its ability to break pieces of plastic, or keeping track of both circumference and rigidity by means of a sensing device and computer. All tests may have to be repeated if results are equivocal. It is more reliable but also more expensive to have them performed in a sleep laboratory under controlled conditions.

BEFORE THE TEST

Avoid nonessential medications, alcohol, narcotics, and medications as directed by your doctor.

AFTER THE TEST

No special aftercare is needed.

SIGNIFICANCE OF RESULTS

The general principle is that if you get "normal" erections while you sleep there is nothing wrong with your blood vessels and nerves and that your impotence is psychological. Results can be borderline, however, and some urologists consider these tests to have limited value unless performed in a sleep laboratory. The **penile injection test, penile blood flow,** and penile **ultrasound** may be helpful.

SYNONYMS AND INCLUDED TESTS

Nocturnal penile tumescence test.

□ □ □

☐ **Sleep study**

WHAT IT IS AND WHY IT'S OBTAINED

Sleep studies comprise a range of tests designed to study the working of the body during sleep. They are usually used to determine the cause of excessive daytime sleepiness and to evaluate the disorder known as sleep apnea, in which an interference with normal nighttime breathing creates decreased oxygen in the blood. Disturbances in heart rhythm (arrhythmias) may result. This test is not for simple fatigue or restlessness during sleep.

HOW IT WORKS

The complexity of the study depends upon your symptoms and what information is being sought. Exactly what is done in a specific laboratory may vary greatly, as new methods and technology are developed. Tests may include the **electroencephalogram,** electrooculogram **(electrophysiologic eye testing), electromyogram,** and **electrocardiogram.** Many different techniques for measuring your breathing may be used, including **carbon dioxide** analyzers, microphones, and sensors in the esophagus. The amount of oxygen in your blood may be estimated with a device attached to your ear. Sleep studies are best done at night but may be performed during the daytime if you are able to sleep for the several hours which are necessary.

BEFORE THE TEST

Follow the instructions of your doctor carefully regarding medications.

AFTER THE TEST

No special aftercare is needed.

SIGNIFICANCE OF RESULTS

Interpretation of sleep studies is difficult because the most accurate methods for measuring your breathing and the amount of oxygen you are getting are the most uncomfortable and thus the most difficult to sleep with. Good sleep studies will take into consideration the different stages of sleep, the position of your body, and the pattern of your breathing, and will correlate them to your heart rate and rhythm.

SYNONYMS AND INCLUDED TESTS

Cardiopulmonary sleep study, sleep apnea study, polysomnography.

□ □ □

□ Slit-lamp examination

WHAT IT IS AND WHY IT'S OBTAINED

The slit lamp is a type of microscope which is used to examine the various portions of the eye: the conjunctiva, cornea, sclera, iris, lens, vitreous, and retina. It is commonly employed as part of a routine eye examination by ophthalmologists.

HOW IT WORKS

You will be asked to sit in a chair leaning forward with your chin on a chin rest. The examiner will be seated across from you looking into a binocular microscope and will direct a beam of light into your eye. The device has the ability to make the transparent structures of the eye appear as layers. Each eye will be examined separately and you may be asked to look in different directions, to blink, and so forth. The examination is painless. A slit-lamp examination may be used in conjunction with drops to dilate the pupils, dye to help visualize the ocular surface, or special lenses to obtain better views of certain structures, including the area between the iris and cornea which is the main exit site for eye fluid. The last named examination is called gonioscopy and may be used to evaluate the potential for glaucoma. Other lenses can be used to view the retina in three dimensions.

BEFORE THE TEST

No special preparation is required.

AFTER THE TEST

If dilating eyedrops were used your vision will be blurry for several hours. Some doctors instill another drop which will reverse the dilation, usually within an hour. These drops may sting when instilled.

SIGNIFICANCE OF RESULTS

A wide variety of abnormalities may be seen, including cataracts, corneal abrasions, foreign bodies, conjunctivitis, and iritis.

□ □ □

□ Small bowel biopsy

WHAT IT IS AND WHY IT'S OBTAINED

As its name implies, this test is used to obtain tissue from the small intestine. It is used to evaluate symptoms such as diarrhea, especially if malabsorption (in which the intestines fail to absorb nutrients properly) is suspected.

HOW IT WORKS

There are several techniques for obtaining tissue from the small intestine. One technique, called a capsule biopsy, is carried out in a special room equipped with **X-ray** equipment. You will be asked to sit upright and usually a local anesthetic will be sprayed on to the back of your throat. If you are anxious you may be given a mild sedative. A lubricated tube with a capsule on the end of it will be guided into your mouth and down your throat. Follow instructions and swallow the tube. Try to remain relaxed; you will not choke on it. After it has been advanced into your stomach you will be placed on your right side in order for it to pass into the small intestine. After a time its position will be checked with fluoroscopy*. This will be repeated in small steps with each advance being followed by fluoroscopy. When it is in the desired position suction will be used to pinch off a small portion of the intestinal lining. This is painless. Several specimens may be taken and the tube will be withdrawn. Another technique is similar to that of **upper endoscopy** except that a special device called an enteroscope is used. Some gastroenterologists employ a pediatric colonoscope (used for **colonoscopy** in children) for the same purpose.

BEFORE THE TEST

You should fast overnight. Avoid aspirin for at least a week and ibuprofen, ketoprofen, or naproxen for one day.

AFTER THE TEST

You should not eat or drink until your gag reflex returns in one to two hours. If you received sedation you should have someone drive you home. This procedure is generally safe but bleeding can occur. Report any abdominal pain or rectal bleeding immediately.

SIGNIFICANCE OF RESULTS

Many diseases may be diagnosed by intestinal biopsy. A negative biopsy may be helpful in ruling out certain diseases, such as celiac disease (gluten enteropathy). Negative biopsies, however, must be interpreted with caution, since small bowel biopsy is "blind" in that the best site cannot always be chosen. Although this can be circumvented in part by taking a biopsy with **upper gastrointestinal endoscopy,** small bowel biopsy can reach farther into the intestine.

☐ ☐ ☐

☐ Smooth muscle antibody

WHAT IT IS AND WHY IT'S OBTAINED

Smooth muscle is that which is not under voluntary control, such as is found in the intestines. Blood levels of antibody (a blood protein important to the immune system) to these muscles is used to evaluate liver disease.

HOW IT WORKS

You will be asked to provide a **venous blood sample** from which serum* will be separated. Immunoassay* is used for the laboratory analysis.

BEFORE THE TEST

No special preparation is required.

AFTER THE TEST

Follow **venous blood sample** aftercare.

SIGNIFICANCE OF RESULTS

The presence of smooth muscle antibody is found in chronic active hepatitis, an autoimmune liver disease (in which the immune system reacts against the body's own tissues). A **liver biopsy** and other more specialized tests (such as antibodies against liver/kidney microsomes and against soluble liver antigen) should also be obtained to diagnose chronic active hepatitis. The results of other **liver function tests** will be taken into consideration in evaluating your case.

☐ ☐ ☐

☐ Sodium

WHAT IT IS AND WHY IT'S OBTAINED

Sodium is one of the major **electrolytes** in the blood and has important functions throughout the body. Blood levels are used to evaluate acid-base balance and water balance.

HOW IT WORKS

You will be asked to provide a **venous blood sample** from which serum* will be separated. Several methods may be used in the laboratory for measurement. Urine may also be tested.

BEFORE THE TEST

No special preparation is required.

AFTER THE TEST

Follow **venous blood sample** aftercare.

SIGNIFICANCE OF RESULTS

Blood levels of sodium usually depend more on the amount of water in the body than the amount of sodium. Thus, dehydration is the most common cause of a high blood sodium. High sodium also may occur in Cushing's syndrome, diabetes insipidus, and primary aldosteronism (Conn's syndrome). Low sodium may be found in excessive fluid intake, malnutrition, heart failure, hypothyroidism, the syndrome of inappropriate secretion of antidiuretic hormone, kidney failure, liver disease, adrenal insufficiency (Addison's disease), and pituitary insufficiency. The evaluation of a high or low sodium will often take into account the other electrolytes, **osmolality, liver function tests,** and **kidney function tests.**

☐ ☐ ☐

☐ Somatomedin-C

WHAT IT IS AND WHY IT'S OBTAINED

Somatomedin-C (SC) is produced in the liver in response to stimulation by **growth hormone** secreted by the pituitary gland. Blood levels are used to evaluate disturbances of growth such as abnormally short or large stature. It is also used to monitor treatment with growth hormone.

HOW IT WORKS

You will be asked to provide a **venous blood sample** from which serum* will be separated. Immunoassay* is used for the laboratory analysis.

BEFORE THE TEST

You should fast overnight.

AFTER THE TEST

Follow **venous blood sample** aftercare.

SIGNIFICANCE OF RESULTS

High SC is found in acromegaly, adolescence, obesity, pituitary gigantism, and pregnancy. Low values are seen in pituitary insufficiency, Laron dwarfism (due to inadequate action of growth hormone), malnutrition, liver disease, hypothyroidism, in children, and in the very old.

SYNONYMS AND INCLUDED TESTS

Insulinlike growth factor.

☐ ☐ ☐

☐ Somatosensory response studies

WHAT IT IS AND WHY IT'S OBTAINED

The somatosensory system carries information about vibration, pain, temperature, touch, and the sense of position from the nerves through the spinal cord and to the brain. Somatosensory response studies of the upper and lower extremities are used to evaluate this system.

HOW IT WORKS

Electrodes as for an **electroencephalogram** will be placed on your scalp, along your spine, and on your extremities. The position of the electrodes on your arms and legs depends upon the information being sought. A series of mild electric shocks will then be delivered to one of the extremity electrodes. This is painless, but you may feel your muscles twitch. The time and nature of your response to this stimulus will be detected by the electrodes along your spine and scalp and will be sent to a computer which will produce a graph of the results.

BEFORE THE TEST

No special preparation is required.

AFTER THE TEST

No special aftercare is needed.

SIGNIFICANCE OF RESULTS

Results may help to determine the nature and location of a nerve disease or injury. Characteristic patterns are often found in disorders of the nerves, spinal cord, or brain.

Somatosensory-evoked potentials.

□ □ □

□ Spinal tap

WHAT IT IS AND WHY IT'S OBTAINED

A spinal tap is used to obtain a specimen of cerebrospinal fluid (CSF), the fluid which envelops and cushions the brain and spinal cord. This test is most valuable in meningitis and other infectious diseases of the brain, although it is also used to evaluate a variety of symptoms related to the nervous system.

HOW IT WORKS

A spinal tap may be performed in a hospital, clinic, or private doctor's office. You may be asked to lie on your side or sit up, but in either event you should try to flex your back as much as possible, to place your chin on your chest, and to draw your knees to your chest in order to open up the spaces between your vertebrae. The doctor will feel for the space between your fourth and fifth lumbar vertebrae by palpating the top of your pelvic bone. The skin over this area will be cleansed with an antiseptic and you will feel a slight amount of burning or stinging as it is injected with a local anesthetic. You should feel no discomfort as the spinal needle is introduced and as the CSF pressure is measured and fluid withdrawn. Report any tingling or shooting pains down your legs. This is not a serious complication, and the needle will simply be repositioned. You may be asked to extend your legs at some point in order to get a more accurate pressure reading. The CSF will be sent to the laboratory and may be analyzed for cells, **glucose,** glutamine, **lactic acid, lactic dehydrogenase,** or **protein.** If warranted it may also be tested by **bacterial culture, viral culture,** or **fungal culture.**

BEFORE THE TEST

You will be given a neurological examination and an eye examination and possibly **computed tomography** of your skull. No other special preparation is required.

AFTER THE TEST

You will be kept on strict bed rest for several hours during which time your vital signs (pulse, blood pressure, respiration, and temperature) will be taken frequently. The most common complication is headache. Rarely, a blood clot (hematoma) may develop in the spinal cord or persistent pain may result. Although rare, the most serious complication is herniation of the brain through the base of the skull, which may be fatal. Since it is almost always caused by a brain abscess or tumor, many hospitals require computed tomography before a spinal tap.

SIGNIFICANCE OF RESULTS

Although a number of abnormalities may be detected by spinal tap, the most important are those related to meningitis, in which an increase in white blood cells is found in the CSF. In this event, the exact nature of the germ causing it can be found by culture. Except for meningitis, a spinal tap usually gives nonspecific results, although the information may be valuable when your symptoms and the results of other tests are taken into consideration.

SYNONYMS AND INCLUDED TESTS

Lumbar puncture, LP.

□ □ □

☐ Sputum culture

WHAT IT IS AND WHY IT'S OBTAINED

Sputum is the matter which is expelled when you cough.
Sputum culture is a type of **bacterial culture** and is used to
determine the cause of pneumonia.

HOW IT WORKS

You will be given a plastic container in which to place
sputum which you cough up. Sputum should be from a *deep*
cough. The material will be incubated with a nutrient and
any organisms will be allowed to grow.

BEFORE THE TEST

No special preparation is required.

AFTER THE TEST

No special aftercare is needed.

SIGNIFICANCE OF RESULTS

If bacteria grow on culture they will be further tested to find
out what type they are. Not all bacteria, however, cause
disease, and some are normally present. A negative result
does not rule out the presence of bacterial pneumonia, only
that bacteria were not cultured from the specimen in
question.

☐ ☐ ☐

☐ Sputum induction

WHAT IT IS AND WHY IT'S OBTAINED

Sputum is the matter which you expel when you cough.
Sputum induction refers to the stimulation of coughing and

sputum production and is used in those who have difficulty in providing sputum for testing, such as in the investigation of persistent cough, difficulty breathing, chest pain, or abnormal findings on chest **X ray, computed tomography,** or **magnetic resonance imaging.**

HOW IT WORKS

You will be asked to breathe through a nebulizer. A salt solution will liquefy your sputum and lead to coughing. You will be provided with a sterile plastic container in which to collect the specimen. It may analyzed by **acid fast smear, cytology,** or **sputum culture.**

BEFORE THE TEST

Brush your teeth and rinse thoroughly to provide as clean a specimen as possible.

AFTER THE TEST

No special aftercare is needed.

SIGNIFICANCE OF RESULTS

A negative result means that no malignant cells and no disease-causing organisms were found. Positive results may reveal bacterial pneumonia, tuberculosis, or findings suspicious for cancer.

SYNONYMS AND INCLUDED TESTS

Sputum collection.

□ □ □

□ Stomach saline load test

WHAT IT IS AND WHY IT'S OBTAINED

This test is used to evaluate the ability of the stomach to empty itself.

HOW IT WORKS

You will be seated comfortably and a small, flexible, lubricated tube will be inserted into one of your nostrils and gently passed down your throat. Follow instructions and do not fight the tube; you can swallow it down without discomfort. You may have a slight gagging sensation but you will not choke. The tube will then be advanced slowly into your stomach. The contents of your stomach will next be evacuated by suction, after which a quantity of salt solution (normal saline) will be dripped in. After a time your stomach will again be emptied by suction and the volume of this fluid measured. You will be asked to move into different positions in order to make sure your stomach has been completely evacuated.

BEFORE THE TEST

You should fast overnight.

AFTER THE TEST

No special aftercare is needed. Complications are uncommon, but if you have heart problems you should be aware of the increased salt intake. You may have a mild sore throat for a day or two and some nausea. Aspiration of saline solution into the lungs has occurred but is rare.

SIGNIFICANCE OF RESULTS

A normal test means that most of the saline was emptied from your stomach. Fluid retention means either that there is an obstruction, such as a tumor, or that the stomach movement itself is impaired, such as occurs in some cases of diabetes.

SYNONYMS AND INCLUDED TESTS

Saline load test for gastric emptying.

◻ ◻ ◻

☐ Stool for muscle fiber

WHAT IT IS AND WHY IT'S OBTAINED

This test is used to screen for malabsorption (in which the intestines fail to absorb nutrients properly).

HOW IT WORKS

You will be provided with a plastic container into which you should place a random sample of stool. Do not place toilet paper in the container. In the laboratory a portion of the specimen is placed on a glass slide, stained, and examined under the microscope for undigested meat fibers.

BEFORE THE TEST

Eat an adequate amount of meat for three days. Avoid laxatives for one week.

AFTER THE TEST

No special aftercare is needed.

SIGNIFICANCE OF RESULTS

Muscle fibers in the stool are evidence for intestinal malabsorption. A positive test, however, does not identify whether the source of the problem is in the intestine or the pancreas, both of which can cause similar symptoms.

☐ ☐ ☐

☐ Stool for occult blood

WHAT IT IS AND WHY IT'S OBTAINED

This is a very common screening test for colon and rectal cancer. It is inexpensive and painless and should be performed routinely as part of every physical examination.

HOW IT WORKS

The best results are obtained from several different stool samples. If performed in the hospital the specimens may be placed in a plastic container. If you have been given one of the commercial kits to take home, read the instructions which come with it and return it to the doctor's office or laboratory. The assay in most cases is based upon guaiac, but other and more expensive methods are available.

BEFORE THE TEST

Follow the instructions given by the laboratory. For the guaiac-based test eat a high fiber diet and avoid apples, artichokes, bananas, bean sprouts, broccoli, cantaloupe, cauliflower, fish, grapes, horseradish, meat, mushrooms, oranges, radishes, and turnips for three days. Avoid aspirin, alcohol, and nonessential medications for the same amount of time. If the HemoQuant kit is used, ignore the vegetable restrictions.

AFTER THE TEST

No special aftercare is needed.

SIGNIFICANCE OF RESULTS

A positive test is more significant than a negative test, but there are many false positives as well as false negatives. A positive result means that further testing is indicated, usually a **colonoscopy** or **barium enema.** If the bleeding continues and its source cannot be identified, a **blood loss localization** study may prove helpful.

SYNONYMS AND INCLUDED TESTS

Stool guaiac, fecal occult blood test.

□ □ □

☐ Stool for ova and parasites

WHAT IT IS AND WHY IT'S OBTAINED

This test is used to diagnose intestinal parasites. These parasites can cause many symptoms, including skin rashes, weight loss, fatigue, abdominal pain, fever, cramps, diarrhea, or constipation. At times the symptoms are related to different organs, such as the lungs or liver.

HOW IT WORKS

Most of the time you will be asked to provide a random stool specimen. This should *not* be refrigerated. The method of identification depends upon the specific organism being sought. Sometimes fresh, warm stool is smeared on a microscope slide and examined directly under a microscope. Immunoassay* may also be used for different organisms. Multiple tests are advisable to rule out the presence of parasites. The procedure for one parasite, *Entamoeba histolytica,* is different. For this organism you will have to submit a series of stool specimens obtained by enema. Follow the directions given to you and collect the specimens.

BEFORE THE TEST

Avoid laxatives for one week. Do not try to obtain a stool specimen with mineral oil, bismuth, or magnesium-containing enemas.

AFTER THE TEST

No special aftercare is needed.

SIGNIFICANCE OF RESULTS

The presence of parasites in a stool specimen is virtual proof that they are causing the symptoms in question (except for one organism, *Blastocystis hominis,* which may be normally present). The real significance of finding a specific organism in your stool may depend upon your general health. *Cryptosporidium,* for example, causes mild diarrhea if you are healthy, but more severe symptoms if you have problems with your immune system.

□ □ □

□ Streptozyme

WHAT IT IS AND WHY IT'S OBTAINED

The streptozyme test is used to screen for recent infections with *Streptococcus,* such as "strep throat."

HOW IT WORKS

You will be asked to provide a **venous blood sample** from which serum* will be separated. Immunoassay* is used for the laboratory analysis.

BEFORE THE TEST

No special preparation is required.

AFTER THE TEST

Follow **venous blood sample** aftercare.

SIGNIFICANCE OF RESULTS

This test includes the antibodies which are detected by other tests for recent streptococcal infections, such as **antistreptolysin O, antideoxyribonuclease-B,** and **antihyaluronidase,** although the specific antibody cannot be discerned. The concentration of antibody (titer) is significant as is a determination as to whether the level is rising, falling, or remaining the same.

□ □ □

◻ Stress test

WHAT IT IS AND WHY IT'S OBTAINED

The stress test is used to evaluate the heart, specifically the effect of exercise on heart rhythm and blood flow through the coronary arteries. It is also used to monitor treatment for heart disease and to determine how much physical activity can be engaged in safely.

HOW IT WORKS

The procedure is performed in a special room or laboratory. **Electrocardiogram** (ECG) electrodes will first be applied to your chest and a blood pressure cuff will be attached to your upper arm, and a baseline ECG and blood pressure will be taken. You will then be asked to step on a treadmill and told to walk. The ECG will be monitored continuously and your blood pressure taken at intervals as the speed of the treadmill and its incline are gradually increased in stages. You will be asked to report any chest pain or other discomfort or sudden shortness of breath. The length of the test depends upon your stamina. It is terminated if you report significant discomfort, if your ECG or blood pressure becomes abnormal, or if you reach the level appropriate for your age. If you cannot walk or run, bicycle or upper arm ergometers can be used.

BEFORE THE TEST

Follow your doctor's instructions regarding medications. Bring exercise attire and running or walking shoes to the test site. Do not eat or drink for four hours before the test.

AFTER THE TEST

You will be allowed to return home when your pulse has become normal. You may take a lukewarm shower but avoid extremes of water temperature, either hot or cold. Avoid strenuous physical activity for a day afterward.

SIGNIFICANCE OF RESULTS

A normal stress test is good evidence that your heart is functioning adequately but does not rule out heart disease. If a heartbeat irregularity was precipitated by the exercise, its nature can be further investigated, if needed, by **invasive electrophysiologic studies** or a **Holter monitor.** If the test showed evidence of coronary artery disease, an **echocardiogram, cardiac catheterization,** or **heart scan** may be indicated.

SYNONYMS AND INCLUDED TESTS

Exercise tolerance test.

□ □ □

□ Sugar water test

WHAT IT IS AND WHY IT'S OBTAINED

This test is used to screen for paroxysmal nocturnal hemoglobinuria, a rare type of anemia.

HOW IT WORKS

You will be asked to provide a **venous blood sample** which will be incubated with a solution of sugar (sucrose) in water and observed for breakdown (hemolysis) of red blood cells.

BEFORE THE TEST

No special preparation is required.

AFTER THE TEST

Follow **venous blood sample** aftercare.

SIGNIFICANCE OF RESULTS

A positive result should be confirmed with the **Ham test.**

Paroxysmal nocturnal hemoglobinuria test screen, PNH test screen.

□ □ □

□ Sweat test

WHAT IT IS AND WHY IT'S OBTAINED

The sweat test measures the amounts of **electrolytes** in sweat and is used to diagnose cystic fibrosis, an inherited disease which causes problems in many areas of the body, including the lungs, liver, pancreas, and intestines. Symptoms may range from mild to severe

HOW IT WORKS

Since this test is usually done in children it is helpful for parents to be present. The process involves the stimulation and collection of sweat and there are many variations to it. The following is a typical scenario. A site on the right forearm or leg is usually selected. After the site is washed and dried, an electrode similar to that used for an **electrocardiogram** and a gauze pad impregnated with pilocarpine are placed on the skin. Another electrode and gauze impregnated with a salt solution is then placed close to the first one. Both electrodes are hooked up to a device which produces a low level of electricity at intervals. During this time you will feel a slight tingling or tickling, but no pain. If you experience a burning sensation, however, tell the technician and the electrode position will be adjusted. After about five minutes, the electrodes will be removed and a dry piece of gauze or paper will be placed over the pilocarpine site and covered with plastic and tape. After about thirty minutes the gauze or paper will be removed, weighed, and sent to the laboratory for analysis. Some tests are performed in heated rooms and involve collection of sweat in capillary tubes for analysis.

BEFORE THE TEST

No special preparation is required. The sweat test should not be performed after heavy exercise or on skin which is inflamed.

AFTER THE TEST

A slight redness at the site is normal but burns have resulted from improper electrode placement. If this occurs, follow your doctor's instructions for treatment.

SIGNIFICANCE OF RESULTS

A high sweat **chloride** and high **sodium** indicate cystic fibrosis, with a high chloride being somewhat more reliable. Other diseases, such as Addison's disease, may cause moderate elevations of sodium or chloride. Because of technical complexity, sweat tests are often repeated, whether positive or negative. Cystic fibrosis is inherited as a recessive trait which may be caused by any one of over two dozen different mutations to a certain gene. The sweat test does not detect the genetic carrier state of this gene, which is about one in every twenty people. For genetic counseling, the **polymerase chain reaction** and DNA identification for the cystic fibrosis gene should be used. The latter test, which can be performed on blood or amniotic fluid obtained from an **amniocentesis,** will eventually replace the sweat test for the diagnosis of cystic fibrosis in all cases.

□ □ □

□ TA-4

WHAT IT IS AND WHY IT'S OBTAINED

TA-4 is a protein found in the type of cancer called squamous cell carcinoma. Blood levels of it are used to evaluate and monitor the treatment of this cancer.

HOW IT WORKS

You will be asked to provide a **venous blood sample** from which serum* will be separated. Immunoassay* is used for the laboratory analysis.

BEFORE THE TEST

No special preparation is required.

AFTER THE TEST

Follow **venous blood sample** aftercare.

SIGNIFICANCE OF RESULTS

Elevated levels of TA-4 are found in squamous cell carcinomas anywhere in the body, particularly if the disease is advanced. A rising level of TA-4 after treatment indicates recurrence.

SYNONYMS AND INCLUDED TESTS

Tumor-antigen 4.

□ □ □

□ Teichoic acid antibody

WHAT IT IS AND WHY IT'S OBTAINED

Teichoic acid is a substance present in bacteria. Blood levels of antibody (a blood protein important to the immune system) to it are used to evaluate serious infections, particularly those of the heart or bones.

HOW IT WORKS

You will be asked to provide a **venous blood sample** from which serum* will be separated. Immunoassay* is used for the laboratory analysis.

BEFORE THE TEST

No special preparation is required.

AFTER THE TEST

Follow **venous blood sample** aftercare.

SIGNIFICANCE OF RESULTS

The presence of this antibody in significant amounts is evidence for continuing bacterial infection and the possible need for further treatment.

□ □ □

□ Testosterone

WHAT IT IS AND WHY IT'S OBTAINED

Testosterone is a hormone which causes male characteristics. It is manufactured in the testicles of men in large amounts and in the ovaries and adrenal glands in women in smaller amounts. Blood levels are used most often to evaluate virilization (the appearance of male characteristics) in women but may be obtained in men to investigate abnormal sexual development and sexual dysfunction.

HOW IT WORKS

You will be asked to provide a **venous blood sample** from which serum* will be separated. Immunoassay* is used for the laboratory analysis.

BEFORE THE TEST

No special preparation is required.

AFTER THE TEST

Follow **venous blood sample** aftercare.

SIGNIFICANCE OF RESULTS

In men low testosterone is found in testicular insufficiency, pituitary insufficiency, Klinefelter's syndrome, and some cases of impotence. In women high values are seen in hirsutism (excessive hair growth), the polycystic ovary syndrome (Stein-Leventhal syndrome), and congenital adrenal hyperplasia. In both sexes testosterone-secreting tumors may cause high blood levels. Other tests for virilization in women are **dehydroepiandosterone, 17-hydroxyprogesterone,** and **androstenedione.**

□ □ □

□ Thoracentesis

WHAT IT IS AND WHY IT'S OBTAINED

Thoracentesis is the withdrawal of an abnormal fluid collection—called a pleural effusion—in the space between the lung and the wall of the chest. It is performed either to find out why the fluid formed or to relieve breathing.

HOW IT WORKS

The procedure can be carried out in a doctor's office, emergency room, or hospital bed. You will usually be asked to sit and lean over, possibly hugging a pillow, in order to widen the spaces between your ribs. Before the test a chest **X ray** will have been performed in order to localize the fluid, and percussion (the tapping of the chest) will be done to confirm the level of fluid. A local anesthetic will sting or burn slightly as it is injected into your skin over the site to be tapped, which is usually on your back toward one side. It is important to keep as still as possible during the procedure and not to cough or breathe deeply. Avoid in particular any sudden movements. The thoracentesis needle will be introduced above one of your ribs in order to avoid the blood vessels and nerves, which are located just below the rib. As the needle is advanced the doctor will apply suction in an attempt at removing the fluid. Once fluid is found and removed, the needle will be replaced with a plastic tube and fluid is removed to the desired amount. If you were having difficulty breathing you should experience rapid relief. The fluid will be sent to the laboratory and may be analyzed for **cytology, protein, glucose,** and enzymes. **Bacterial culture** or other cultures may be obtained if indicated.

BEFORE THE TEST

Avoid aspirin for at least a week and ibuprofen, ketoprofen, or naproxen for one day.

AFTER THE TEST

You may experience mild shortness of breath, light-headedness, and a mild cough but these symptoms are transient. The major complication of thoracentesis is collapse of the of the lung (pneumothorax). For this reason a chest X ray will be obtained immediately after the procedure and your vital signs (pulse, blood pressure, respiration, and temperature) will be measured until they are stable. Rarer complications are puncture of the liver, spleen, or an artery beneath a rib. Infection is also uncommon. You should report any significant pain, fever, sudden shortness of breath, or anxiety to your doctor.

SIGNIFICANCE OF RESULTS

By its nature, a pleural effusion is abnormal, but analysis does not always determine its cause. The more common possibilities include heart failure, liver disease, kidney disease, cancer, tuberculosis, and pneumonia. Rarely it may also be caused by pancreatitis (inflammation of the pancreas), rupture of the esophagus, autoimmune diseases (in which the immune system reacts against the body's own tissues), or sarcoidosis.

SYNONYMS AND INCLUDED TESTS

Pleural fluid analysis.

□ □ □

☐ Thorn test

WHAT IT IS AND WHY IT'S OBTAINED

The Thorn test is used to diagnose diseases of the adrenal gland, specifically adrenal insufficiency (Addison's disease).

HOW IT WORKS

You will be asked to provide a **venous blood sample** upon which an **eosinophil count** will be performed. You will then receive an injection of **adrenocorticotropic hormone** (ACTH) and four hours later the eosinophil count will be repeated.

BEFORE THE TEST

No special preparation is required.

AFTER THE TEST

Follow **venous blood sample** aftercare.

SIGNIFICANCE OF RESULTS

Under normal conditions the eosinophil count will drop by about half after the injection of ACTH. If it stays the same the adrenal gland is not working. A better test, however, is the **cosyntropin test,** and most specialists consider the Thorn test to be out of date.

☐ ☐ ☐

☐ Throat swab for strep throat

WHAT IT IS AND WHY IT'S OBTAINED

Throat swab for strep throat is used to screen for "strep throat" (infection with Group A *Streptococcus).* Strep throat is important to recognize and treat because it can be associated with serious complications such as rheumatic fever and kidney disease.

HOW IT WORKS

You will be asked to open your mouth and stick out your tongue. A swab will then be used to vigorously swab your throat and tonsils, after which it will be immersed in a chemical which extracts streptococcal antigen*. Immunoassay* is used for the laboratory analysis.

BEFORE THE TEST

No special preparation is required.

AFTER THE TEST

No special aftercare is needed.

SIGNIFICANCE OF RESULTS

A positive result is very good evidence of a strep throat and indicates the need for specific treatment. A negative result, however, does not rule out infection. **Bacterial culture** provides a more definite answer.

□ □ □

□ Thrombin time

WHAT IT IS AND WHY IT'S OBTAINED

Thrombin is an enzyme which is important to the blood clotting system. (It causes **fibrinogen** to split into the fragments known as fibrin, the substance which forms the meshwork of a blood clot.) The thrombin time (TT) is used to evaluate bleeding disorders, particularly disseminated intravascular coagulation, a serious disease in which the substances responsible for blood clotting—mainly fibrinogen—are used up, leading to excessive bleeding from multiple sites.

HOW IT WORKS

You will be asked to provide a **venous blood sample** from which plasma* will be separated. In the laboratory thrombin will be added and the time it takes for the plasma* to clot will be noted.

BEFORE THE TEST

No special preparation is required.

AFTER THE TEST

Follow **venous blood sample** aftercare.

SIGNIFICANCE OF RESULTS

A long TT is seen in disseminated intravascular coagulation, abnormal fibrinogen, liver disease, and in those taking the blood thinner heparin.

□ □ □

□ Thyroglobulin

WHAT IT IS AND WHY IT'S OBTAINED

Thyroglobulin is a **protein** which is formed in the thyroid gland and which stores thyroid hormone. Blood levels are used to monitor the treatment of thyroid cancer. Thyroglobulin is not the same as **thyroid binding globulin.**

HOW IT WORKS

You will be asked to provide a **venous blood sample** from which serum* will be separated. Immunoassay* is used for the laboratory analysis.

BEFORE THE TEST

No special preparation is required.

AFTER THE TEST

Follow **venous blood sample** aftercare.

SIGNIFICANCE OF RESULTS

The presence of any amount of thyroglobulin in the blood is taken to mean that thyroid tissue is present in the body. Since thyroid cancer is usually treated by complete removal of the thyroid gland, the presence of thyroglobulin after treatment signifies that further surgery is indicated.

□ □ □

□ Thyroid antibodies

WHAT IT IS AND WHY IT'S OBTAINED

Blood levels of antibodies to the thyroid gland are used to diagnose Hashimoto's disease. Hashimoto's disease is a type of inflammation caused by autoimmunity, in which the immune system reacts against the body's own tissues, in this case the thyroid gland.

HOW IT WORKS

You will be asked to provide a **venous blood sample** from which serum* will be separated. Immunoassay* is used for the laboratory analysis.

BEFORE THE TEST

No special preparation is required.

AFTER THE TEST

Follow **venous blood sample** aftercare.

SIGNIFICANCE OF RESULTS

Two antibodies are included in this test, and the presence of both of them in significant amounts strongly indicates

Hashimoto's thyroiditis. Other autoimmune diseases, however, can cause false positives.

□ □ □

□ Thyroid binding globulin

WHAT IT IS AND WHY IT'S OBTAINED

Thyroid binding globulin (TBG) is a protein which binds thyroid hormone and transports it in the blood. Blood levels are used to evaluate thyroid function. This test should be distinguished from **thyroglobulin.**

HOW IT WORKS

You will be asked to provide a **venous blood sample** from which serum* will be separated. Immunoassay* is used for the laboratory analysis.

BEFORE THE TEST

No special preparation is required.

AFTER THE TEST

Follow **venous blood sample** aftercare.

SIGNIFICANCE OF RESULTS

TBG is high in pregnancy, with estrogen or tamoxifen therapy, and can be inherited as a harmless trait. It is decreased in kidney disease, in those taking steroids, and also in certain genetic conditions. Low levels of TBG are not serious but may produce abnormal thyroid function test results. Liver disease may cause an increased or decreased TBG.

□ □ □

☐ Thyroid biopsy

WHAT IT IS AND WHY IT'S OBTAINED

Thyroid **biopsy** is the surgical removal of a portion of the thyroid gland for analysis. It is used to evaluate thyroid enlargement which may have been detected by physical examination, **thyroid scan,** or thyroid **ultrasound.**

HOW IT WORKS

This procedure may be performed in a special room in an outpatient facility or hospital and under local or general anesthesia. Discuss these options with your doctor. For a needle biopsy you will be asked to lie on your back with a pillow beneath your shoulder blades. The skin over your neck will be cleansed with an antiseptic, and a small amount of local anesthetic will be injected into your skin. This will sting or burn slightly. The doctor will insert a special biopsy needle into your neck being careful to avoid blood vessels. This will cause transient discomfort. Thyroid biopsies performed under general anesthesia are done in an operating room in a hospital. In this case the skin over your neck will be incised and the gland visualized before the specimen is taken.

BEFORE THE TEST

Avoid aspirin for at least a week and ibuprofen, ketoprofen, or naproxen for one day. Your blood clotting ability should be checked with a **platelet count, prothrombin time,** and **partial thromboplastin time.**

AFTER THE TEST

Since the thyroid gland is filled with blood vessels, hemorrhage is always a potential problem. Pressure will be applied to the site for a number of minutes and should be continued as directed. Avoid strenuous physical activity and report any undue pain, redness, or bleeding in your neck.

SIGNIFICANCE OF RESULTS

A negative test means that no abnormality was found. This usually rules out cancer, but not always, since thyroid cancer can be small and scattered throughout the gland. A variety of benign or malignant tumors may be diagnosed, in addition to the findings characteristic of different types of thyroiditis (inflammation).

❑ ❑ ❑

❑ Thyroid function tests

WHAT IT IS AND WHY IT'S OBTAINED

The thyroid gland, located in the neck, produces two hormones, **thyroxine** (T_4) and **triiodothyronine** (T_3). Both stimulate metabolism and are the most commonly evaluated hormones in medicine. Indeed, every person born in the United States has theoretically had at least one thyroid function test, the one which is required by law shortly after birth. This is used to detect an underactive thyroid (hypothyroidism), which leads to cretinism. In adults thyroid tests are usually performed as part of a routine physical. Over the years the best way to screen for thyroid disease has changed along with technology and it still remains controversial. In the past, most screening was with blood levels of T_3 and T_4, but today most doctors prefer the **thyroid stimulating hormone** (TSH). Symptoms of an underactive thyroid are fatigue, weight gain, intolerance to cold, depression, constipation, dry skin, and muscle cramps. Symptoms of an overactive thyroid (hyperthyroidism) are fatigue, weight loss, intolerance to heat, anxiety, increased bowel movements, tremor, heart palpitations, and rapid pulse. Mild thyroid dysfunction of any type, however, may not be picked up by blood tests.

HOW IT WORKS

You will be asked to provide a **venous blood sample** from which serum* will be separated. There are several methods available for various assays.

BEFORE THE TEST

See individual test listings.

AFTER THE TEST

See individual test listings.

SIGNIFICANCE OF RESULTS

Thyroid function tests should be evaluated along with your symptoms because there are a number of situations in which the tests are abnormal in the face of normal thyroid function. This can occur, for example, when **protein** or **thyroid binding globulin** is abnormal (high or low). The thyroid may be visualized by means of thyroid **ultrasound** or a **thyroid scan** and thyroid tissue may be sampled with a **thyroid biopsy. Thyroid uptake** with suppression or stimulation tests may also be useful.

SYNONYMS AND INCLUDED TESTS

Thyroid profile.

□ □ □

□ Thyroid scan

WHAT IT IS AND WHY IT'S OBTAINED

This is a type of **radionuclide scan** which is used to evaluate thyroid function, particularly an overactive thyroid (hyperthyroidism), thyroid nodules, goiter (general enlargement), and inflammation (thyroiditis).

HOW IT WORKS

The test takes about one hour and is carried out in the nuclear medicine department of a hospital, clinic, or private physician's office, sometimes as part of a radiology facility.

You will be given a radioactive tracer compound, either by injection or orally. The substance will be allowed to disperse (about thirty minutes for injections and twenty-four hours for oral forms) and your neck will be scanned with a computer-driven device called a gamma camera that detects the compound's radioactive emissions. The actual scanning is painless and takes from ten to twenty minutes. You should try to remain as still as possible.

BEFORE THE TEST

Numerous foods and medications may interfere with interpretation of thyroid scanning, especially those containing iodides, such as seafood, vitamin pills, kelp, Ovaltine, cough syrups, iodized salt, tranquilizers, steroids, antihistamines, anticoagulants, and thyroid medications. Your doctor or the laboratory should provide you with a list of substances which may cause problems. Avoid those for the specified time periods. There is no other special preparation if the isotope is injected. If the oral form is used, however, you should fast for at least two hours before taking the iodine tracer.

AFTER THE TEST

If you were given an intravenous tracer, follow **venous blood sample** aftercare. Resume your regular diet and medications. Although safe, this test does involve the injection of a radioactive compound.

SIGNIFICANCE OF RESULTS

A negative result means that the thyroid appeared normal. Positive results are generally of two types. These may be "hot spots," in which metabolism is increased, or "cold spots," in which it is decreased. In either event further testing is necessary, such as a **thyroid uptake** with suppression for hot spots, or a **thyroid biopsy** for cold spots.

□ □ □

☐ Thyroid stimulating hormone

WHAT IT IS AND WHY IT'S OBTAINED

Thyroid stimulating hormone (TSH) is produced by the pituitary gland and stimulates the thyroid gland to produce thyroid hormone. The amount of thyroid hormone is controlled through feedback, in which an increase in thyroid hormone causes the pituitary to slow down production of TSH. Conversely, if thyroid hormone is low, the pituitary is stimulated to produce more TSH. Blood TSH is used as a screening test, both for an underactivity (hypothyroidism) and overactivity (hyperthyroidism). The use of a thyroid test is mandatory on newborns to detect hypothyroidism.

HOW IT WORKS

You will be asked to provide a **venous blood sample** from which serum* will be separated. Immunoassay* is used for the laboratory analysis. In infants a **heelstick blood sample** is used.

BEFORE THE TEST

No special preparation is required.

AFTER THE TEST

Follow **venous blood sample** or **heelstick blood sample** aftercare.

SIGNIFICANCE OF RESULTS

In general, high TSH is found in hypothyroidism and a low TSH is found in hyperthyroidism. The situation, however, is not so simple because of the complex interplay between the nervous system, brain, and endocrine glands. In brief the TSH is a very good but not a perfect test for thyroid function. For example, if the pituitary gland itself is overactive or underactive, causing the thyroid problem by producing either too much TSH or not enough TSH, the results will be opposite to those one would expect. For this reason, abnormal TSH results must be confirmed by other tests such as **thyroxine, triiodothyronine,** and **thyroid binding globulin.** Suspected pituitary gland disease may be tested by **visual fields** and skull imaging techniques such as **X rays, magnetic resonance imaging,** or **computed tomography.**

□ □ □

□ Thyroid uptake

WHAT IT IS AND WHY IT'S OBTAINED

This thyroid function test is often obtained along with the **thyroid scan** in order to distinguish among thyroid disorders, mainly to diagnose an overactive thyroid (hyperthyroidism).

HOW IT WORKS

The test is carried out in the nuclear medicine laboratory of a hospital, clinic, or private physician's office. You will be given an oral dose of a radioactive iodine compound. After several hours the outside of your neck will be measured for radioactivity. It will usually be measured again in twenty-four hours. The test is painless. The *thyroid suppression test* is a thyroid uptake obtained after you have taken an oral dose of a synthetic **triiodothyronine** (Cytomel) for about a week. The *thyroid stimulation test* is a thyroid uptake after you have taken an oral dose of **thyroid stimulating hormone** for about three days.

BEFORE THE TEST

Numerous foods and medications may interfere with this test, including seafood, vitamin pills, kelp, Ovaltine, cough syrups, iodized salt, tranquilizers, steroids, antihistamines, anticoagulants, and thyroid medications. Your doctor or the laboratory will provide you with an updated list of substances which may cause problems. Avoid those for the specified time periods. You should fast for at least two hours before taking the oral isotope.

AFTER THE TEST

Resume your normal diet and medications. Although this test involves absorbing a radioactive compound, the actual amount of radiation you will receive is small.

SIGNIFICANCE OF RESULTS

A low thyroid uptake indicates an underactive thyroid (hypothyroidism) or excess iodine in your diet. A high uptake may mean hyperthyroidism, decreased blood **protein,** or enlargement of the thyroid (goiter). Inflammation of the thyroid (thyroiditis) produces variable results. The suppression and stimulation variants of this test may help clarify the problem.

SYNONYMS AND INCLUDED TESTS

Radioactive iodine uptake test, RAIU.

□ □ □

□ Thyrotropin receptor antibody

WHAT IT IS AND WHY IT'S OBTAINED

Thyrotropin receptor antibody is an antibody directed against the thyroid gland. When present, it usually stimulates the thyroid to produce excess amounts of thyroid hormone and produces symptoms of an overactive thyroid (hyperthyroidism or Graves' disease). Blood levels are used to evaluate thyroid function.

HOW IT WORKS

You will be asked to provide a **venous blood sample** from which serum* will be separated. In the laboratory the serum will be injected into a radioactive mouse. The assay is performed by measuring how much radioactive thyroid hormone the mouse produces over a period of time. A positive test is signified by prolonged stimulation of the mouse thyroid.

BEFORE THE TEST

No special preparation is required.

AFTER THE TEST

Follow **venous blood sample** aftercare.

SIGNIFICANCE OF RESULTS

High levels are found in Graves' disease, but may be present in otherwise normal individuals. This test must be interpreted along with other **thyroid function tests.**

□ □ □

□ Thyroxine

WHAT IT IS AND WHY IT'S OBTAINED

Thyroxine (T_4) is one of the two forms of thyroid hormone, the other being **triiodothyronine** (T_3). The general effect of thyroid hormone is to stimulate metabolism. Blood levels of T_4 are used to evaluate thyroid function. As a screening test, however, **thyroid stimulating hormone** is more economical and probably better.

HOW IT WORKS

You will be asked to provide a **venous blood sample** from which serum* will be separated. Several methods of laboratory analysis are possible. Either *free* or *total* levels may be measured.

BEFORE THE TEST

No special preparation is required.

AFTER THE TEST

Follow **venous blood sample** aftercare.

SIGNIFICANCE OF RESULTS

In general, T_4 is high in an overactive thyroid (hyperthyroidism) and low in an underactive thyroid (hypothyroidism). But because T_4 exists in two forms in the blood, both free (active) and bound to **protein** (inactive), it is possible, if protein is high, that total T_4 will be high also, but the thyroid function may be normal. This condition exists, for example, in pregnancy. In such cases *free* T_4 should be obtained as well as **thyroid binding globulin.** It is also possible for T_4 to be normal in cases of hyperthyroidism due to increased **triiodothyronine.**

□ □ □

□ Tissue typing

WHAT IT IS AND WHY IT'S OBTAINED

Although tissue typing is usually used in organ or bone marrow transplantation, it is also used in legal matters and as an aid in diagnosing certain diseases. The principle of the test lies in finding out which types of four antigens (substances which provoke the immune system to react), termed A, B, C, and D, are present on white blood cells. These are called human leukocyte antigens (HLA).

HOW IT WORKS

You will be asked to provide a **venous blood sample.** Antigens A, B, and C are analyzed by immunoassay*. Antigen D is analyzed by a **mixed lymphocyte culture.**

BEFORE THE TEST

No special preparation is required.

AFTER THE TEST

Follow **venous blood sample** aftercare.

SIGNIFICANCE OF RESULTS

Tissue typing is similar to **blood typing** except that in this case white blood cells rather than red blood cells are used. HLA types are most useful when matching organ donors to organ recipients, in disproving paternity, and in differentiating between various forms of arthritis.

SYNONYMS AND INCLUDED TESTS

Lymphocyte crossmatch, human leukocyte antigen test, HLA typing.

□ □ □

□ Tonometry

WHAT IT IS AND WHY IT'S OBTAINED

Tonometry is used to measure the pressure of the fluids within the eyeball in order to diagnose glaucoma, which is often associated with increased pressure within the eye.

HOW IT WORKS

There are several methods of tonometry, the most widely used being applanation tonometry with the Goldmann tonometer. It is often performed as part of the **slit-lamp examination.** Your eye will be anesthetized with a few drops of a local anesthetic and stained with fluorescein* dye by touching your eyelid with an impregnated paper strip. The examiner will then move the tonometer forward until it gently touches your cornea. The pressure necessary to flatten your cornea is read off a gauge. A second method is called indentation tonometry, using the Schiötz tonometer. Again your eye will be anesthetized, you will be asked to look up, and a handheld instrument will be lowered onto your cornea. A small plunger in the center of the footplate indents the cornea and allows the examiner to read the pressure off a gauge. A third type of instrument does not require anesthesia and uses a puff of air to indent the cornea. A fourth type is a handheld electronic instrument which is placed against the cornea and gives a digital reading of the pressure.

BEFORE THE TEST

No special preparation is required.

AFTER THE TEST

No special aftercare is needed.

SIGNIFICANCE OF RESULTS

High pressure inside the eyeball may indicate glaucoma, which is a leading cause of blindness. Further testing with **ophthalmoscopy** and **visual fields** can confirm the diagnosis and evaluate its extent.

SYNONYMS AND INCLUDED TESTS

Intraocular pressure, intraocular tension, ocular pressure.

□ □ □

□ TORCH

WHAT IT IS AND WHY IT'S OBTAINED

TORCH stands for TOxoplasma, Rubella, Cytomegalovirus, and Herpes, any of which can be particularly serious in newborn infants. This blood test screens for antibodies to these organisms.

HOW IT WORKS

You will be asked to provide a **venous blood sample** from which serum* will be separated. Immunoassay* is used for the laboratory analysis. A **heelstick blood sample** may be used in infants.

BEFORE THE TEST

No special preparation is required.

AFTER THE TEST

Follow **venous blood sample** or **heelstick blood sample** aftercare.

SIGNIFICANCE OF RESULTS

The presence of any of these antibodies in significant amounts is evidence for the infection in question. A rising concentration (titer) of the antibody is particularly incriminating.

□ □ □

□ Transesophageal echocardiography

WHAT IT IS AND WHY IT'S OBTAINED

This procedure is a type of **echocardiography** in which the sensing device is placed in the esophagus. It is used in certain cases of heart disease in order to provide a more detailed image of the heart and particularly of the heart valves.

HOW IT WORKS

You will be asked to disrobe from the waist up. Electrodes for an **electrocardiogram** will be pasted to your chest and a blood pressure cuff will be placed on your arm. You will be given a mild sedative orally or intravenously and asked to lie on your left side. A local anesthetic will be sprayed into your throat and a flexible tube inserted into your mouth and guided slowly into your esophagus. You will be instructed to allow saliva to run out of the side of your mouth and into a basin. Follow instructions carefully, relax, and breathe normally. You will not choke on the tube. There is only minor discomfort and no real pain. The transducer will be moved up and down your esophagus during the course of the examination but this too should cause no pain.

BEFORE THE TEST

You should fast overnight.

AFTER THE TEST

Do not eat or drink until your gag reflex has returned. If the test was done as an outpatient you should arrange to have someone drive you home because of the sedation. Your throat might be slightly sore for a day, but should not require treatment.

SIGNIFICANCE OF RESULTS

Many abnormalities may be detected by this study, such as heart valve dysfunction, septal defects ("holes" in the heart), pericardial effusion, cardiac enlargement, tumors of the heart, and cardiomyopathy*.

□ □ □

□ Transferrin

WHAT IT IS AND WHY IT'S OBTAINED

Transferrin is the main **protein** which transports iron in the blood. Blood levels are used to evaluate anemia and iron deficiency.

HOW IT WORKS

You will be asked to provide a **venous blood sample** from which serum* will be separated. Immunoassay* is used for the laboratory analysis.

You should fast overnight.

AFTER THE TEST

Follow **venous blood sample** aftercare.

SIGNIFICANCE OF RESULTS

High transferrin levels are found in iron deficiency, pregnancy, and in those taking birth control pills. It is low in liver disease, kidney disease, cancer, chronic inflammation, hereditary transferrin deficiency, or when there are excessive amounts of iron in the body. **Ferritin** is the best single test for evaluating iron deficiency.

❏ ❏ ❏

❏ **Trichomonas preparation**

WHAT IT IS AND WHY IT'S OBTAINED

Trichomonas vaginalis is a parasite which causes a yellow, foamy vaginal discharge in women and, less commonly, a milky white discharge from the penis in men. This test is designed to detect it.

HOW IT WORKS

Several sources of specimen may be used. If you are a woman a cervical smear may be taken at the same time as a **Pap smear,** but your vagina may be swabbed separately. If you are a man, urine or a sample of the discharge from your penis may be used. The specimen will be placed on a glass slide and examined under a microscope.

BEFORE THE TEST

Women should not douche for three days.

AFTER THE TEST

No special aftercare is needed.

SIGNIFICANCE OF RESULTS

The presence of *Trichomonas* organisms along with symptoms confirms the diagnosis. False negatives, however, are common, and repeated tests may be called for. Cultures for this organism are available but they are expensive.

❑ ❑ ❑

❑ Triglycerides

WHAT IT IS AND WHY IT'S OBTAINED

Triglycerides are the form in which most body fat is stored. Blood levels are used to evaluate the risk of coronary artery disease (CAD) and to investigate disorders of fat (lipid) metabolism.

HOW IT WORKS

You will be asked to provide a **venous blood sample** from which serum* will be separated. Several methods of assay are available.

BEFORE THE TEST

You should fast overnight and avoid alcohol for several days before the test. It is also helpful to be on your normal, preferably stable, diet for a few weeks beforehand.

AFTER THE TEST

Follow **venous blood sample** aftercare.

SIGNIFICANCE OF RESULTS

The triglyceride value should be evaluated along with the other values in the **lipid screen.** A decreased high-density lipoprotein (HDL) **cholesterol,** for example, along with a high triglyceride often means increased risk of CAD, whereas the risk is less if the HDL cholesterol is elevated. High triglyceride is found in underactivity of the thyroid (hypothyroidism), kidney disease, alcoholism, liver disease, obesity, diabetes, pregnancy, and genetic disorders of fat metabolism (hyperlipoproteinemias). Triglycerides are also increased in those taking certain medications, such as birth control pills.

□ □ □

□ Triiodothyronine

WHAT IT IS AND WHY IT'S OBTAINED

Triiodothyronine (T_3) is one of two hormones produced by the thyroid gland, the other being **thyroxine** (T_4). The general effect of thyroid hormone is to stimulate metabolism. Blood levels of T_3 are used to evaluate thyroid function, in particular to confirm the diagnosis of the disease called T_3 thyrotoxicosis, which is a type of overactivity of the thyroid (hyperthyroidism).

HOW IT WORKS

You will be asked to provide a **venous blood sample** from which serum* will be separated. Immunoassay* is used for the laboratory analysis.

BEFORE THE TEST

No special preparation is required.

AFTER THE TEST

Follow **venous blood sample** aftercare.

High T_3 is found in hyperthyroidism, both the usual type, in which both T_3 and T_4 are increased, as well as in the type in which only T_3 is increased. T_3 is also high in pregnancy and in those taking birth control pills.

☐ ☐ ☐

☐ Triiodothyronine uptake

WHAT IT IS AND WHY IT'S OBTAINED

The triiodothyronine uptake (TU) is a test of thyroid gland function which is sometimes used to distinguish between true and apparent thyroid dysfunction. Thyroid blood tests are sometimes abnormal because of blood **protein** abnormalities; this test measures thyroid hormone "binding sites" on protein.

HOW IT WORKS

You will be asked to provide a **venous blood sample** from which serum* will be separated. In the laboratory, radioactive triiodothyronine (T_3) and a resin are added to the serum*, the resin is separated, and the amount of radioactivity remaining in the serum* or bound to the resin is measured.

BEFORE THE TEST

No special preparation is required.

AFTER THE TEST

Follow **venous blood sample** aftercare.

SIGNIFICANCE OF RESULTS

This test has mostly been replaced by **thyroxine (T_4)**, **triiodothyronine** and **thyroid stimulating hormone (TSH)**. The

TU is only of value when interpreted along with the T_4 blood level. In general, if both the TU and the T_4 are high, an overactive thyroid (hyperthyroidism) is indicated; if both are low, an underactive thyroid (hypothyroidism) is more likely. If one is high and the other is low, a protein problem is probably at fault. The latter **(thyroid binding globulin)**, however, can be measured directly if needed.

SYNONYMS AND INCLUDED TESTS

T_3 resin uptake.

□ □ □

□ Troponin

WHAT IT IS AND WHY IT'S OBTAINED

Troponin is a protein found in muscle. Blood levels are used to help diagnose heart attacks.

HOW IT WORKS

You will be asked to provide a **venous blood sample** from which serum* will be separated. There are three forms of troponin which can be separated by immunoassay*.

BEFORE THE TEST

No special preparation is required.

AFTER THE TEST

Follow **venous blood sample** aftercare.

SIGNIFICANCE OF RESULTS

High troponin levels are associated with recent heart muscle injury. Several measurements should be obtained, as well as other tests, such as **creatine kinase, electrocardio-gram,** and **lactic dehydrogenase,** if a heart attack is suspected.

□ □ □

□ Tuberculin skin test

WHAT IT IS AND WHY IT'S OBTAINED

The tuberculin skin test determines if your immune system has ever responded to infection with the tuberculosis germ (bacterium). It is a standard test which should be performed about every three years, unless there are occupational or other risk factors, in which case it should be repeated yearly. The only exception to this is if the tuberculin skin test has ever been positive, in which case it should not be repeated. The reason is that subsequent reactions can be severe. Tuberculin skin testing is becoming more important as tuberculosis becomes more prevalent.

HOW IT WORKS

The skin of your forearm will be cleansed with an antiseptic and a small needle will be introduced just under your skin to [inject a tiny amount of test material, forming a small bleb.] Discomfort is minimal. Although the test can be read by you, it is better to have a health professional do it, especially if you aren't sure of the results. The main sign of a positive reaction is firmness (induration), which develops in two or three days. No induration means the test is negative. If there is induration its extent is estimated with a reference card or ruler.

BEFORE THE TEST

No special preparation is needed.

AFTER THE TEST

Keep the test site open; do not cover with a Band-Aid. Wash normally and pat dry. Don't scratch or manipulate the test site. If it itches put a cool plain tap water compress on it.

SIGNIFICANCE OF RESULTS

A negative test result means one of two things. Either you have never been infected with tuberculosis or you have been infected but your immune system is impaired and cannot respond. A positive test also means one of two things. Either you have been infected with tuberculosis at some point in the past or you have been inoculated with BCG (bacillus Calmette Guerin), an outmoded form of tuberculosis immunization. If you have previously tested negative and have recently "converted" to positive, an investigation will be launched to see if the tuberculosis is active. This starts with a chest **X ray.** If positive, further tests, such an **acid fast smear** or **bacterial culture** of your sputum will be obtained. If the tests for active tuberculosis prove negative you will probably be placed on antituberculous medication as a precaution. Make sure you follow up with recommended treatment, since the cause of the current problem with multiple drug resistant varieties of tuberculosis is due to not taking medications properly.

□ □ □

□ Ultrasound

WHAT IT IS AND WHY IT'S OBTAINED

Ultrasound is used to take pictures of internal organs by bouncing sound waves off them. It can be used for virtually any area of the body, such as the chest, abdomen, pelvis, neck, breast, extremities, eye, or penis. It is performed extensively during pregnancy. Ultrasound has provided a major advance in medical diagnosis by providing noninvasive images which have in many cases replaced more hazardous procedures. Some organs, however, most notably the brain, cannot be visualized adequately, and in general the clarity (degree of resolution) is not so good as with **magnetic resonance imaging** or **computed tomography.**

HOW IT WORKS

Sound waves travel through the body and are reflected from internal organs depending upon the type of tissue and contents (air or water). Although reflected sound waves can be seen on a screen and recorded on film, no **X rays** are employed. Typically, you will uncover the site to be studied and a gel will be smeared over your skin. A device called a transducer will then be moved over your skin, "painting" an image. In the case of the eye, no gel is used, but the surface of the eye is anesthetized. In the case of the prostate, a rectal probe is employed. Ultrasound is painless. The devices are so small that many doctors have them in their offices. A variant called high-definition ultrasound provides more detailed images and can be used to investigate breast masses which have been detected by **mammography.** In colorflow Doppler ultrasound a computer translates the velocity and direction of blood flow within blood vessels into a rainbow of colors on a screen and allows for the investigation of circulatory problems.

BEFORE THE TEST

Preparation for these tests depends upon the organ studied but in general little or no preparation is required.

AFTER THE TEST

No special aftercare is needed. Ultrasound is safe. No radiation is used at any time.

SIGNIFICANCE OF RESULTS

Many abnormalities may be detected by this method. Tumors, cysts, fluid collections, organ enlargement, and organ atrophy (shrinkage) can be seen. The status of the fetus in pregnancy can be checked. Blood vessel narrowing, widening, or leakage can be visualized. The length of the eye can be calculated for intraocular lenses. The heart and its action can be evaluated by the type of ultrasound called the **echocardiogram.**

SYNONYMS AND INCLUDED TESTS

Ultrasonography, sonogram.

□ □ □

□ Unstable hemoglobin

WHAT IT IS AND WHY IT'S OBTAINED

The unstable hemoglobin test attempts to identify certain rare abnormal hemoglobins which may not be detected by **hemoglobin electrophoresis.** Symptoms of these diseases may include jaundice (yellowing of the skin), enlarged spleen, and anemia.

HOW IT WORKS

You will be asked to provide a **venous blood sample.** In the laboratory the red cells will be washed and disrupted to free up the hemoglobin. The mixture is either heated or treated with alcohol and observed for cloudiness.

BEFORE THE TEST

Avoid nonessential medications or do as your doctor directs.

AFTER THE TEST

Follow **venous blood sample** aftercare.

SIGNIFICANCE OF RESULTS

A positive result indicates the presence of an abnormal, unstable hemoglobin, which may produce symptoms ranging from mild to severe. These hemoglobins may be further evaluated with sophisticated laboratory techniques. Certain drugs and other substances may interefere with this test.

□ □ □

□ Upper gastrointestinal endoscopy

WHAT IT IS AND WHY IT'S OBTAINED

Upper gastrointestinal endoscopy is used to examine the esophagus, stomach, and duodenum (first part of the small intestine). It is indicated in evaluating intestinal symptoms such as bleeding, difficulty swallowing, and chest or abdominal pain.

HOW IT WORKS

The procedure usually takes place in a special room devoted to the purpose and is performed by a gastroenterologist or surgeon. You will have your vital signs (pulse, blood pressure, respiration, and temperature) taken and an intravenous fluid drip will be started, after which you will be given a sedative and a painkiller. This will make you feel relaxed but you will still be conscious. You will usually be asked to lie on your left side, although other positions are possible, and you will be given a plastic mouthpiece to protect your teeth. A local anesthetic will then be sprayed on to the back of your throat. At this point you will be unable to swallow your saliva and will be told to let it drain out of the side of your mouth into a basin. The examiner will next guide a flexible tube into your mouth with the aid of his finger. The sensation is unusual but not painful, and you should remember that you will not choke on the tube. At first you will be instructed to swallow, then the tube will be slowly advanced without your swallowing. At times you will feel pressure, fullness, or other sensations in your chest or abdomen but no real pain. This is from tube movement and air or water being introduced into your stomach. Although the main purpose of this test is to look at the lining of your intestines, there are a number of small channels in the fiber-optic endoscope which allow for biopsy, culture, or brushing specimens to be taken. You will usually be unaware that this is happening.

BEFORE THE TEST

Follow instructions carefully with regard to food and medications. It is usual to fast overnight for an early morning test and to be without food for eight hours in any event. Antacids should be discontinued as directed.

AFTER THE TEST

Your vital signs will be monitored in a recovery area depending upon your physical condition. After about an hour your gag reflex will be tested by a nurse or technician touching the back of your throat with a tongue depressor. After the reflex has returned you can eat and drink. You may burp or belch excessively for a few hours and have a sore throat for a few days. If this procedure has been performed as an outpatient have someone drive you home since you will be groggy for a number of hours. Although generally safe, upper gastrointestinal endoscopy can produce complications such as perforation of the esophagus or stomach and aspiration of fluid into the lungs. Report any abnormal pain, difficulty breathing, black stool, or vomiting blood.

SIGNIFICANCE OF RESULTS

A negative test means that the portion of the intestine observed was free of disease. Not all areas can be seen, however, and it is possible to miss abnormalities. Many diseases may be diagnosed by endoscopy, including ulcers, gastritis, esophagitis, tumors, enlarged veins (varices), polyps, diverticula (outpouchings), hiatal hernia, and pyloric stenosis (narrowing of the opening which leads out of the stomach). Culture or biopsy reports may take a week or more.

SYNONYMS AND INCLUDED TESTS

EGD, esophagogastroduodenoscopy, peroral endoscopy, upper endoscopy.

□ □ □

□ Uric acid

WHAT IT IS AND WHY IT'S OBTAINED

Uric acid is a waste product of the metabolism of purines, compounds which are involved in the chemistry of DNA. Blood levels are used mainly to diagnose and monitor gout.

HOW IT WORKS

You will be asked to provide a **venous blood sample** from which serum* will be separated. Several methods using the enzyme* uricase are available for analysis. A **24-hour urine sample** may also be analyzed.

BEFORE THE TEST

You should fast overnight.

AFTER THE TEST

Follow **venous blood sample** aftercare.

SIGNIFICANCE OF RESULTS

Although a high uric acid is associated with gout, many other conditions may cause it, including dehydration, cancer, chemotherapy, heart failure, heart attacks, mononucleosis, lead poisoning, thyroid disease, and parathyroid disease. It is also high in those on weight loss diets and in those taking many drugs and medications, including aspirin and water pills (diuretics). Actually, the most common cause of a high uric acid is something *other* than gout, and many times no reason can be found for it. Low uric acid is seen with liver disease and with many drugs, including steroids and outdated tetracycline. Kidney disease may produce either high or low uric acid, depending on the problem.

□ □ □

□ Urinalysis

WHAT IT IS AND WHY IT'S OBTAINED

The examination of urine to detect disease is the oldest and most common medical test. Doctors actually used to taste the urine as part of the clinical examination. This is how the common type of diabetes, diabetes *mellitus,* got its name: *mel* in Latin means "honey," and the urine of diabetics is sweet because of sugar. Urinalysis is a routine test which should be part of every physical examination. It is inexpensive, painless, and provides a wealth of information about the kidneys and the general state of health. The term urinalysis refers to "routine urinalysis." Urine itself can be used as a specimen source for a wide variety of examinations.

HOW IT WORKS

If you are a woman you should be careful in the collection technique if you are in the middle of a your menstrual period or if you are suffering from a vaginal discharge. In order to avoid contamination, follow the instructions for a clean catch specimen under **urine culture.** Examination of the urine specimen may be performed initially by your doctor or nurse and then sent to the laboratory. Many quick and inexpensive commercial methods of office analysis are possible through the use of "dipsticks," which are strips of firm paper or plastic which are impregnated with bands of colored indicator chemicals. The strip is dipped into the urine and any color change is matched to a chart. Dipsticks are available in different forms. Some, such as Tes-Tape, are used to detect **glucose** only and are commonly used by diabetics. Others, such as Chemstrip-8, test for **bilirubin,** blood, glucose, ketones, nitrite, pH, **protein,** and urobilinogen. The sample may also be centrifuged to concentrate solid matter and examined under a microscope for red blood cells, white blood cells, other cells, crystals, and germs. Computerized machines are available which can perform the entire test.

BEFORE THE TEST

No special preparation is required.

AFTER THE TEST

No special aftercare is needed.

SIGNIFICANCE OF RESULTS

Interpretation of abnormal urine findings is a science unto itself. The examination may be broken down into categories:

Color. Urine is normally clear and straw-colored or light yellow. Lighter than normal color may result from excessive fluid intake, diuretic (water pill) use, or diabetes. Darker than normal color may be caused by liver disease, porphyrias, and certain drugs. Cloudy or hazy urine is sometimes seen in infections, but can also be due to a very alkaline urine or contamination with vaginal fluid. Red urine may indicate blood, which can be caused by diseases of the kidney, bladder, prostate, urethra, or blood clotting system. It can also occur after eating large amounts of beets.

Odor. Urine has a characteristic odor which can change dramatically with dietary intake such as asparagus or onions or with concentration of urine (which can vary with how much fluid you drink). Diabetes often produces a fruity odor, whereas infections with certain bacteria can cause an unpleasant smell. Maple syrup urine disease vividly describes the characteristic finding in that genetic disorder.

Glucose. The presence of sugar (glucose) in urine is the hallmark of diabetes but may be seen in kidney disease and other diseases. The dipstick method for glucose also detects other sugars which may be found in certain inherited disorders.

Protein. Protein in urine may be found in kidney disease, multiple myeloma (a cancer of plasma cells, a type of cell which is usually found in the bone marrow), heart failure, and after stress or surgery; it may be normal in some individuals.

pH. This varies with diet, but usually is acidic in the range of pH 5–6. Alkaline urine is associated with a vegetarian diet (especially citrus fruits), vomiting, diuretics, and excess ingestion of antacids such as baking soda (sodium bicarbonate).

Specific gravity. Urine specific gravity is high (the urine is concentrated) in dehydration, diabetes, adrenal insufficiency, and in conditions in which there is excess protein in the urine. It is low (dilute urine) with excessive fluid intake and some kidney diseases.

Nitrite or leukocyte esterase. The presence of either strongly suggests bacterial infection of the urinary tract.

Ketones. These are found in diabetes, malnutrition, alcoholism, vomiting, diarrhea, and in those on high protein diets.

Bile*. Bile in urine is seen in liver disease, gallstones, and cancers which obstruct the flow of bile.

Casts. These are molds of the kidney tubules. Several types can be detected under the microscope. Some are insignificant whereas others indicate kidney disease.

Crystals. Some are normally present in urine whereas others may indicate diseases such as gout or kidney stones.

Urobilinogen. High levels indicate liver damage. Low levels signify obstruction of the flow of bile. If you use home dipsticks and find an abnormal reading you should bring it to your doctor's attention.

□ □ □

□ Urine culture

WHAT IT IS AND WHY IT'S OBTAINED

The urine culture is a type of **bacterial culture** which is used to detect infections of the urinary tract, most often the urinary bladder. **Fungal culture** for urine may also be obtained, but it is less common.

HOW IT WORKS

The general technique for both men and women is to provide a "midstream clean-catch" specimen which is as free from external bacterial contamination as possible. The following instructions or similar ones provided by your doctor or the laboratory should be followed as carefully as possible.

If you are a man you should retract your foreskin and clean the tip of your penis with an antiseptic solution or warm soapy water on a sponge, wiping away from the urinary opening in a circular motion. If you are using an antiseptic solution, discard each swab after use. If you are using a soapy sponge, use a separate sponge for each wiping motion, then clean off any excess soap with plain tap water.

If you are a woman, squat over the toilet and separate the lips of your vulva with your thumb and forefinger. Clean around the urinary opening—located above the opening of the vagina—with a towelette containing antiseptic solution or with warm soapy water on a sponge, wiping downward and away from the urinary opening. If you are using an antiseptic solution, discard each swab or towelette after use. If you are using a soapy sponge, use a separate sponge for each wiping motion, then clean off any excess soap with plain tap water.

In both cases, to obtain the specimen itself, begin to void into the toilet. Then stop, position the container, and catch the rest of the urine in it. Do not touch the inner surface of the container. Replace the cap. If you are not submitting the specimen directly to the laboratory, refrigerate it. In the laboratory the specimen is incubated with a bacterial nutrient and any growth is noted.

BEFORE THE TEST

No special preparation is required.

AFTER THE TEST

No special aftercare is needed.

SIGNIFICANCE OF RESULTS

In women, contamination of urine during collection by bacteria normally found in vaginal fluid or on the skin is very common. This is why the collection technique is so important. In men, if bacteria grow significantly it virtually proves a urinary tract infection, but in women results are less certain and repeat cultures may be necessary. A repeat specimen collected by a small catheter is sometimes required since many women have difficulty providing uncontaminated specimens.

□ □ □

□ Uroflowmetry

WHAT IT IS AND WHY IT'S OBTAINED

Uroflowmetry evaluates urinary bladder function and is used to investigate frequent urination, urgent urination, incontinence, or difficulty in starting or stopping one's stream.

HOW IT WORKS

This test is painless and easy and is often considered as part of a basic examination by a urologist. You will be left alone in the testing room and asked to urinate through a funnel; men standing, women sitting. The funnel leads to a container which calculates the rate of urine flow. The results are recorded on a strip of paper.

BEFORE THE TEST

Discontinue medications which may interfere with bladder function, such as antihistamines. Drink extra fluids and do not void, if possible, for several hours in order to have a full bladder before beginning the test.

AFTER THE TEST

No special aftercare is needed.

SIGNIFICANCE OF RESULTS

Abnormally fast or slow rates are found with bladder muscle weakness, obstruction, and some types of urinary incontinence.

☐ ☐ ☐

☐ Urogram

WHAT IT IS AND WHY IT'S OBTAINED

A urogram is an **X-ray contrast study** which visualizes the kidneys, bladder, and the tubes which which lead from the kidneys to the bladder (ureters). It is used to evaluate blood in the urine, back pain, or abnormal **kidney function tests.** Kidney **ultrasound** will often have been performed first.

HOW IT WORKS

The test is performed in the X-ray department of a hospital or clinic or in a private radiologist's office. You will be asked to undress from the waist up, to put on a hospital gown, and to lie on your back on a table. **X rays** of your abdomen will then be taken, after which you will receive an intravenous injection of a contrast agent or "dye." This will produce a feeling of warmth, possibly associated with a metallic taste and nausea. After about a minute a series of X rays will be taken at varying intervals. At some point a belt with rubber balloons may be strapped around your midsection and inflated in order to slow the excretion of the contrast agent. This is not painful.

BEFORE THE TEST

Drink plenty of fluids the day before but you should fast overnight. Some doctors recommend a mild laxative in order to improve the images.

AFTER THE TEST

The contrast agent has the potential for causing a variety of allergic reactions, ranging from mild to severe, and from immediate to delayed. This often occurs in those with a history of allergy to iodine. The symptoms are transient but if uncomfortable may be treated with antihistamines or steroids. Follow **venous blood sample** aftercare at the site of injection.

SIGNIFICANCE OF RESULTS

Many abnormalities may be detected by urography, including kidney stones, obstruction in the blood vessels feeding the kidneys, cysts, tumors, inflammations, and anatomical irregularities.

SYNONYMS AND INCLUDED TESTS

Excretory urography, intravenous pyelogram, IVP.

□ □ □

☐ Vanillylmandelic acid

WHAT IT IS AND WHY IT'S OBTAINED

Vanillylmandelic acid (VMA) is a waste product of **catecholamines** which are produced by the adrenal glands. Blood levels are used to evaluate high blood pressure, specifically to diagnose certain tumors which produce excessive amounts of catecholamines.

HOW IT WORKS

You will be asked to provide a **24-hour urine sample.** Several laboratory methods are available for analysis.

BEFORE THE TEST

Avoid coffee, tea, bananas, citrus fruits, chocolate, and vanilla for the time specified by your doctor or the laboratory. Avoid excessive physical activity during the collection period. Check with your doctor for medications you are taking which may influence the test.

AFTER THE TEST

Resume normal diet, activity, and medications.

SIGNIFICANCE OF RESULTS

A positive result means that the level of VMA was high, signifying the overproduction of catecholamines. This may be caused by a pheochromocytoma, neuroblastoma, or ganglioneuroma. Further testing, such as urine **homovanillic acid,** is then required.

☐ ☐ ☐

☐ Vasoactive intestinal peptide

WHAT IT IS AND WHY IT'S OBTAINED

Vasoactive intestinal peptide (VIP) is a substance found in the intestines which can be produced in large amounts by some tumors. Symptoms often include severe diarrhea which leads to dehydration. Blood levels of VIP are used to diagnose this condition.

HOW IT WORKS

You will be asked to provide a **venous blood sample** from which serum* will be separated. Immunoassay* is used for the laboratory analysis.

BEFORE THE TEST

You should fast overnight. This fast, unlike most, should be complete, i.e., not even water. Discontinue all nonessential medications for one or two days before the test, particularly antacids and laxatives.

AFTER THE TEST

Follow **venous blood sample** aftercare.

SIGNIFICANCE OF RESULTS

High levels are seen with VIP-secreting tumors which may arise in the pancreas, intestines, lung, thyroid, or nervous system, among other sites. VIP may also be elevated in those who take a lot of laxatives.

☐ ☐ ☐

☐ Venogram

WHAT IT IS AND WHY IT'S OBTAINED

A venogram is an **X-ray contrast study** which visualizes veins. Venograms may be obtained of the arms, legs, pelvis, or internal organs in the abdomen. The venogram is used to detect impaired circulation

HOW IT WORKS

The test is performed in a procedure room with surgical and X-ray equipment. The technique depends upon which veins are to be visualized. For most of the studies involving internal organs, the femoral vein in the groin is used. You will be asked to undress from the waist down and to put on a hospital gown. Your vital signs (pulse, blood pressure, respiration, and temperature) will be taken and an intravenous fluid drip will be started. The skin of your groin will be cleansed with an antiseptic and shaved if necessary. You will feel a slight burning sensation as a local anesthetic is injected. A needle will then be inserted into the femoral vein and a catheter introduced through it. With the aid of fluoroscopy (a type of X ray in which images appear on a screen) the catheter will be guided to the desired site. As the contrast agent is injected you will feel a generalized warmth, a salty or metallic taste in your mouth, and possibly nausea. **X rays** will be taken at intervals. If your groin is not suitable, the jugular vein in your neck can be substituted. For an arm or leg venogram, a superficial vein on the back of the hand or foot is used.

BEFORE THE TEST

Preparation depends upon the site being studied. Follow instructions regarding diet and medications.

AFTER THE TEST

You will be placed on bed rest for a number of hours while your vital signs are taken and the puncture site is checked for signs of bleeding. Unlike an **angiogram,** however, the pressure within veins is not so great as that in arteries and bleeding is less likely a problem. Allergic reactions to the contrast dye are possible, ranging from mild to severe, and from immediate to delayed. This often occurs in those with a history of allergy to iodine. The symptoms are transient, but if uncomfortable may be treated with antihistamines or steroids. Kidney failure may occur if you are dehydrated, so drink plenty of fluids.

SIGNIFICANCE OF RESULTS

Possible abnormalities detectable by a venogram include blood clots, narrowing, growths, aneurysms, injury, or leakage.

□ □ □

□ Venous blood sample

WHAT IT IS AND WHY IT'S OBTAINED

Venous blood collection is the most common way of obtaining blood for analysis.

HOW IT WORKS

The blood sample may be taken in a laboratory, doctor's office, hospital, or clinic. Usually you will be asked to sit, either in a special chair with an armrest or on a table. If you are very anxious or if you faint or sweat or get light-headed easily at the mere thought of a needle, tell the doctor, nurse, or technician, and ask to be allowed to lie down. It is virtually impossible to faint when lying flat and you will be much more comfortable. Next, a vein will be selected, usually one in the crook of your elbow, either the basilic vein, cephalic vein, or median cubital vein. In difficult cases, however, other veins can be used, such as those on the backs of your hands or feet. In infants a scalp vein may be used. A rubber tourniquet will then be placed above the site and your veins will be allowed to fill from below. Opening and closing your fist will help. Your skin will be cleansed with an antiseptic, usually alcohol, unless blood is being drawn for alcohol. Your skin will be punctured and the vein entered. There is usually very little discomfort associated with this. Most commonly a Vacutainer tube and holder are employed. The Vacutainer tube contains a vacuum and blood is automatically sucked into it. Different tubes have different colored stoppers depending upon whether they contain anticoagulants. The most common stopper color is red (no anticoagulant), which allows for serum* or plasma* separation. The next most common color is lavender, which contains the anticoagulant EDTA and which is used for a **complete blood count.**

BEFORE THE TEST

Preparation for a venous blood collection depends entirely upon the analyses to be performed. An "overnight fast" is generally considered to mean twelve hours without food. Water, coffee, or tea without sugar or milk, however, is permitted. Other tests may have different requirements.

AFTER THE TEST

Apply pressure to the puncture site and elevate your arm slightly until bleeding stops. If you have been taking aspirin, ibuprofen, ketoprofen, or naproxen or if you suffer from liver disease you may note prolonged bleeding and may need increased pressure. If you have been taking anticoagulants such as warfarin (Coumadin) or heparin or if you suffer from a bleeding disorder you will almost always require additional pressure. A black and blue mark, or hematoma (collection of blood beneath the skin), sometimes develops but will go away by itself. Infection is rare. A Band-Aid or piece of cotton will be placed over the wound and may be removed in a few hours. No other treatment is needed.

SIGNIFICANCE OF RESULTS

See individual test listings.

SYNONYMS AND INCLUDED TESTS

Blood collection, phlebotomy, venipuncture.

□ □ □

☐ Vestibular test

WHAT IT IS AND WHY IT'S OBTAINED

The term "vestibular" refers to the vestibule of the inner ear and the balance portion of the inner ear. The vestibular test is used to evaluate symptoms related to the inner ears, such as dizziness or vertigo.

HOW IT WORKS

This test is performed in a special laboratory. You will be asked to lie down on a special table and electrodes will be placed on your forehead and around your eyes. This is painless. From this point on, individual testing procedures vary according to the information being sought. In general you will be asked to perform a variety of tasks, such as staring at an object, keeping your eyes closed, following a light, moving your head rapidly, lying flat on your back or on one side or the other, and leaning backward quickly. In one portion of the test, called *calorics,* water or air of different temperatures will be introduced into your ears. This portion of the test may be uncomfortable, but the discomfort is usually transient.

BEFORE THE TEST

Follow any instructions you have been given with regard to avoiding certain medications, stimulants, and depressants. Discontinue smoking, alcohol, and caffeine for one to two days and do not eat heavily just before the test.

AFTER THE TEST

Resume medications as directed.

SIGNIFICANCE OF RESULTS

The results of this test are interpreted by an ear, nose, and throat specialist, neurologist, or audiologist. By studying the electrical patterns it is often possible to determine whether the symptoms in question arise from the ear or the brain.

SYNONYMS AND INCLUDED TESTS

Calorics, electronystagmography

□ □ □

□ Viral antibodies

WHAT IT IS AND WHY IT'S OBTAINED

Blood levels of antibody (a blood protein important to the immune system) to a virus are used to assist in the diagnosis of viral infections. Many infections may be tested for in this way, including various types of encephalitis, herpes, German measles, influenza, polio, mumps, chickenpox, Epstein-Barr virus, and others. **HIV tests** and most hepatitis tests use viral antibodies.

HOW IT WORKS

You will be asked to provide a **venous blood sample** from which serum* will be separated. Various methods of immunoassay* are available in the laboratory.

BEFORE THE TEST

No special preparation is required.

AFTER THE TEST

Follow **venous blood sample** aftercare.

SIGNIFICANCE OF RESULTS

An elevated level of antibody to a specific virus is indirect evidence of infection with that virus, but multiple tests which show a rise in concentration (titer) are much more significant. Many antibodies, however, cross react with other antibodies, and positive serology tests should be confirmed by **viral culture,** if possible.

SYNONYMS AND INCLUDED TESTS

Viral serology.

□ □ □

□ **Viral culture**

WHAT IT IS AND WHY IT'S OBTAINED

Viruses differ from most other germs by being much smaller and needing a host cell in which to live. Viral culture is more difficult than **bacterial culture** or **fungal culture,** for example, because the latter only need nutrients. Viral culture has progressed greatly in the past several years and continues to improve. Cultures can now be taken of the viruses which cause polio, mononucleosis, herpes, AIDS, influenza, mumps, German measles, chickenpox, and many others.

HOW IT WORKS

Any body fluid or tissue can be a source of the specimen, including blood, fluid from a **spinal tap,** skin, tears, secretions, stool, urine, fluid from an **amniocentesis,** or material from a surgical biopsy. The sample is inoculated into living cells and observed over the course of days or weeks. If the virus is present the cells are changed in a characteristic way which is different for each virus. The type of cell used in the culture varies according to the virus, some of which have strict requirements. A variation of the standard culture is the "rapid" culture. In this technique, the source of the sample is the same, but the inoculation is made into the cells by spinning the mixture to concentrate it. This enhances the infection. Then immunoassay* is used. The rapid technique usually provides results overnight whereas the standard technique may take days to weeks for a final report.

BEFORE THE TEST

No special preparation is required.

AFTER THE TEST

This depends on the source of the specimen. Follow your doctor's instructions.

SIGNIFICANCE OF RESULTS

A positive culture for a virus, unless there has been contamination, is proof that the virus is most likely causing the symptoms in question. A negative result, however, does not necessarily mean the absence of the virus, only that it did not grow. **Viral direct detection** is more rapid but less sensitive than viral culture. **Viral antibodies** can be of help, but sometimes, as in the case of **herpes blood tests,** they can be confusing. The **polymerase chain reaction** and **DNA probe testing** hold promise for the future.

◻ ◻ ◻

◻ Viral direct detection

WHAT IT IS AND WHY IT'S OBTAINED

Direct detection can be used for rapid identification of several viruses, including those that cause herpes, influenza, mumps, measles, rabies, and chickenpox, among others.

HOW IT WORKS

Several sources of specimen may be used, including tissue, smears from tissue, pus, swabs, or scrapings. The material is placed on a glass slide and the analysis is performed by immunoassay*.

BEFORE THE TEST

No special preparation is required.

AFTER THE TEST

No special aftercare is needed.

SIGNIFICANCE OF RESULTS

Because this test relies upon a lot of virus in the specimen, it is not so sensitive as **viral culture**. A positive result is more significant, therefore, than a negative result. **Viral antibodies** may be helpful in evaluating suspected viral infections.

□ □ □

□ Visual acuity

WHAT IT IS AND WHY IT'S OBTAINED

Visual acuity tests are used to diagnose and monitor visual impairment, and to evaluate the need for corrective lenses or corrective surgery.

HOW IT WORKS

Tests are designed for both distance and near vision, and are performed with and without your glasses. The distance test uses the familiar Snellen chart, which consists of rows of letters or numbers, larger at the top, smaller at the bottom. For people who are illiterate or for young children, the "E" chart has multiple E's aimed in different directions. In the standard distance test you will be placed about twenty feet away from the chart and asked to read the letters with each eye. Each line has a number associated with it, such as 15, 20, 40, 80, etc. The report is given as a fraction, such as 20/20, the top number referring to the distance to the chart in feet and the bottom number referring to the size of the test object. If you make one mistake on your lowest line, say the 40 line, the report would read 20/40−1. If you read the 40 line correctly and were able to read 2 letters on the line below it, the report would read 20/40+2. If you can read only the large letter on top your vision is 20/200. If you are unable to see this letter, you will be asked to walk toward the chart until it becomes visible. If this distance is

10 feet, your vision would be 10/200. The tests are standardized so that a person with normal vision can read the 20 line at 20 feet, the 40 line at 40 feet, and so on. In the "pinhole" variant of this test you will again be asked to read the letters, but looking through a tiny hole in a card. This negates a refractive error to a large degree. For near vision a handheld chart is commonly used. This is designed to be read at about 14 inches, and normal values are read off in "Jaeger" equivalents (J1, J2, J3, etc.)

BEFORE THE TEST

Bring any corrective lenses with you.

AFTER THE TEST

No special aftercare is needed.

SIGNIFICANCE OF RESULTS

The vast majority of visual problems occur because light rays do not focus exactly on the retina. These defects are called refractive errors. Nearsightedness (myopia) is usually due to an eyeball which is too long, and the rays of light focus in front of the retina. Farsightedness (hyperopia) is due to an eyeball which is too short. Presbyopia occurs with age, the prefix "presby-" meaning old. In this case the problem is loss of flexibility of the lens of the eye and weakening of the muscles which control it. In all cases vision may be impaired to a variable extent. If the eye is otherwise healthy, refractive errors can be corrected by glasses or contact lenses. The process of finding out what strength of corrective lenses you need is called **refraction.** Refractive surgery using incisions or lasers may also be used to correct some refractive errors permanently.

□ □ □

☐ Visual evoked responses

WHAT IT IS AND WHY IT'S OBTAINED

Visual evoked responses are used to detect diseases of the optic nerves and the parts of the brain which receive messages from the eyes.

HOW IT WORKS

This test is similar in principle to the **electroencephalogram,** but utilizes more sophisticated and powerful equipment to amplify brain electrical activity. It is conducted in a special room. You will be seated in a chair and electrodes will be applied to your scalp, forehead, and ear. Then you will be asked to gaze at a checkerboard pattern in front of you. The pattern will shift rapidly, and as it does, the electrical activity in your brain will be recorded on a strip of paper. The test is painless.

BEFORE THE TEST

No special preparation is required.

AFTER THE TEST

No special aftercare is needed.

SIGNIFICANCE OF RESULTS

Abnormal patterns are seen in multiple sclerosis, brain tumors, and optic neuritis.

SYNONYMS AND INCLUDED TESTS

Pattern-shift visual evoked responses.

☐ ☐ ☐

☐ Visual fields

WHAT IT IS AND WHY IT'S OBTAINED

Visual field tests are designed to evaluate central peripheral vision: the area which is visible when gazing at a central point. These tests are used to diagnose and monitor some diseases which cause visual impairment.

HOW IT WORKS

There are several ways to test visual fields. The simplest, called the "confrontation test," is performed during a standard physical examination. One eye is examined at a time. You and the examiner look at each other's eye while the examiner's wiggling fingers are gradually brought in from outside of the area where you both can see them moving toward the center. You will be asked to report when you first see the wiggling fingers. The fingers are moved in from four directions. The tangent screen test employs a black screen and white or colored objects of different sizes which are moved from the periphery toward the center. The general principle is the same, except that a map of your field of vision can be drawn. Computerized devices are now very prevalent and rely upon test objects being projected upon an illuminated background throughout the field at varying intensities. The results of recent tests may be compared with the results of older tests which have been stored in the computer's memory. All visual field tests depend entirely upon your cooperation and the accuracy of your reporting.

BEFORE THE TEST

Bring any corrective lenses if you have them.

AFTER THE TEST

No special aftercare is needed.

SIGNIFICANCE OF RESULTS

Abnormal visual field tests occur in many ocular, optic nerve, and brain disorders, and include glaucoma, optic neuritis, detached retina, retinitis pigmentosa, strokes, aneurysms, and brain tumors.

SYNONYMS AND INCLUDED TESTS

Perimetry, tangent screen examination, field of vision, automated perimetry.

□ □ □

□ Vitamin A

WHAT IT IS AND WHY IT'S OBTAINED

Vitamin A is a fat soluble vitamin essential to many organs, including the skin and eyes. Blood levels are used to evaluate nutritional status. Symptoms of low vitamin A include dry eyes and decreased night vision. Severe vitamin A deficiency causes blindness. Vitamin A is one of the few vitamins which can cause toxicity if taken in excess. Symptoms of this include dry skin, liver enlargement, joint pain, hair loss, and visual disturbances. Fatalities, however, have not been reported.

HOW IT WORKS

You will be asked to provide a **venous blood sample** from which serum* will be separated. Several methods of assay are available.

BEFORE THE TEST

You should fast overnight.

AFTER THE TEST

Follow **venous blood sample** aftercare.

SIGNIFICANCE OF RESULTS

Low vitamin A is found with inadequate dietary intake or malabsorption (in which the intestines fail to absorb nutrients properly). High vitamin A occurs with increased dietary intake, diabetes, underactive thyroid (hypothyroidism), and kidney disease. **Carotene** may also be used to evaluate vitamin A.

□ □ □

□ Vitamin B₁

WHAT IT IS AND WHY IT'S OBTAINED

Vitamin B₁ is important to general metabolism. Blood or urine levels are used to evaluate nutritional status. There are many symptoms associated with deficiency, the classic disorder being called beriberi, which is associated with nerve and heart problems.

HOW IT WORKS

You will be asked to provide either a **venous blood sample** or a **24-hour urine sample** which will be analyzed in the laboratory by chromatography*.

BEFORE THE TEST

No special preparation is required.

AFTER THE TEST

No special aftercare is needed.

SIGNIFICANCE OF RESULTS

Low levels of vitamin B₁ can result from malnutrition, alcoholism, liver disease, and chronic diarrhea.

SYNONYMS AND INCLUDED TESTS

Thiamine.

❒❒❒

❒ Vitamin B_2

WHAT IT IS AND WHY IT'S OBTAINED

Vitamin B_2 is important to many body functions. Blood levels are used to evaluate nutritional status. Symptoms of deficiency include inflammation of the mouth, tongue, throat, skin, and eyes, but often there are other problems related to deficiencies of the other B vitamins.

HOW IT WORKS

You will be asked to provide a **venous blood sample** from which serum* will be separated. Chromatography* is used in the laboratory.

BEFORE THE TEST

No special preparation is required.

AFTER THE TEST

Follow **venous blood sample** aftercare.

SIGNIFICANCE OF RESULTS

Low vitamin B_2 may be seen with malnutrition and malabsorption (in which the intestines fail to absorb nutrients properly).

SYNONYMS AND INCLUDED TESTS

Riboflavin.

❒❒❒

☐ Vitamin B₆

WHAT IT IS AND WHY IT'S OBTAINED

Vitamin B_6 is a water-soluble vitamin important to many body functions, including the immune system, nervous system, and blood. Blood levels are used mainly to evaluate nutritional status and diagnose vitamin B_6 deficiency, which can cause many symptoms. In infants symptoms such as colic, irritability, and seizures may be due to vitamin B_6 deficiency, particularly if formula has been heated excessively. Vitamin B_6 toxicity may cause numbness, tingling, and clumsiness.

HOW IT WORKS

You will be asked to provide a **venous blood sample** from which serum* will be separated. Chromatography* is used for the assay.

BEFORE THE TEST

No special preparation is required.

AFTER THE TEST

Follow **venous blood sample** aftercare.

SIGNIFICANCE OF RESULTS

Low vitamin B_6 occurs with inadequate dietary intake, malabsorption (in which the intestines fail to absorb nutrients properly), pregnancy, birth control pills, alcoholism, and some drugs. Increased levels are seen in those ingesting abnormally large amounts.

SYNONYMS AND INCLUDED TESTS

Pyridoxine.

☐ ☐ ☐

☐ Vitamin B₁₂

WHAT IT IS AND WHY IT'S OBTAINED

Vitamin B_{12} is central to a wide variety of biological processes. Blood levels are used to diagnose deficiency of the vitamin, symptoms of which include weakness, numbness, tingling, and loss of certain sensations. This test, along with **folic acid,** is usually obtained to evaluate abnormal **red blood cell indices,** particularly if the results show large red blood cells.

HOW IT WORKS

You will be asked to provide a **venous blood sample** from which serum* will be separated. Immunoassay* is used for the laboratory analysis.

BEFORE THE TEST

You should fast overnight. Avoid nonessential medications or do as directed by your doctor.

AFTER THE TEST

Follow **venous blood sample** aftercare.

SIGNIFICANCE OF RESULTS

Low vitamin B_{12} is seen in pernicious anemia, decreased stomach acid, malabsorption (in which the intestines fail to absorb nutrients properly), inflammatory bowel disease, tapeworm infestation, after stomach or intestinal surgery, and in those taking a variety of medications, including sedatives, antibacterials, diuretics, anticonvulsants, and birth control pills. Poor nutrition—except in strict vegetarians—is rarely a cause of deficiency, however, since this vitamin is so widely distributed in nature. Rather, the problem is usually poor absorption. The **Schilling test** is designed to study vitamin B_{12} absorption, and **instrinsic factor antibody** can be helpful. Increased vitamin B_{12} levels are associated with leukemia, kidney failure, congestive heart failure, diabetes, obesity, emphysema, and some cases of liver disease.

SYNONYMS AND INCLUDED TESTS

Cyanocobalamin.

◻ ◻ ◻

◻ Vitamin C

WHAT IT IS AND WHY IT'S OBTAINED

Vitamin C is important in the manufacture of collagen, one of the main structural components of the body. Blood levels are used to evaluate nutritional status and to diagnose scurvy, which can cause fatigue, muscle aches, bleeding gums, and bleeding into the skin.

HOW IT WORKS

You will be asked to provide a **venous blood sample** from which serum* will be separated. Chromatography* is used for the analysis.

BEFORE THE TEST

You should fast overnight.

AFTER THE TEST

Follow **venous blood sample** aftercare.

SIGNIFICANCE OF RESULTS

Low vitamin C levels are seen in scurvy, malabsorption (in which the intestines fail to absorb nutrients properly), alcoholism, pregnancy, overactivity of the thyroid (hyperthyroidism), and kidney disease. High levels are found in those ingesting large amounts of the vitamin.

SYNONYMS AND INCLUDED TESTS

Ascorbic acid.

❐ ❐ ❐

❐ Vitamin D

WHAT IT IS AND WHY IT'S OBTAINED

Vitamin D is a fat-soluble vitamin which has many important functions, particularly in calcium and bone metabolism. Blood levels are used to evaluate nutritional status, diseases of the bone, and abnormal blood **calcium** levels.

HOW IT WORKS

You will be asked to provide a **venous blood sample** from which serum* will be separated. Several methods are available for the assay.

BEFORE THE TEST

You should fast overnight.

AFTER THE TEST

Follow **venous blood sample** aftercare.

SIGNIFICANCE OF RESULTS

Increased levels of vitamin D are found after exposure to sunlight, in sarcoidosis, overactivity of the parathyroid glands (hyperparathyroidism), and in some cases of cancer. It is low in malnutrition, rickets, and underactivity of the parathyroids (hypoparathyroidism). **Parathyroid hormone** and blood calcium are usually evaluated along with vitamin D.

SYNONYMS AND INCLUDED TESTS

Vitamin D_3.

❐ ❐ ❐

☐ Vitamin E

WHAT IT IS AND WHY IT'S OBTAINED

Vitamin E is a fat-soluble vitamin which is important to the nervous system. Blood levels are used to diagnose vitamin E deficiency, which may cause a variety of symptoms, including difficulty in sensing one's body position.

HOW IT WORKS

You will be asked to provide a **venous blood sample** from which serum* will be separated. Chromatography* is used for the assay.

BEFORE THE TEST

No special preparation is required.

AFTER THE TEST

Follow **venous blood sample** aftercare.

SIGNIFICANCE OF RESULTS

Low vitamin E is associated with malabsorption (in which the intestines fail to absorb nutrients properly), cystic fibrosis, and intestinal bypass surgery. Deficiency of this vitamin is almost never due to inadequate intake because it is so plentiful in nature, but rather as result of poor absorption.

SYNONYMS AND INCLUDED TESTS

Tocopherol.

☐ ☐ ☐

☐ Water deprivation test

WHAT IT IS AND WHY IT'S OBTAINED

The water deprivation test is used to distinguish among the causes of excessive urination (after diabetes mellitus has been eliminated as a possibility).

HOW IT WORKS

There are several ways to conduct this test. Usually, after an overnight fast you will be weighed and a urine sample and a **venous blood sample** will both be obtained and tested for **osmolality.** All oral fluids will then be discontinued and you will be weighed and your blood sampled the same way every hour. All of your urine will also be collected, measured, and tested. The test will be discontinued if you lose more than a certain percentage of your body weight or if the osmolality of your urine or blood reaches a predetermined level. You may be given an injection or nasal instillation of vasopression (a pituitary hormone) during the test.

BEFORE THE TEST

In most cases you will be instructed not to have anything by mouth overnight, unless you have been urinating a very large amount. Follow any instructions *very* carefully.

AFTER THE TEST

Follow **venous blood sample** aftercare.

SIGNIFICANCE OF RESULTS

A completed test will usually point to one of the three main causes for excessive urination (other than diabetes mellitus): excessive fluid intake, diabetes insipidus due to pituitary disease, or diabetes insipidus due to kidney disease.

Urine concentration test, Fishberg concentration test.

□ □ □

□ White blood cell competence

WHAT IT IS AND WHY IT'S OBTAINED

Neutrophils are a type of white blood cell whose primary job is to kill bacteria. This test is used to evaluate neutrophil function in those with recurrent bacterial infections.

HOW IT WORKS

You will be asked to provide a **venous blood sample** from which serum* will be separated. Many methods of analysis are available.

BEFORE THE TEST

No special preparation is required.

AFTER THE TEST

Follow **venous blood sample** aftercare.

SIGNIFICANCE OF RESULTS

Poor white blood cell competence is found in the rare disease called chronic granulomatous disease of childhood and several other diseases caused by poorly functioning neutrophils.

SYNONYMS AND INCLUDED TESTS

Phagocytic cell immunocompetence profile, neutrophil phagocytosis.

□ □ □

☐ White blood cell count

WHAT IT IS AND WHY IT'S OBTAINED

White blood cells (WBC) are crucial to the immune system. The WBC count is a part of the **complete blood count** and is used routinely in a wide variety of situations to assess general health and to screen, diagnose, and monitor infections, inflammations, cancer (particularly leukemia), and chemotherapy for cancer.

HOW IT WORKS

You will be asked to provide a **venous blood sample.** The count may be performed manually by examining blood under a microscope in a counting chamber, but it is most often done by machine. A **heelstick blood sample** may be used in infants.

BEFORE THE TEST

No special preparation is required.

AFTER THE TEST

Follow **venous blood sample** or **heelstick blood sample** aftercare.

SIGNIFICANCE OF RESULTS

Elevated WBC counts usually indicate an infection of some type. Further clues as to the type of infection can be obtained from the **white blood cell differential.** High WBC counts may also be seen in leukemia, heart attacks, and burns. The **leukocyte alkaline phosphatase** may help in differentiating the cause of high WBC counts. Low counts may occur in autoimmune diseases (in which the immune system reacts against the body's own tissues), some viral infections (such as mononucleosis, hepatitis, and influenza), and some blood disorders. Many substances, such as drugs, poisons, medications, and chemicals influence WBC counts, some depressing it, such as chemotherapy drugs, others elevating it, such as steroids.

□ □ □

□ White blood cell differential

WHAT IT IS AND WHY IT'S OBTAINED

White blood cells (WBC) consist of neutrophils, eosinophils, basophils, lymphocytes, and monocytes. The WBC differential counts these groups. This test is widely and routinely used to evaluate a variety of infections, inflammations, leukemias, and blood disorders.

HOW IT WORKS

You will be asked to provide a **venous blood sample.** The differential count may be done manually or by machine, and in certain cases by a combination of both.

BEFORE THE TEST

No special preparation is required.

AFTER THE TEST

Follow **venous blood sample** aftercare.

SIGNIFICANCE OF RESULTS

There are many abnormal variations which may be seen in the differential count, and most findings are only *suggestive* of certain diseases. The most common causes of each variable are as follows:

High neutrophils are caused by infections (particularly due to bacteria), burns, heart attacks, physical stress, and inflammation. Low neutrophils are seen with chemotherapy, radiation exposure, autoimmune disease (in which the immune system reacts against the body's own tissues), and some infections.

High eosinophils are associated with allergic diseases, parasites, cancer, and autoimmune diseases. Low eosinophils are found in physical stress and Cushing's syndrome.

High basophils occur in leukemia, polycythemia (in which red blood cells are increased), Hodgkin's disease, and kidney disease. Low basophils occur in thyroid overactivity, pregnancy, and physical stress.

High lymphocytes are caused by infections (particularly due to viruses), tuberculosis, thyroid disease, and ulcerative colitis. Low lymphocytes are associated with AIDS, heart failure, Hodgkin's disease, chronic diseases of any type, and in those taking steroids.

High monocytes are found in tuberculosis, hepatitis, certain infections (such as with protozoa and rickettsia), autoimmune diseases, cancer, leukemia, and lymphomas.

□ □ □

□ White blood cell scan

WHAT IT IS AND WHY IT'S OBTAINED

This is a type of **radionuclide scan** which is designed to a detect hidden infection.

HOW IT WORKS

The test is carried out in the nuclear medicine department of a hospital, clinic, or private physician's office, sometimes as part of a radiology facility. First you will be asked to provide a **venous blood sample.** In the laboratory your blood will be incubated with a radioactive isotope, called a "tracer," to label the white blood cells. The labeled blood will then be reinjected into a vein. After several hours, and often again the next day, the actual scanning takes place. The images are taken with a gamma camera, a computerized device which detects the tracer's emissions. This is painless and you should try to remain as still as possible.

BEFORE THE TEST

No special preparation is required.

AFTER THE TEST

No special aftercare is needed. Although safe, this test involves the administration of a radioactive substance.

SIGNIFICANCE OF RESULTS

Active sites of infection show up as sites of increased uptake of the white blood cells. This test may be performed with a **bone scan** for detection of bone infections and with a **gallium scan** for detection of infection in other sites.

SYNONYMS AND INCLUDED TESTS

Indium leukocyte scan, infection scintigraphy.

□ □ □

□ X ray

WHAT IT IS AND WHY IT'S OBTAINED

The X-ray examination is a common noninvasive method for demonstrating internal structures. It is used to diagnose broken bones, joint problems, tumors, infections, and many other diseases. Sometimes these studies indicate the need for other testing. Variations of the X ray include **computed tomography, X-ray contrast studies,** and fluoroscopy, in which the image appears on a screen rather than on film. Although virtually any organ can be X-rayed, exposure of the abdomen during pregnancy, especially during the first three months, should be avoided if possible. Fewer screening X rays are done now than formerly because of concerns about radiation exposure.

HOW IT WORKS

X rays may be taken in the X-ray or radiology department of a hospital, in the offices of private radiologists, or in the offices of private doctors who have X-ray machines. Portable X-ray units may be taken to the bedside if you are too ill to be transported to the X-ray department, but the images are inferior to those provided by the larger equipment. An X ray is a portion of the electromagnetic spectrum located between ultraviolet and gamma rays. These invisible rays penetrate the body and are absorbed differently by various internal structures. The method is to transmit X rays from one side of your body to the other side and then onto photographic film. Bone, for example, is good at absorbing X rays and so shows up white on the X-ray film. Air and water absorb little, and so show up darker. Internal organs, such as the heart, liver, and blood vessels, have moderate uptake of X rays and thus show up as varying shades of gray.

BEFORE THE TEST

In general there is no special preparation for routine X rays.

AFTER THE TEST

There is no special aftercare needed. Although safe, each X ray delivers a certain amount of radiation to your tissues. In general, however, the benefits of diagnostic X rays far outweigh the risks.

SIGNIFICANCE OF RESULTS

The interpretation of X rays may be performed by anyone who has the requisite training. Definitive reports are given by radiologists, but there are many specialists, such as orthopedic surgeons, urologists, and neurosurgeons, who rely largely upon their own readings, since they are the ones who are ultimately responsible for your care. Multiple X rays taken over time are helpful in difficult cases because they can be compared with one another, making it possible to follow the course of a medical problem.

SYNONYMS AND INCLUDED TESTS

Radiography, roentgenographic examination.

□ □ □

☐ X-ray contrast study

WHAT IT IS AND WHY IT'S OBTAINED

The **X-ray** contrast study is used to enhance visualization of structures within the body by using a substance called contrast agent. Substances include air, carbon dioxide, barium sulfate, and organic compounds containing iodine. Contrast agents are sometimes referred to as "dyes" and are not radioactive. When air or carbon dioxide is used (most commonly in joints), the gas will create an outline effect of the particular area. When barium sulfate or organic iodine is used, the agent will block X rays from penetrating. The main uses for these studies are in the digestive tract, blood vessels, lymph channels, brain, and spinal cord.

HOW IT WORKS

Individual tests include the **angiogram, arthrogram, barium enema, barium meal, barium swallow, hysterosalpinogram, lymphangiogram, myelogram, urogram,** and **venogram.**

BEFORE THE TEST

Preparation depends upon the individual study.

AFTER THE TEST

Posttest care depends upon the individual study.

SIGNIFICANCE OF RESULTS

The introduction of contrast dyes represented a great advance in X-ray imaging, and although many of these techniques are considered "invasive," the degree of invasion is much less than that required if a surgical operation were needed to find out the same information.

☐ ☐ ☐

◻ Xylose absorption test

WHAT IT IS AND WHY IT'S OBTAINED

Xylose is a sugar which is normally absorbed into the bloodstream and excreted unchanged. In other words, it is neither digested nor metabolized. How well it is absorbed is used to evaluate intestinal malabsorption, the symptoms of which may include diarrhea, weakness, and weight loss. In infants malabsorption causes a failure of normal development.

HOW IT WORKS

The actual mechanics of the test vary from laboratory to laboratory, but a typical sequence is as follows. First, you will be asked to provide a **venous blood sample.** You will then be given an oral dose of xylose. At intervals more blood samples will obtained, up to about five hours. During this time your urine will also be collected and all specimens will be analyzed for xylose. You will be asked to remain lying flat on your back for the duration of the test and will be encouraged to drink water.

BEFORE THE TEST

You should fast overnight. In addition, for several days prior to the test you should avoid jams, jellies, and fruits, all of which contain xylose. Follow directions from the laboratory and your doctor regarding medications. In general, all medications, including aspirin and over the counter pain medications, should be discontinued for twenty-four hours. You should continue, however, to drink plenty of water.

AFTER THE TEST

No special aftercare is needed. You may have mild diarrhea which will go away on its own.

SIGNIFICANCE OF RESULTS

If your kidneys are working normally this is a good test for intestinal function. Low absorption is seen in celiac disease (gluten enteropathy) and tropical sprue. It may also be decreased in gastroenteritis, intestinal parasites, and bacterial overgrowth in the intestine. Results may be misleading in children owing to the difficulty in collecting a five-hour urine sample. A **small bowel biopsy** may be indicated for further investigation of intestinal malabsorption.

SYNONYMS AND INCLUDED TESTS

D-xylose tolerance test.

◻ ◻ ◻

◻ Zinc

WHAT IT IS AND WHY IT'S OBTAINED

Although normally present in small amounts, zinc is crucial to numerous bodily functions. Blood levels are used to evaluate suspected zinc deficiency or toxicity. Zinc deficiency is characterized by poor wound healing, retarded growth, and atrophy (shrinkage) of the reproductive organs. Zinc toxicity can cause nausea, vomiting, and diarrhea.

HOW IT WORKS

You will be asked to provide a **venous blood sample** from which serum* will be separated. Special zinc-free equipment will be used. The assay is performed by atomic absorption. Urine may also be tested.

BEFORE THE TEST

No special preparation is required.

AFTER THE TEST

Follow **venous blood sample** aftercare.

SIGNIFICANCE OF RESULTS

Low blood levels of zinc may represent actual low levels, but may also be due to what is called redistribution of zinc from the blood to the rest of the body, where it cannot be detected. This is what can happen in serious infections or burns. True low zinc (which is more reliably diagnosed with urine levels) can be found in malnutrition, malabsorption (in which the intestines fail to absorb nutrients properly), or those in whom there is increased excretion (as in liver or kidney diseases). Low zinc can also be present in AIDS, premature infants, and after heart attacks. A normal zinc does not entirely rule out mild zinc deficiency. If strongly suspected, sophisticated tests may be performed to find out. High zinc may be found in cases of industrial exposure or after increased ingestion.

Cross-reference Tables

□ □ □

Acid-base and water balance

Anion gap
Bicarbonate
Blood gas
Calcium
Carbon dioxide
Chloride
Electrolytes
Osmolality
Phosphates
Potassium
Sodium

Blood clotting (coagulation)

Activated clotting time
Bleeding time
Capillary fragility test
Clot lysis time
Coagulation factor screen
Fibrin split products
Fibrinogen
Partial thromboplastin time
Plasminogen
Platelet adhesion
Platelet aggregation

Platelet count
Platelet sizing
Protein C
Prothrombin time
Thrombin time

Blood disorders

Antineutrophil antibody
Autohemolysis test
Blood typing
Blood viscosity
Blood volume
Bone marrow
Complete blood count
Erythropoietin
Ferritin
Folic acid
Glucose-6-phosphate dehydrogenase
Ham test
Haptoglobin
Heinz bodies
Hematocrit
Hemoglobin
Hemoglobin electrophoresis
Human T-cell leukemia virus antibody
Intrinsic factor antibody
Iron and iron binding capacity
Leukemia and lymphoma panel
Leukocyte alkaline phosphatase
Methemoglobin
Osmotic fragility
Parietal cell antibody
Paroxysmal cold hemoglobinuria test
Pyruvate kinase
Red blood cell count
Red blood cell indices
Red blood cell mass
Red blood cell survival
Reticulocyte count
Schilling test
Sedimentation rate

Sickle cell test
Sugar water test
Transferrin
Unstable hemoglobin
White blood cell count
White blood cell differential

Bones and joints

Antinuclear antibody
Arthrogram
Arthroscopy
Bone biopsy
Bone scan
Joint fluid analysis
Joint tap
Magnetic resonance imaging
Uric acid
X ray

Cancer

Acid phosphatase
Alpha fetoprotein
Carcinoembryonic antigen
CA 125
CA 15-3
CA 19-9
Prostate specific antigen

Carbohydrate metabolism

Fructosamine
Glucagon
Glucose
Glucose tolerance test
Glycohemoglobin
Insulin
Insulin antibody
Lactic acid
Lactose tolerance test
Postprandial glucose

Ear, nose, and throat

Acoustic admittance test
Brain stem auditory evoked responses
Computed tomography
Hearing test
Magnetic resonance imaging
Nasal endosocopy
Otoscopy
Vestibular test
X ray

Esophagus, stomach, liver, and intestines

Acid reflux test
Alaninine aminotransferase
Alkaline phosphatase
Ammonia
Anal rectal motility
Anoscopy
Aspartate aminotransferase
Barium enema
Barium meal
Barium swallow
Bernstein test
Bilirubin
Blood loss localization
Ceruloplasmin
Cholecystogram
Colonoscopy
Computed tomography
Endomysial antibodies
Endoscopic retrograde cholangiopancreatography
Esophageal motility
Esophageal pH study
Fecal fat
Gamma glutamyl transferase
Gastric intubation
Gastrin
Helicobacter pylori antibody
Hepatitis screening tests
Hollander test

Lactose tolerance test
Laparoscopy
Leucine aminopeptidase
Lipase
Liver and spleen scan
Liver biopsy
Liver function tests
Magnetic resonance imaging
Pancreatic peptide
Paracentesis
Sigmoidoscopy
Small bowel biopsy
Stomach saline load test
Stool for muscle fiber
Stool for occult blood
Stool for ova and parasites
Ultrasound
Upper gastrointestinal endosccpy
Vasoactive intestinal peptide
X ray

Eye

Amsler grid test
Color vision testing
Computed tomography
Corneal topography
Electrophysiologic eye testing
Endothelial photography
Exophthalmometry
Fluorescein angiography
Ophthalmoscopy
Refraction
Schirmer test
Slit-lamp examination
Tonometry
Ultrasound
Visual acuity
Visual fields
X ray

Heart and blood vessels

Apolipoprotein A and B
Cardiac catheterization
Cardiac enzymes
Catecholamines
Cholesterol
Computed tomography
Creatine kinase
Echocardiogram
Electrocardiogram
Heart scan
Holter monitor
Homocysteine
Homovanillic acid
Invasive electrophysiologic studies
Lactic dehydrogenase
Lipid profile
Magnetic resonance imaging
Metanephrines
Pericardiocentesis
Renin
Renin stimulation test
Right heart catheterization
Sleep study
Stress test
Transesophageal echocardiography
Triglycerides
Ultrasound
Vanillylmandelic acid

Hormones (Endocrine system)

Adrenal antibody
Adrenocorticotropic hormone
Aldosterone
Calcitonin
Cortisol
Cosyntropin test
Dehydroepiandosterone
Dexamethasone suppression test
Estradiol

486

Estriol
Estrogens
Follicle stimulating hormone
Glucagon
Growth hormone
Human chorionic gonadotropin
Insulin
17-ketogenic steroids
17-ketosteroids
Luteinizing hormone
Parathyroid hormone
Parathyroid scan
Placental lactogen
Progesterone
Prolactin
Testosterone
Thorn test
Thyroid stimulating hormone
Thyroxine
Triiodothyronine
Triiodothyronine uptake
Water deprivation test

Immune system

Allergy skin testing
Anergy skin testing
Anti-DNA
Antimitochondrial antibody
C-reactive protein
Cold agglutinins
Complement
Cryoglobulin
Eosinophil count
Eosinophil smear
Food allergy tests
Immunofixation electrophoresis
Immunoglobulin A
Immunoglobulin E
Immunoglobulin G
Immunoglobulin G subclasses
Immunoglobulin M

LE cell test
Lip biopsy for Sjögren's syndrome
Lymphocyte transformation test
Lymphocyte typing
Mixed lymphocyte culture
Patch test
Pemphigus/pemphigoid antibody
Radioallergosorbent test
Rheumatoid factor
Scleroderma antibody
Sjögren's antibodies
Skeletal muscle antibody
Smooth muscle antibody
Thyroid antibodies

Infectious diseases

Acid fast smear
Antibacterial activity
Antideoxyribonuclease-B
Antihyaluronidase
Bacterial antibodies
Bacterial antigens
Bacterial culture
Bacterial sensitivity
Blood culture
Buffy coat bacteremia detection
Darkfield examination
Febrile agglutinins
FTA-ABS
Fungal antibodies
Fungal culture
Fungal sensitivity
Fungal skin testing
Gram stain
Hepatitis A antibody
Hepatitis B tests
Hepatitis C antibody
Hepatitis D antibody
Hepatitis screening tests
Herpes antigen
Herpes blood tests

HIV tests
Infectious mononucleosis screen
Lyme disease antibody
Malaria smear
Parasite antibodies
Pinworm identification
Serologic test for syphilis
Sputum culture
Stool for ova and parasites
Streptozyme
Throat swab for strep throat
TORCH
Trichomonas preparation
Urine culture
Viral antibodies
Viral culture
Viral direct detection
White blood cell competence
White blood cell scan

Kidneys and urinary bladder (urinary tract)

Blood urea nitrogen
BUN/creatinine ratio
Computed tomography
Creatinine
Creatinine clearance
Cystogram
Cystometry
Cystoscopy
Electromyogram
Glomerular basement membrane antibody
Kidney biopsy
Kidney function tests
Kidney scan
Kidney stone analysis
Magnetic resonance imaging
Ultrasound
Urinalysis
Urine culture
Uroflowmetry
Urography

X ray
X-ray contrast study

Lungs and respiratory system

Allergic lung antibodies
Blood gas
Bronchography
Bronchoscopy
Computed tomography
Lung scan
Magnetic resonance imaging
Pleural biopsy
Pulmonary function tests
Sputum culture
Sputum induction
Sweat test
Thoracentesis
Tuberculin skin test
X ray

Nervous system

Acetylcholine receptor antibody
Brain scan
Cholinesterase
Computed tomography
Dibucaine number
Electroencephalogram
Electromyogram
Magnetic resonance imaging
Myelogram
Nerve conduction studies
Somatosensory response studies
Spinal tap
Ultrasound
X ray
X-ray contrast study

Reproductive system

MALE
Penile blood flow

Penile injection test
Prostate biopsy
Semen analysis
Sleep erection monitoring
Testosterone
Ultrasound

FEMALE
Amniocentesis
Breast biopsy
Cervical punch biopsy
Colposcopy
Estrogens
Follicle stimulating hormone
Hysterosalpingogram
Laparoscopy
Luteinizing hormone
Mammogram
Pap smear
Pregnancy test

Thyroid gland

Magnetic resonance imaging
Radioactive iodine uptake test
Thyroglobulin
Thyroid antibodies
Thyroid binding globulin
Thyroid biopsy
Thyroid function tests
Thyroid scan
Thyroid stimulating hormone
Thyroid uptake
Thyroxine
Triiodothyronine
Triiodothyronine uptake
Ultrasound

Vitamins, minerals, and nutritional status

Albumin
Albumin/globulin ratio
Aluminum

Calcium
Carotene
Chromium
Copper
Folic acid
Magnesium
Manganese
Molybdenum
Phosphate
Protein
Vitamin A
Vitamin B$_1$
Vitamin B$_2$
Vitamin B$_6$
Vitamin B$_{12}$
Vitamin C
Vitamin D
Vitamin E
Zinc

Glossary

□ □ □

Acid-base balance. The study of the pH* of the blood and the ions (charged particles) in the body. The pH of the blood must be controlled within a narrow range in order for biochemical processes to function normally. In general, metabolism tends to make the blood more acidic (decreases the pH). The lungs (by means of carbon dioxide) and kidneys (by means of ammonium and bicarbonate ions) compensate for this by excreting or reabsorbing the appropriate ions to make the blood more alkaline (increasing the pH). Certain conditions upset this balance and as a result change the values of the **electrolytes** in the bloodstream.

Acidosis. A condition in which acidic ions accumulate in the blood or in which basic ions are lost from the blood. It may be "respiratory," in which carbon dioxide is abnormally retained, or "metabolic," in which either too much acid is produced (as in severe diabetes), too much base is excreted (as in severe diarrhea), or not enough acid is excreted (as in severe kidney disease).

Acute. Short-lived or sudden in onset. Contrast with chronic*.

Alkalosis. A condition in which basic (alkaline) ions accumulate in the blood or in which acidic ions are lost from the blood. It may be "respiratory," in which hyperventilation causes excessive carbon dioxide excretion, or "metabolic," in which either large amounts of acidic ions are lost (as in severe vomiting) or large amounts of basic ions are ingested (as in taking too many antacids).

Amino acid. A class of biochemicals which are widely distributed in plants and animals and which form peptides*, the building blocks of **protein.**

Amniotic fluid. The liquid which cushions and protects the fetus during pregnancy. A sample can be obtained by **amniocentesis.**

Androgen. A hormone which produces male characteristics, such as facial hair, deep voice, increased muscle mass, and aggression. The most powerful is **testosterone.**

Antibody. A protein which is an essential part of the immune system. Antibodies are produced by the B-lymphocytes and react with specific antigens*.

Anticoagulant. A blood "thinner." Heparin* and warfarin Coumadin are the best known therapeutic anticoagulants. There are also naturally occurring anticoagulants which help break down blood clots.

Antigen. A substance which is recognized, or should be recognized, by the immune system as being foreign. Antigens take many forms: ragweed pollen, proteins in shellfish, drugs such as penicillin, bacteria such as *Streptococcus,* and viruses such as HIV. Antigens provoke an immune response which includes formation of an antibody*.

Arrhythmia. Irregularity of the heartbeat.

Autoimmune. Referring to the immune system reacting to the body's own tissues. It is usually used in the term "autoimmune disease." Synonyms for the latter are "connective tissue disease" or "collagen vascular disease." Examples include lupus erythematosus*, rheumatoid arthritis, rheumatic fever, scleroderma, dermatomyositis, Hashimoto's thyroiditis, mixed connective tissue disease, and many cases of hemolytic anemia*.

Bile. A chemically complex liquid which is produced by the liver and secreted into the small intestine. Bile is concentrated in the gallbladder and is important to digestion, particularly of fats.

Cardiomyopathy. A heart disease caused by progressive deterioration of the heart muscle.

Cerebrospinal fluid. The fluid which envelops and cushions the brain and spinal cord. A sample may be obtained and analyzed with a **spinal tap.**

Chromatography. A laboratory method for separating the components of a mixture by using differences based on physical or chemical properties. Types of chromatography include paper, liquid, gel, gas, thin layer, and ion exchange. In high performance liquid chromatography, the unknown solution is pumped through a column of glass beads under pressure.

Chronic. Persisting for a long time. Contrast with acute*.

Colon. The portion of the large intestine which extends from the end of the small intestine to the rectum.

Colorimetry. A laboratory technique for measuring differences in color between test substances and reference standards.

Congenital adrenal hyperplasia. A disease caused by a deficiency of an enzyme in the adrenal gland and which leads to an accumulation of androgens*. It may cause a number of symptoms of varying severity.

Cushing's syndrome. A disease caused by overproduction of **cortisol** by the adrenal glands. Symptoms include acne, fat accumulations of the face ("moon face") and upper back ("buffalo hump"), high blood pressure, and diabetes*.

Diabetes. A condition characterized by increased excretion of urine. There are two types, the more common by far being diabetes *mellitus,* which is caused by inadequate *insulin* metabolism. The rarer type is diabetes *insipidus,* caused by disease of the pituitary gland.

Disseminated intravascular coagulation. A serious disease in which the substances responsible for blood clotting—mainly **fibrinogen**—are depleted, leading to excessive bleeding from multiple sites.

Diuretic. A substance which causes an increased volume of urine. Commonly called a "water pill."

Duodenum. The first portion of the small intestine, extending from the stomach to the jejunum.

Electrophoresis. A laboratory technique in which a substance is analyzed by placing it in an electric field. Either a gel or paper strip may be used. The various components migrate at different rates and show up as distinct bands.

Endocarditis. A serious disease caused by inflammation of the valves of the heart, usually by bacteria. Often called bacterial endocarditis.

Endocrine. Referring to the complex system of glands which produce hormones*.

Endoscopy. A visualizing technique in which a tube is passed into a hollow organ. Examples include **colonoscopy, sigmoidoscopy, upper gastrointestinal endoscopy,** and **cystoscopy.**

Enzyme. A protein which causes another substance (called a substrate) to change its form. Many of the blood tests in this book, such as **liver function tests,** measure blood levels of enzymes.

Esophagus. The part of the intestine from the throat (pharynx) to the stomach.

Flow cytometry. Cytometry refers to the physical characteristics of cells, such as their diameter, volume, weight, or staining properties. Flow refers to sending the cells through a machine one at a time where they can be measured automatically. Flow cytometry, therefore, is a system of counting and classifying cells in a computer-driven machine.

Fluorescein. A dye which is of use in helping to visualize certain body processes or laboratory results.

Fluoroscopy. An **X ray** in which the image is seen as it is being produced on a screen rather than on film which has to be developed. It is most useful in guiding the placement of biopsy needles, catheters, and surgical instruments.

Globulin. A **protein** which is widely distributed in plants and animals and which is important to the production of antibodies*.

Graves' disease. A type of hyperthyroidism* which is associated with bulging eyes, an enlarged thyroid gland (goiter), nervousness, and a rapid pulse. It is an autoimmune* disease produced by **thyrotropin receptor antibody.**

Hematoma. A collection of blood.

Hemolysis. Disruption of a red blood cell and release of **hemoglobin** into the blood.

Hemolytic anemia. An anemia characterized by premature destruction of red blood cells* and hemolysis*.

Heparin. A commonly prescribed anticoagulant* which is given intravenously.

Hirsutism. Male-pattern hair growth in women.

Hormone. A biochemical produced by one part of the body, usually a gland, which affects another part of the body. Hormones usually have significant and sometimes profound effects, even though they are produced in minute quantities. Testing for diseases of the endocrine* system can be very complex because of the numerous glands which are involved (see table). The hormones produced are often regulated by intricate feedback loops.

Glands and their hormones	
Pituitary	**Adrenocorticotropic hormone, follicle stimulating hormone, human growth hormone, luteinizing hormone, prolactin, thyroid stimulating hormone**
Thyroid	**Thyroxine, triiodothyronine**
Adrenal	**Aldosterone, cortisol, catecholamines**
Pancreas	**Insulin**
Ovaries	**Estrogens, progesterone**
Testicles	**Testosterone**
Parathyroid	**Parathyroid hormone**

Hyperparathyroidism. A condition of overactivity of the parathyroid glands. It may be primary, due to a tumor or simple enlargement, in which case large amounts of **parathyroid hormone** cause an increase in blood **calcium.** Symptoms include weakness, nausea, vomiting, abdominal pain, bone pain, and bone thinning. Secondary hyperparathyroidism is a reaction caused by conditions which tend to lower blood calcium, such as some cases of kidney disease.

Hyperthyroidism. An overactive thyroid gland. Symptoms such as in Graves' disease* may be produced or it may be detected only by testing.

Hypoglycemia. Low blood sugar (**glucose**). Symptoms may include headache, shivering, sweating, and confusion. If severe, seizures and coma may result.

Hypoparathyroidism. A condition caused by diminished or absent production of **parathyroid hormone,** often as a result of surgery. The resulting low blood **calcium** may cause muscle twitching and cramping.

Hypothalamus. A portion of the brain which controls many vital and basic functions and which is closely linked to the pituitary gland.

Hypothyroidism. An underactive thyroid gland. Symptoms may include weight gain, dry skin, slowed speech, and intolerance to cold. If this occurs in infancy it can lead to cretinism. If mild, symptoms may be absent and the condition detectable only by testing.

Idiopathic. Of unknown cause.

Idiopathic thrombocytopenic purpura. An autoimmune* disease in which a low **platelet count** leads to abnormal bleeding.

Immunoassay. A class of many laboratory techniques which analyze for the presence of unknown substances by means of reactions between antigen* and antibody*. The reaction may be detected directly, as when particles of antigen or antibody clump together and form a cloudy solution or precipitate (agglutination, immunodiffusion), or indirectly, as when an enzyme* (enzyme immunoassay), radioactive isotope (radioimmunoassay), or fluorescein dye (immunofluorescence) are combined with an antibody or antigen.

Immunoglobulin. A protein whose main function is as an antibody*.

Infarction. Local tissue death caused by an interruption of the blood supply. A heart attack is the result of infarction of heart muscle.

Intrinsic factor. A substance produced in the stomach which allows **vitamin B$_{12}$** to be absorbed into the blood.

Ion. An atom or group of atoms with a positive or negative charge.

Lupus erythematosus. An autoimmune* disease which may cause many symptoms, such as weakness, fatigue, fever, skin rash, and kidney problems.

Lymphocyte. A type of white blood cell which is crucial to the immune system. May be classified by **lymphocyte typing.**

Lymphoma. A cancer of the lymphatic system. The best known is Hodgkin's disease.

Malabsorption. Failure to absorb nutrients properly from the intestines.

Multiple myeloma. A cancer of plasma cells, a type of cell which is usually found in the bone marrow and which is important to the immune system.

Osteomyelitis. Infection within a bone.

Oximetry. Measurement of blood oxygen.

Parathyroid. Four small glands which secrete **parathyroid hormone.** They are located in the neck near the thyroid*.

Peptide. A biochemical composed of two or more amino acids* which form the building blocks of **protein.**

Pernicious anemia. A type of anemia caused by faulty absorption of **vitamin B$_{12}$.**

pH. A symbol used to denote the acidity or alkalinity of a solution. The pH ranges from 0 to 14, with pure water being 7. The pH of the blood must be kept between 7.35 and 7.45.

Phagocytosis. Engulfing of a substance by white blood cells in order to destroy and eliminate it from the body.

Pheochromocytoma. A tumor, usually located in the abdomen, which produces **catecholamines.**

Plasma. The liquid portion of blood in which the particles, such as red blood cells* and white blood cells*, are suspended.

Platelet. A particle in the blood which is crucial to the development of blood clotting.

Polycythemia. An increase in the number of red blood cells*. The opposite of anemia.

Porphyria. Any of a number of diseases in which porphyrin* metabolism is disturbed.

Porphyrin. A group of chemical compounds widely disbursed in nature which form the building blocks of chlorophyll and hemoglobin.

Pseudohypoparathyroidism. A hereditary disease caused by the failure of organs to respond to normal levels of **parathyroid hormone.**

Pseudo-pseudohypoparathyroidism. A form of pseudohypoparathroidism* in which blood **calcium** and **phosphorus** are within normal limits.

Rectum. The portion of the large intestine which extends from the sigmoid* to the anus.

Red blood cell. A disk-shaped cell without a nucleus whose main function is to carry **hemoglobin.**

Retina. The back of the eyeball upon which light rays converge.

Rh. An antigen* on red blood cells*. Most individuals (about 85 percent) have the Rh factor already, and so do not recognize it as foreign, but the remainder—called Rh negative—may develop hemolytic anemia* if they receive a transfusion with Rh positive blood. Hemolytic disease of the newborn, also called erythroblastosis fetalis or Rh disease, is due to Rh incompatibility between a mother and fetus.

Sarcoidosis. A disease of unknown cause which can affect virtually any organ of the body, but which is most serious when affecting the lungs, kidneys, or eyes.

Scleroderma. An autoimmune* disease in which the skin and internal organs are progressively replaced by firm unyielding tissue.

Serum. Plasma* from which **fibrinogen** has been removed through the formation of a blood clot.

Sickle cell anemia. A hereditary disease which causes red blood cells* to become distorted into crescentic shapes when oxygen is low.

Sigmoid. The portion of the large intestine which extends from the colon* to the rectum*.

Southern blot. A method for analyzing the structure of DNA. The general procedure is to release DNA from cells and to process it with various enzymes* designed to break apart the molecule in specified regions. Electrophoresis* is then used to separate the fragments. By adding radioactive probes, then exposing the result to film, a pattern of DNA is obtained and analyzed visually.

Spectrophotometry. A laboratory method for analyzing a substance by determining the wavelengths of light it absorbs.

Spherocytosis. A hereditary disease which causes red blood cells* to become distorted into spheres rather than disks. This leads to hemolytic anemia*.

Steatorrhea. Increased fat in the stool. Found in intestinal malabsorption* and other disorders of digestion.

Stylet. 1. A wire which fits inside a needle or catheter either to provide stiffness or to prevent debris from accumulating. 2. A small pointed piece of metal used to make a superficial puncture in the skin.

Thalassemia. A form of hereditary hemolytic anemia* which may vary in severity according to the specific type.

Thrombolytic. A substance which dissolves blood clots.

Thyroid. A gland located in the neck which produces **thyroxine** and **triiodothyronine.**

Thyroiditis. Inflammation of the thyroid*. It may be due to infection with various organisms, autoimmune* disease, or for unknown reasons. The usual end result is diminished thyroid function.

Titer. A common method of measuring and reporting the concentration of a substance in solution by progressively diluting it. If a blood test for a certain antibody*, for example, is found to be positive, it is diluted with an equal volume of saline and tested again. If still positive, it is diluted again and retested, until the test is negative. The titer is then reported as the last dilution which was positive, e.g., 1:2, 1:4, 1:8, 1:16, and so forth.

Tumor. The general term for any abnormal growth. It may be benign or malignant.

Vasculitis. Inflammation of blood vessels. Symptoms may range from mild to severe.

Virus. The smallest known microorganism. Viruses need a host cell in which to live since they are not capable of reproducing by themselves.

Vital signs. A common method for determining the general state of your health. It includes pulse, temperature, blood pressure, and respiratory rate.

Wegener's granulomatosis. A severe form of vasculitis*.

Western blot. A laboratory method for determining the presence of certain proteins. Known proteins are separated by electrophoresis* and the test serum is added. Any adhering antibody* is then labeled with another antibody (radioactive or enzyme linked) in order to be visualized. Diagnostic patterns show up as bands of varying intensity.

White blood cell. One of the two main types of cells in the blood, the other being **red blood cells***. There are several types—neutrophils, basophils, eosinophils, monocytes, and lymphocytes—each of which has a different function. They can be distinguished by means of the **white blood cell differential.**

Wilson's disease. An inherited disease caused by faulty **copper** metabolism and causing widespread disease, most seriously of the brain and liver.

Synonyms and Included
Tests Index

□ □ □

A

5-HT, 379
5-hydroxytryptamine, 379
12- or 24-hour pH study, 172
2 D echo, 157
A_1AT, 21
Acetylcholinesterase, 116
Acid elution for fetal hemoglobin, 261
Acid hemolysis test, 207
Acid infusion test, 65
Acid perfusion test, 65
Acoustic immitance, 8
Acoustic reflexes, 8
Activated coagulation time, 9
Activated partial thromboplastin time, 323
Acute phase proteins, 21
Acute phase reactant, 94
AIDS antibody, 225
AIDS screen, 225
Air conditioner lung test, 17

Alk phos, 16
Allergy screen, 357
Alpha fetoprotein tumor marker, 20
Ambulatory electrocardiography, 228
ANCA, 43
Anorectal manometry, 29
Anti HAV, 217
Anticardiolipin antibody, 45
Antiglobulin test, 131
Antiparietal cell antibody, 321
Antistreptococcal DNase B, 39
Antistreptococcal hyaluronidase, 40
APTT, 323
ARM, 29
ART, 378
Arterial blood gasses, 73
Arteriogram, 33
Arthrocentesis, 254
Arylamidase, 269
Ascites fluid tap, 317

Ascorbic acid, 467
ASLO, 46
ASPA, 43
Aspiration of pericardial
fluid, 329
Audiogram, 209
Automated perimetry, 461

B

Bacterial serology, 56
Bacterial smear, 205
Balloon manometry, 29
Basal acid output, 197
Basal gastric secretion test,
197
Beta carotene, 107
Blood collection, 452
Blood loss scan, 74
Blood sugar, 201
Bone scintigram, 83
Brain scintigram, 84
Brain stem auditory
evoked potentials, 85
Breast X ray, 294
Breath analysis, 234
Breath hydrogen analysis,
234
Bronchogram, 88

C

Calorics, 454
Cancer antigen 125, 95
Capillary blood collection,
182, 212
Carbohydrate antigen
15-3, 96
Carbohydrate antigen
19-9, 97

Carbon monoxide, 103
Cardiac blood pool
imaging, 211
Cardiac positron emission
tomography, 211
Cardiac scan, 211
Cardiac scintigram, 211
Cardiopulmonary sleep
study, 387
CAT scan, 130
Cervical smear, 316
Cervical/vaginal cytology,
316
Chromium-51 RBC
survival, 362
Clomid test, 119
Closed pleural biopsy, 339
Closed renal biopsy, 257
Cold hemolysin test, 322
Cold spot myocardial
imaging, 211
Colon X ray, 61
Color Doppler, 157
Complete blood count and
differential, 128
Computed transaxial
tomography, 130
Connecting peptide insulin,
93
Contact dermatitis skin
test, 324
Coronary heart disease risk
index, 275
Corticotropin, 11
Creatine phosphokinase,
137
Crit, 214
Cyanocobalamin, 466
Cyclic adenosine
monophosphate, 141
Cystometrogram, 143
Cystourethroscopy, 145
Cytopathology, 146

D

Delta agent serology, 220
Diluted whole blood clot
  lysis, 120
DNA fingerprinting, 152
Doppler echo, 157
D-xylose tolerance test, 478

E

EGD, 440
EKG, 158
Electronystagmography,
  454
Electrooculogram, 163
Electroretinogram, 163
Endothelial cell count, 167
EOG, 163
ERG, 163
Erythrocyte sedimentation
  rate, 373
Esophageal manometry,
  171
Esophageal pH study with
  intraluminal electrode,
  172
Esophagogastroduodeno-
  scopy, 440
Esophagram, 64
ESR, 373
Euglobin clot lysis time,
  120
Excretory urography, 447
Exercise tolerance test, 404

F

Factor assay, 122
Farmer's lung disease, 17

Farnworth-Munsell test, 125
Fasting blood sugar, 201
Fasting glucose, 201
FBS, 201
Fecal occult blood test, 400
Fibrin breakdown
  products, 180
Fibrin degradation
  products, 180
Fibrinolysis time, 120
Field of vision, 461
Fine needle aspiration, 54
Fingerstick blood
  collection, 182
Fishberg concentration
  test, 470
FNA, 54
Folate level, 184
Fungal serology, 189

G

Gall bladder X ray, 113
Gamma glutamyl
  transpeptidase, 195
Gastrointestinal bleed
  localization study, 74
Glycated albumin, 187
Glycosylated hemoglobin,
  204
Goodpasture's antibody, 199
Granulocyte antibody, 42
Ground glass clotting time,
  9
Guthrie test, 330

H

Heelstick blood collection,
  212

Herpes antibody, 223
Herpes serology, 223
Heterophile test, 246
HIS bundle recordings, 251
HLA typing, 425
Hot spot myocardial
    imaging, 211
HTLV antibody, 232
Human immunodeficiency
    virus test, 225
Human leukocyte antigen
    test, 425
Hydrocortisone, 134
Hypersensitivity
    pneumonitis serology, 17

I

IgE specific antibody, 357
Immunodeficiency profile,
    289
Immunoelectrophoresis,
    240
Impedence audiometry, 8
Inborn errors of
    metabolism screen, 23
Indium leukocyte scan, 474
Infarct avid imaging, 211
Infection scintigraphy, 474
Infertility screen, 375
Injection of the corpus
    cavernosum, 327
Insulin induced peak acid
    output, 227
Insulinlike growth factor,
    392
Intraocular pressure, 426
Intraocular tension, 426
Intravenous pyelogram,
    447
Ishihara plates, 125
IVP, 447

J

Joint study, 51

K

Kahn test, 378
Kidney profile, 258
Kline test, 378

L

Labial salivary gland
    biopsy, 272
Lactogen, 347
Lactogenic hormone, 347
LDH, 264
LE prep, 268
Lipoprotein phenotyping,
    276
Liver battery, 281
Liver panel, 281
Liver profile, 281
Liver scan, 278
Liver screen, 281
Lower gastrointestinal X
    rays, 61
Lower GI, 61
LP, 395
Lumbar puncture, 395
Lupus anticoagulant, 45
Lupus test, 268
Lyme arthritis serology,
    284
Lymph gland biopsy, 286
Lymphangiography, 287
Lymphocyte crossmatch,
    425
Lymphocyte subset
    enumeration, 289

M

M mode echo, 157
Magnetic resonance scan, 292
Mazzini test, 378
Mono test, 247
Monospot, 246

N

Nagel anomaloscope, 125
NBT test, 308
Needle biopsy of the liver, 280
Needle pleural biopsy, 339
Nerve conduction velocity, 306
Neutrophil phagocytosis, 470
Nocturnal penile tumescence test, 385
Nuclear medicine, 358

O

Ocular pressure, 426
Oral glucose tolerance test, 202

P

PAP, 5
Papaverine test, 327
Parathormone, 319
Paroxysmal nocturnal hemoglobinuria, 207, 405
Paternity testing, 152

Pattern-shift evoked responses, 459
Penile Doppler studies, 326
Pericardial effusion tap, 329
Perimetry, 461
Peritoneal endoscopy, 267
Peritoneoscopy, 267
Peroral endoscopy, 440
Persantine-thallium imaging, 211
Phagocyte immunocompetence profile, 470
Phenylalanine screen, 330
Phlebotomy, 452
Phosphorus, 331
Pleural fluid analysis, 410
PNH, 207, 405
Polysomnography, 387
Preoperative corneal evaluation, 167
Pro time, 354
Proctoscopy, 36
Prostatic acid phosphatase, 5
Protein bound glucose, 187
Pseudocholinesterase, 116
Pulmonary artery catheterization, 369
Pure tone audiometry, 209
Pyridoxine, 464

R

Radioactive iodine uptake test, 422
Radiography, 475
RAIU, 422
Rapid ACTH test, 135
Rapid plasma reagin, 377

RFLP analysis for parentage, 152
Riboflavin, 463
Roentgenographic examination, 475
RPR, 378
Rumpel-Leede test, 100

S

Saline load for gastric emptying, 398
Scintigram, 358
Scl-1 antibody, 372
Scl-70 antibody, 372
Scotch tape test, 332
Sed rate, 373
Serum glumatic pyruvate transaminase, 12
Serum glutamic oxaloacetic transaminase, 43
Serum protein electrophoresis, 353
SGOT, 43
SGPT, 12
Skin puncture blood collection, 182, 212
Sleep apnea study, 387
SMA, 376
SMAC, 376
Small bowel series, 63
Somatosensory-evoked potentials, 394
Somatotropin, 206
Sonogram, 437
SPECT scan, 84
Specular microscopy, 167
Speech discrimination, 209
Speech reception threshold, 209
Speech testing, 209

Sperm count, 375
Sperm examination, 375
Spirometry, 355
Spleen scan, 278
Sputum collection, 397
SS-A and SS-B, 382
Standard acid reflux test, 6
Stool fat, 167
Stool for white cells, 298
Stool guaiac, 400
Swan-Ganz catheterization, 369
Synovial fluid analysis, 253

T

T- and B-cell count, 289
Tangent screen examination, 461
Thallium imaging, 211
Thallium scintigraphy, 211
Thiamine, 463
Thyrocalcitonin, 98
Thyroid profile, 418
Tocopherol, 468
Total urinary estrogens, 175
Tourniquet test, 100
Tumor-antigen 4, 407
Tuttle test, 6
Two-hour postprandial blood glucose, 343
Tympanometry, 8

U

Ultrasonography, 437
Upper endoscopy, 440
Upper gastrointestinal series, 63

Upper GI, 63
Urea nitrogen, 76
Urinary calculus
    composition, 260
Urine concentration
    test, 470
Urodynamic testing for
    bladder function, 143
Uterogram, 239

V

VDRL, 378
Venipuncture, 452

Ventilation/perfusion scan,
    282
Viral serology, 455
Vitamin B_{12} absorption
    test, 370
Vitamin D_3, 467
Voiding cystourethrogram,
    142

W

Wasserman test, 378
Wet mount for fungus, 262
Whole blood clot lysis, 120
Whole body bone scan, 83

NOTES

NOTES

NOTES

NOTES

THE ◆ PDR

PDR
FAMILY
GUIDES

POCKET GUIDE
TO PRESCRIPTION DRUGS™

REVISED AND UPDATED
WITH THE LATEST NEW DRUGS
THE SAME INFORMATION YOUR DOCTOR RELIES ON

*Based on Physicians' Desk Reference,
the Nation's Leading Professional Drug Handbook*

◆ Side effects, drug interactions, dosages—all in everyday English

◆ Quick, easy alphabetical references by familiar brand names—with convenient generic cross-references

◆ Hundreds of actual-size full-color drug photographs

◆ 40 new entries, including protease inhibitors, Redux,™ Allegra,™ and drugs for asthma, acne, and more

Coming mid-September from Pocket Books

POCKET
B O O K S

1275-01

PRESCRIPTION AND NONPRESCRIPTION MEDICATIONS FOR

Children

WHAT PARENTS NEED TO KNOW

An Alphabetized, Lifesaving Guide
To More Than 100 Commonly Used Drugs

MAX VAN GILDER, M.D. AND
SHELAGH RYAN MASLINE

A LYNN SONBERG BOOK

Now available from Pocket Books

POCKET
B O O K S

1414

American Medical Association

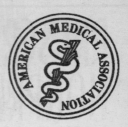

FAMILY

HEALTH

COOKBOOK

Good Food That's Good For You

**Melanie Barnard and Brooke Dojny with
Mindy Hermann, R.D. and
C. Wayne Callaway, M.D.**

Coming mid-October in Hardcover
From Pocket Books

POCKET
BOOKS

1409